Urology

Editor

JOSEPH W. BARTGES

VETERINARY CLINICS OF NORTH AMERICA: SMALL ANIMAL PRACTICE

www.vetsmall.theclinics.com

July 2015 • Volume 45 • Number 4

ELSEVIER

1600 John F. Kennedy Boulevard • Suite 1800 • Philadelphia, Pennsylvania, 19103-2899

http://www.vetsmall.theclinics.com

VETERINARY CLINICS OF NORTH AMERICA: SMALL ANIMAL PRACTICE Volume 45, Number 4
July 2015 ISSN 0195-5616, ISBN-13: 978-0-323-39148-1

Editor: Patrick Manley

Developmental Editor: Meredith Clinton

Veterinary Clinics of North America: Small Animal Practice (ISSN 0195-5616) is published bimonthly by Elsevier Inc., 360 Park Avenue South, New York, NY 10010-1710. Months of issue are January, March, May, July, September, and November. Business and Editorial Offices: 1600 John F. Kennedy Blvd., Ste. 1800, Philadelphia, PA 19103-2899. Customer Service Office: 3251 Riverport Lane, Maryland Heights, MO 63043. Periodicals postage paid at New York, NY and additional mailing offices. Subscription prices are $310.00 per year (domestic individuals), $500.00 per year (domestic institutions), $150.00 per year (domestic students/residents), $410.00 per year (Canadian individuals), $621.00 per year (Canadian institutions), $455.00 per year (international individuals), $621.00 per year (international institutions), and $220.00 per year (international and Canadian students/residents). To receive student/resident rate, orders must be accompanied by name of affiliated institution, date of term, and the *signature* of program/residency coordinator on institution letterhead. Orders will be billed at individual rate until proof of status is received. Foreign air speed delivery is included in all *Clinics* subscription prices. All prices are subject to change without notice. **POSTMASTER:** Send address changes to *Veterinary Clinics of North America: Small Animal Practice*, Elsevier Health Sciences Division, Subscription Customer Service, 3251 Riverport Lane, Maryland Heights, MO 63043. Customer Service (orders, claims, online, change of address): Elsevier Periodicals Customer Service, Elsevier Health Sciences Division Subscription **Customer Service 3251 Riverport Lane Maryland Heights, MO 63043. Tel: 1-800-654-2452 (U.S. and Canada); 314-447-8871 (outside U.S. and Canada). Fax: 314-447-8029. E-mail: journalscustomerservice-usa@elsevier.com (for print support); journalsonlinesupport-usa@elsevier.com (for online support)**.

Reprints. For copies of 100 or more of articles in this publication, please contact the Commercial Reprints Department, Elsevier Inc., 360 Park Avenue South, New York, NY 10010-1710. Tel.: 212-633-3874; Fax: 212-633-3820; E-mail: reprints@elsevier.com.

Veterinary Clinics of North America: Small Animal Practice is also published in Japanese by Inter Zoo Publishing Co., Ltd., Aoyama Crystal-Bldg 5F, 3-5-12 Kitaaoyama, Minato-ku, Tokyo 107-0061, Japan.

Veterinary Clinics of North America: Small Animal Practice is covered in *Current Contents/Agriculture, Biology and Environmental Sciences, Science Citation Index, ASCA, MEDLINE/PubMed (Index Medicus), Excerpta Medica, and BIOSIS.*

Contributors

EDITOR

JOSEPH W. BARTGES, DVM, PhD
Diplomate, American College of Veterinary Internal Medicine (Small Animal Internal Medicine); Diplomate, American College of Veterinary Nutrition; Veterinary Internist and Nutritionist and Academic Director, Cornell University Veterinary Specialists, Stamford, Connecticut

AUTHORS

SARA D. ALLSTADT, DVM
Diplomate, American College of Veterinary Internal Medicine (Oncology); Medical Oncologist, BluePearl Veterinary Partners, Louisville, Kentucky

JOSEPH W. BARTGES, DVM, PhD
Diplomate, American College of Veterinary Internal Medicine (Small Animal Internal Medicine); Diplomate, American College of Veterinary Nutrition; Veterinary Internist and Nutritionist and Academic Director, Cornell University Veterinary Specialists, Stamford, Connecticut

ALLYSON C. BERENT, DVM
Diplomate, American College of Veterinary Internal Medicine; Director, Interventional Endoscopy; Staff, Internal Medicine, Department of Internal Medicine, Department of Surgery, The Animal Medical Center, New York, New York

JULIE K. BYRON, DVM, MS
Diplomate, American College of Veterinary Internal Medicine; Associate Professor - Clinical, Department of Veterinary Clinical Sciences, College of Veterinary Medicine, The Ohio State University, Columbus, Ohio

AMANDA J. CALLENS, BS, LVT
Veterinary Technician, Cornell University Veterinary Specialists, Stamford, Connecticut

CLAIRE M. CANNON, BVSc(Hons)
Diplomate, American College of Veterinary Internal Medicine (Oncology); Assistant Professor, Department of Small Animal Clinical Sciences, College of Veterinary Medicine, University of Tennessee, Knoxville, Tennessee

MARNIN FORMAN, DVM
Diplomate, American College of Veterinary Internal Medicine; Head of Internal Medicine, Internal Medicine Department, Cornell University Veterinary Specialists, Stamford, Connecticut

S. DRU FORRESTER, DVM, MS
Diplomate, American College of Veterinary Internal Medicine; Director of Global Scientific Affairs, Department of Global Professional & Veterinary Affairs, Hill's Pet Nutrition Inc, Topeka, Kansas

SILKE HECHT, Dr med vet
Diplomate, American College of Veterinary Radiology; Diplomate, European College of Veterinary Diagnostic Imaging; Associate Professor in Radiology, Department of Small Animal Clinical Sciences, College of Veterinary Medicine, University of Tennessee, Knoxville, Tennessee

MEGAN MORGAN, VMD
Diplomate, American College of Veterinary Internal Medicine; Staff Internist, Internal Medicine Department, Cornell University Veterinary Specialists, Stamford, Connecticut

SHELLY J. OLIN, DVM
Diplomate, American College of Veterinary Internal Medicine; Assistant Professor, Department of Small Animal Clinical Sciences, College of Veterinary Medicine, University of Tennessee, Knoxville, Tennessee

DONNA M. RADITIC, DVM, CVA
Diplomate, American College of Veterinary Nutrition; Clinical Assistant Professor, Integrative Medicine, Nutrition Service, Department of Small Animal Clinical Sciences, College of Veterinary Medicine, University of Tennessee, Knoxville, Tennessee

TODD L. TOWELL, DVM, MS
Diplomate, American College of Veterinary Internal Medicine; Global Veterinary Consulting, Erie, Colorado

Contents

Performing a urinalysis should be part of a minimum database in addition to physical examination, historical information gathering, complete blood cell counts, and serum/plasma biochemical analysis. Urinalysis provides information on function of various organs and information on renal function. It is necessary to interpret blood urea nitrogen and serum/plasma creatinine concentrations and is useful in assessing urine concentrating and diluting ability, glomerular barrier function, tubular function, proteinuria, discolored urine, urolithiasis, and neoplasia. Performing a urinalysis is technically easy and does not require expensive equipment or disposable supplies.

Diagnostic imaging is routinely performed in small animals with lower urinary tract disease. Survey radiographs allow identification of radiopaque calculi, gas within the urinary tract, and lymph node or bone metastases. Cystography and urethrography remain useful in the evaluation of bladder or urethral rupture, abnormal communication with other organs, and lesions of the pelvic or penile urethra. Ultrasonography is the modality of choice for the diagnosis of most disorders. Computed tomography and magnetic resonance imaging are useful in evaluating the ureterovesical junction and intrapelvic lesions, monitoring the size of lesions, and evaluating lymph nodes and osseous structures for metastases.

Cystoscopy has become an important and widely available component of the diagnostic evaluation of diseases of the lower urinary tract in dogs and cats. In addition, a large number of cystoscopic guided procedures have been described that can be used to treat disease processes that were previously treatable only with invasive surgical procedures. This article reviews the indications and contraindications for cystoscopy, cystoscopy equipment and techniques for male and female dogs and cats, potential complications associated with cystoscopy, and management options for these complications.

Congenital lower urinary tract diseases occur with variable frequency and may result in clinical signs of urinary incontinence, urinary obstruction, or

clinical studies to determine the best management options. Current best evidence for initial management of acute, non-obstructive FIC supports a specific nutritional recommendation for a therapeutic urinary food proven to reduce recurrent episodes, environmental enrichment and feeding moist food.

Lower urinary tract neoplasia is uncommon in dogs and cats, though transitional cell carcinoma (TCC) is the most common tumor of the lower urinary tract in both species. Clinical signs are not specific for neoplasia, but neoplasia should be considered in patients that are older, have specific risk factors, or have persistent, severe, or relapsing signs. Local disease is often the cause of death or euthanasia; local control is challenging owing to tumor size and location. Systemic therapy is the mainstay of treatment. Prognosis is generally guarded, but therapy can result in improvement in clinical signs and quality of life.

The use of novel image-guided techniques in veterinary medicine has become more widespread, especially in urologic diseases. With the common incidence of urinary tract obstructions, stones disease, renal disease, and urothelial malignancies, combined with the recognized invasiveness and morbidity associated with traditional surgical techniques, the use of minimally invasive alternatives using interventional radiology and interventional endoscopy techniques has become incredibly appealing to owners and clinicians. This article provides a brief overview of some of the most common procedures done in endourology in veterinary medicine to date, providing as much evidence-based medicine as possible when comparing with traditional surgical alternatives.

Consumer use of integrative health care is growing, but evidence-based research on its efficacy is limited. Research of veterinary lower urinary tract diseases could be translated to human medicine because veterinary patients are valuable translational models for human urinary tract infection and urolithiasis. An overview of complementary therapies for lower urinary tract disease includes cranberry supplements, mannose, oral probiotics, acupuncture, methionine, herbs, or herbal preparations. Therapies evaluated in dogs and cats, in vitro canine cells, and other relevant species, in vivo and in vitro, are presented for their potential use as integrative therapies for veterinary patients and/or translational research.

VETERINARY CLINICS OF NORTH AMERICA: SMALL ANIMAL PRACTICE

THE CLINICS ARE NOW AVAILABLE ONLINE!
Access your subscription at:
www.theclinics.com

Preface

Urology: It's Gold for a Reason!

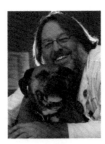

Joseph W. Bartges, DVM, PhD, DACVIM, DACVN
Editor

Urology is literally the "study of urine," but usually infers the study of normal processes and diseases of the lower urinary tract in contrast with nephrology, which infers study of normal processes and diseases of the kidneys. In keeping with that definition, this issue of *Veterinary Clinics of North America: Small Animal Practice* is dedicated to the management of disorders of the lower urinary tract. Dr Don Low, one of the fathers of veterinary nephrology and urology, with Drs Carl Osborne, Del Finco, and Ken Bovee, is credited with the following: "One should strive to practice 30 to 40 years of veterinary medicine and not 1 year 30 or 40 times." In the spirit of that statement, this issue contains reviews and new information concerning diagnostic testing, pathophysiologic processes, and treatment strategies for dogs and cats with lower urinary tract diseases.

Lower urinary tract disorders occur commonly in dogs and cats and can often be frustrating either to treat or to prevent because of their recurrent nature. It is difficult to differentiate many diseases of the lower urinary tract as they present with similar clinical signs. Being familiar with common disorders helps to develop a rational diagnostic and therapeutic plan for your patient. The authors that have written in this issue are experts and provide a wealth of information concerning lower urinary tract disorders. This issue is roughly divided into 3 sections. The first section contains reviews of urinalysis (Ms Amanda Callens and Bartges), imaging (Dr Silke Hecht), and cystoscopy (Drs Megan Morgan and Marnin Forman). These detailed articles excellently set the stage for the second and third sections. The second section is concerned with specific disorders of the lower urinary tract, including congenital lower urinary tract disease (Bartges and Ms Amanda Callens), urinary tract infections (Dr Shelly Olin and Bartges), urolithiasis (Bartges and Ms Amanda Callens), micturition disorders (Dr Julie Byron), feline idiopathic cystitis (Drs Dru Forrester and Todd Towell), and lower urinary tract cancer (Drs Claire Cannon and Sara Allstadt). These outstanding articles contain reviews of the etiopathogenesis, diagnosis, and treatments for these common clinical

Vet Clin Small Anim 45 (2015) ix–x
http://dx.doi.org/10.1016/j.cvsm.2015.03.002
0195-5616/15/$ – see front matter © 2015 Published by Elsevier Inc.

problems. The third section provides new or integrative treatment modalities for diseases of the lower urinary tract, including endourology (Dr Allyson Berent) and complementary and integrative therapies (Dr Donna Raditic). These highly informative articles provide additional information for managing patients with lower urinary tract disorders that owners should be informed of.

I thank the staff, especially Meredith Clinton, at *Veterinary Clinics of North America: Small Animal Practice* for inviting me to edit this issue. Many thanks to the authors, who generously took time out of their busy lives to provide valuable information related to the field of urology. Many of these authors are members of the American Society of Veterinary Nephrology and Urology (http://www.asvnu.org/), which is "a dedicated group of researchers and clinicians working to improve the quality of life of veterinary patients with kidney and urologic diseases by studying the structure, function, and ailments of the urinary system." If you have a similar strong interest in the urinary system (and who doesn't?!?), then you should consider membership. Thank-you to my family, friends, colleagues, and students who support me and inspire me to be the best that I can ("No man is a failure who has friends." —*Clarence*, *It's a Wonderful Life*). Particularly, thank-you to Dr Donna Raditic, who keeps me sane and drives me crazy at the same time ("Have I told you lately that I love you." —*Van Morrison*, "Have I Told You Lately"). I hope that you find this issue useful in your practice and care of your patients.

Joseph W. Bartges, DVM, PhD, DACVIM, DACVN
Cornell University Veterinary Specialists
880 Canal Street
Stamford, CT 06902, USA

E-mail address:
jbartges@cuvs.org

Urinalysis

Amanda J. Callens, BS, LVT, Joseph W. Bartges, DVM, PhD*

KEYWORDS

- Urinalysis • Urine sediment examination • Urine chemistries • Urine specific gravity
- Urine dipstick

KEY POINTS

- Urinalysis is a useful laboratory test in documenting urinary tract diseases, and it can also provide information about other systemic diseases, such as liver failure and hemolysis.
- The collection method and storage time and conditions are the most important preanalytical sample variables.
- Preanalytical patient variables include physiologic variables or introduced variables related to treatment or diagnosis.

Urinalysis is an important laboratory test that can be readily performed in veterinary practice and is considered part of a minimum database. It is useful in documenting various types of urinary tract diseases and may provide information about other systemic diseases, such as liver failure and hemolysis. Preanalytical sample variables and patient variables other than those related to disease may influence urinalysis results. Excellent resources are available for more comprehensive information about urinalysis in small animals.[1-3] Urine may be collected by cystocentesis, urethral catheterization, or voiding and should be evaluated within 30 minutes. If this is not possible, then it may be refrigerated for up to 24 hours or submitted to an outside diagnostic laboratory; however, this may result in crystal precipitation. Refrigeration does not alter urine pH or specific gravity.

IN-HOUSE VERSUS SEND-OUT TESTING

Most veterinary practices can and should do urinalysis in-house, from the standpoint of practice economics and quality of care. The test requires only basic laboratory supplies, including disposable supplies such as a specimen container, disposable pipettes, conical centrifuge tubes, urine dipsticks, glass slides and coverslips, and sediment stain, and equipment, including a centrifuge, a refractometer (preferably

The authors have nothing to disclose.
Department of Internal Medicine, Cornell University Veterinary Specialists, 880 Canal Street, Stamford, CT 06902, USA
* Corresponding author.
E-mail address: Joe.bartges@cuvs.org

a temperature-compensated veterinary model with a feline-specific scale for specific gravity), a microscope, and optionally an automated dipstick reader.[4–6] It can be performed easily by clinic technical staff if they are properly trained, making it an inexpensive, technically feasible test to perform. In-house testing is preferred because of faster turnaround time and greater accuracy of results, because delayed analysis is a potential source of introduced error. Another advantage of in-house testing is that results can be correlated more easily with the rest of the patient's clinical picture.

Performing the Complete Urinalysis

A description of performing a urinalysis is provided. The sample should be identified on the sample container using the patient's clinic number or name and the date and should be matched to the reporting form. The reporting form should include patient identification, date, method and time of collection, and any current or recent medications or diagnostic agents. Transfer 0.5 to 1.0 mL of the sample using sterile technique to a sterile tube after mixing the sample and submit or store for aerobic bacteriologic culture. Record the time the urinalysis is performed and whether the sample was refrigerated on the reporting form. If the sample has been refrigerated, allow it to reach room temperature or warm it with mixing to either known patient body temperature or 38°C (101°F). Gently mix the sample by inverting it several times and transfer 3 to 5 mL to a clear conical centrifuge tube and record the color (yellow, brown, black, red, white), clarity (clear, cloudy, turbid, flocculent), and odor (normal or abnormal and describe if possible) on the reporting form. Perform semiquantitative biochemical analysis by immersing the urine dipstick so that all reagent pads are covered with urine, start timing the reactions, and drag edge of strip against rim of tube to remove excess urine. Perform semiquantitative biochemical analysis using a urine dipstick or automated dipstick reader following manufacturer instructions. Record results on reporting form. If the urine sample is grossly discolored (eg, gross hematuria) or turbid, the pigment discolors the reagent pads on the dipstick, making it difficult to read and giving erroneous interpretation. Attempt to clear the urine by centrifuging the sample first. If centrifugation results in a red sediment at the bottom of the conical tube and a clear supernatant, then the dipstick semiquantitative chemical analysis may be performed on the supernatant after transferring it to another tube using a pipette or by decanting. If the urine sample does not clear with centrifugation, then interpret results cautiously. Record results for protein, pH, glucose, ketones, and bilirubin on reporting form; results for specific gravity, urobilinogen, leukocytes, and nitrite are unreliable, inferior to other tests performed as part of the urinalysis, or of no clinical significance and should not be reported. Using an appropriate refractometer measure the specific gravity of the urine sample and report on form. If the sample is discolored or turbid, then the specific gravity can be measured on the supernatant after centrifugation. Centrifuge 3 to 6 mL of the sample in the conical tube for 5 minutes at 1500 to 2000 rpm (450 g). Do not use the brake to stop the centrifuge as this may result in suspension of the sediment. Transfer all but 0.5 to 1.0 mL of the supernatant depending on the volume of urine in the tube to another tube by using a pipette or by decanting. If the sample cleared with centrifugation, then dipstick semiquantitative chemical analysis and specific gravity determination may be performed as mentioned previously. Suspend the remaining sediment pellet in the 0.5 to 1.0 mL of supernatant by tapping the conical tip of the tube gently on the table top. Use less urine to suspend the sediment pellet if less urine was available for centrifugation. Transfer a drop of the suspension to a clean glass microscope slide using a pipette and place a glass coverslip over it. There should be enough fluid to fill the area under the coverslip, but the coverslip should not float. Examine the slide immediately using bright field light microscopy optimized for contrast by closing the condenser diaphragm if the microscope has one or by lowering the condenser. Using the 10× objective (100× magnification) scan at least 2 edges of the area under the coverslip and note presence of casts and crystals as amount per low power field (#/lpf). Using the 40× objective (400× magnification) scan at least 10 fields of the area under the coverslip for cells (red blood cells [RBCs], white blood cells [WBCs], epithelial cells), amorphous crystalline material, microorganisms (bacteria, yeast, parasites), spermatozoa, and fat droplets and record as amount per high power field (#/hpf). Estimate numbers if it is difficult to quantitate, and if too numerous to count record as such. A second slide may be prepared as described, air dried, stained with a modified Wright stain, Wright-Giemsa stain, or Gram stain, and examined using the 10× and 40× objectives as described and with immersion oil at 100× (1000× magnification) for identification of bacteria.[7–10]

STAINED URINE SEDIMENT EXAMINATION
Preanalytical Sample Variables

A urine sample submitted for analysis should be free of any contaminants, collected into a clean, opaque, airtight, sterile container, and analyzed within 60 minutes of collection; however, as this is not always the case, the clinician should consider the influence of preanalytical sample (ie, nonbiologic) variables when interpreting urinalysis results. The most important of these variables are collection method and storage time and conditions. The collection method is relevant with regard to potential contamination. For example, samples collected by cystocentesis typically have a small amount of iatrogenic blood contamination, voided samples often contain contaminants from the lower urogenital tract (eg, bacteria, epithelial cells, spermatozoa, blood) or the environment (eg, bacteria, plant material, debris), samples obtained by urinary catheterization may contain lower urogenital tract contaminants or iatrogenic hemorrhage, and samples obtained from the floor or examination table or from a litter box lined with nonabsorbent material are often contaminated with microbes and debris. Storage time and conditions may affect urinalysis results. For example, refrigeration may promote crystal formation; prolonged storage of samples at room temperature may result in degeneration of cells and casts, altered crystal formation, or bacterial overgrowth and resultant secondary artifacts (eg, altered pH, decreased glucose concentration); and exposure to light or air may alter the composition of the sample.

Preanalytical Patient Variables

Preanalytical patient variables include physiologic variables or introduced variables related to treatment or diagnosis. Physiologic variables that affect results include diet, time of day, and reproductive factors. For example, diet may influence urine pH or crystal formation, samples collected first thing in the morning tend to be more concentrated and may have altered cellular morphology or microbial viability, and estrus or recent breeding may influence microscopic findings. Introduced patient variables include administration of drugs, fluids, or other exogenous agents. For example, corticosteroids and diuretics interfere with renal concentrating ability, corticosteroids may also cause proteinuria, antimicrobials may mask urinary tract infections or form crystals, hydroxyethyl starch interferes with measurement of specific gravity, and radiographic contrast agents may interfere with measurement of specific gravity or biochemical analytes or may form crystals.

RESULTS OF COMPLETE URINALYSIS
Urine Appearance

Color

Normal urine is typically transparent and yellow or amber on visual inspection. Primarily 2 pigments impart the yellow coloration: urochrome and urobilin. Urochrome is a sulfur-containing oxidation product of the colorless urochromogen. Urobilin is a degradation product of hemoglobin. Because the 24-hour urinary excretion of urochrome is constant, highly concentrated urine is amber in color, whereas dilute urine may be transparent or light yellow color. The intensity of the color is in part related to the volume of urine collected and the concentration of urine produced; therefore, it should be interpreted in the context of the urine specific gravity. Caution must be used not to overinterpret the significance of urine color as part of a complete urinalysis. Significant disease may exist when urine is normal in color. Abnormal urine color may be caused by the presence of several endogenous or exogenous pigments. Although the abnormal color indicates a problem, it provides nonspecific information. Causes of abnormal coloration should be investigated with appropriate laboratory tests and examination of urine sediment. Detection of abnormal urine color should prompt questions related to diet, administration of medication, environment, and collection technique. Knowledge of urine color may also be important in interpreting colorimetric test results because it may induce interference with the test.

Urine color that is anything other than yellow or amber is abnormal. There are many potential causes of discolored urine (**Fig. 1**, **Table 1**). The most common abnormal urine color in dogs and cats is red, brown, or black, which may be caused by hematuria, hemoglobinuria, myoglobinuria, and bilirubinuria.

Pale yellow urine Urine that is pale yellow or clear in appearance may be normal or may indicate a polyuric state. Urine may be appropriately dilute if it is associated with recent consumption or administration of fluids, consumption of a diet containing low quantities of protein or high quantities of sodium chloride, glucocorticoid excess, or administration of diuretics. Urine would be considered to be inappropriately

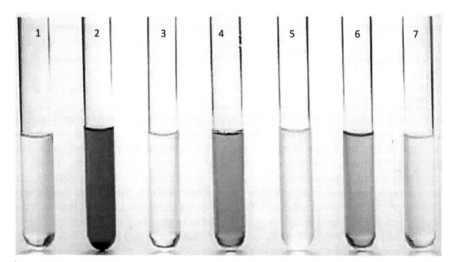

Fig. 1. Urine samples having various colors from clear (3) to pale yellow (1, 5), dark yellow (4, 6, 7), and red due to hematuria (2).

Table 1
Potential causes of discolored urine

Urine Color	Causes	Urine Color	Causes
Yellow or amber	Urochromes Urobilin	Yellow-brown or green-brown	Bile pigments
Deep yellow	Highly concentrated urine Quinacrine[a] Nitrofurantoin[a] Phenacetin[a] Riboflavin (large quantities)[a] Phenolsulfonphthalein (acidic urine)[a]	Brown to black (brown or red-brown when viewed in bright light in thin layer)	Melanin Methemoglobin Myoglobin Bile pigments Thymol[a] Phenolic compounds[a] Nitrofurantoin[a] Nitrites[a] Naphthalene[a] Chlorinated hydrocarbons[a] Aniline dyes[a] Homogentisic acid[a]

(continued on next page)

Table 1
(continued)

Urine Color	Causes	Urine Color	Causes	Urine Color	Causes
Blue	Methylene blue Indigo carmine and indigo blue dye[a] Indicans[a] Pseudomonas infection[a] Water-soluble chlorophyll[a] Rhubarb[a] Toluidine blue[a] Triamterene[a] Amitriptyline[a] Anthraquinone[a] Blue food dye[a]	Colorless	Very dilute urine (diuretics, diabetes mellitus, diabetes insipidus, glucocorticoid excess, fluid therapy, overhydration)		
Green	Methylene blue Dithiazanine Urate crystalluria Indigo blue[a] Evan blue[a] Bilirubin Biliverdin Riboflavin[a] Thymol[a] Phenol[a] Triamterene[a] Amitriptyline[a] Anthraquinone[a] Green food dye[a]	Milky white	Lipid Pyuria Crystals		

Color	
Red, pink, red-brown, red-orange, or orange	Hematuria
	Hemoglobinuria
	Myoglobinuria
	Porphyrinuria
	Congo red
	Phenolsulfonphthalein (following alkalinization)
	Neoprontosil
	Warfarin (orange)[a]
	Food pigments (rhubarb, beets, blackberries)[a]
	Carbon tetrachloride[a]
	Phenazopyridine
	Phenothiazine[a]
	Diphenylhydantoin[a]
	Bromsulphalein (following alkalinization)
	Chronic heavy metal poisoning (lead, mercury)[a]
	Rifampin[a]
	Emodin[a]
	Phenindione[a]
	Eosin[a]
	Rifabutin[a]
	Acetazolamide[a]
	Red food dye[a]
Orange-yellow	Highly concentrated urine
	Excess urobilin
	Bilirubin
	Phenazopyridine
	Sulfasalazine[a]
	Fluorescein sodium[a]
	Flutamide[a]
	Quinacrine[a]
	Phenacetin[a]
	2,4-Dichlorophenoxyacetic acid[a]
	Acetazolamide[a]
	Orange food dye[a]
Brown	Methemoglobin
	Melanin
	Sulfasalazine[a]
	Nitrofurantoin[a]
	Phenacetin[a]
	Naphthalene[a]
	Sulfonamides[a]
	Bismuth[a]
	Mercury[a]
	Feces (rectal-urinary fistula)
	Fava beans[a]
	Rhubarb[a]
	Sorbitol[a]
	Metronidazole[a]
	Methocarbamol[a]
	Anthracin cathartics[a]
	Clofazimine[a]
	Primaquine[a]
	Chloroquine[a]
	Furazolidone[a]
	Copper toxicity

[a] Only observed in human beings.

concentrated if it were dilute in the presence of dehydration. Diseases that may be associated with persistently dilute urine include diabetes mellitus, diabetes insipidus, hyperadrenocorticism, hypoadrenocorticism, hypercalcemia, hyperthyroidism, and renal failure. If urine is pale yellow or clear, the urine specific gravity is often less than 1.015. A simple test to determine whether polyuria is persistent is to determine the urine specific gravity of a sample collected in the morning. Other tests should include serum biochemical analysis and a complete urinalysis. Additional testing may include measurement of serum thyroxine concentration, adrenal function testing, or monitoring urine specific gravity after several days of vasopressin administration.

Red, brown, or black urine Red, brown, or black urine suggests the presence of blood, hemoglobin, myoglobin, or bilirubin. A positive occult blood reaction is obtained when urine contains any of these substances. Discoloration of urine may also result in false-positive reactions on other urine dipstick test pads. Analysis of urine sediment reveals the presence of RBCs if the discoloration is due to hematuria. If no RBCs are present on microscopic examination of urine sediment, presence of hemoglobin, myoglobin, or bilirubin should be suspected. Examination of plasma color may aid in differentiating these. If the urine is discolored because of myoglobin, the plasma is clear because myoglobin in plasma is not bound significantly to a carrying protein, which results in filtration and excretion of myoglobin. If the plasma is pink, it is suggestive of hemoglobin. If the plasma is yellow, it is suggestive of bilirubin; serum bilirubin concentration should also be increased. Myoglobinuria indicates muscle damage; serum creatine kinase activity is often increased in this setting. Hemoglobinemia indicates intravascular hemolysis resulting from immune-mediated, parasite-mediated, or drug-mediated destruction of RBCs. Hyperbilirubinemia may result from liver disease, post–hepatic obstruction, or hemolysis.

Milky white urine Milky white urine may be due to the presence of WBCs (pyuria), lipid, or crystals. The more concentrated the urine sample is the more opaque it may appear. The presence of pyuria secondary to a bacterial urinary tract infection is the most common cause of milky white urine; however, pyuria may occur because of inflammation and not be associated with an infection. Lipiduria may be observed in healthy animals but is frequently observed in cats affected with hepatic lipidosis. Crystalluria if heavy and present in a concentrated urine sample may also result in milky white urine. Microscopic examination of urine sediment aids in differentiation of these causes.

Clarity
Urine is typically clear but may become less transparent with pigmenturia, crystalluria, hematuria, pyuria, lipiduria, or when other compounds such as mucus are present. Depending on the cause, increased turbidity may disappear with centrifugation of the sample.

Odor
Normal urine has a slight odor of ammonia; however, the odor depends on urine concentration. Some species, such as cats and goats, have pungent urine odor because of urine composition. Bacterial infection may result in a strong odor due to pyuria; a strong ammonia odor may occur if the bacteria produce urease.

URINE CHEMICAL ANALYSIS

Urine must be at room temperature for accurate measurement of specific gravity and for chemical analysis. These tests are usually done before centrifugation; however, if urine is discolored or turbid, it may be beneficial to perform these tests on the supernatant.

Specific Gravity

Specific gravity is defined as the ratio of the weight of a volume of liquid to the weight of an equal volume of distilled water; therefore, it depends on the number, size, and weight of particles in the liquid. It is different from osmolality, which depends only on the number of particles in the liquid; measurement of osmolality requires specialized instrumentation. Urine specific gravity is determined using a refractometer designed for veterinary samples, which includes a scale calibrated specifically for cat urine. Urine specific gravity for species other than cats should be determined using the scale for dogs. In healthy animals, urine specific gravity is highly variable, depending on fluid and electrolyte balance of the body. Interpretation of urine specific gravity, therefore, depends on the clinical presentation and findings of serum chemical analysis. An animal that is dehydrated or has other causes of prerenal azotemia has hypersthenuric urine with a specific gravity of 1.025 to 1.040 (depending on the species). Dilute urine in a dehydrated or azotemic animal is abnormal and could be caused by renal failure, hypoadrenocorticism or hyperadrenocorticism, hypercalcemia, diabetes mellitus, hyperthyroidism, diuretic therapy, or diabetes insipidus. Glucosuria increases the urine specific gravity despite increased urine volume.

Semiquantitative, Colorimetric Reagent Strips

Reagent strips such as Multistix (Siemens Healthcare, Erlangen, Germany) or Chemstrip (Roche Diagnostics, Indianapolis, IN) can be used to perform several semiquantitative chemical evaluations simultaneously. They are used routinely to determine urine pH, protein, glucose, ketones, bilirubin/urobilinogen, and occult blood. Some reagent strips include test pads for leukocyte esterase (for detection of WBCs), nitrite (for detection of bacteria), and (urine specific gravity) USG; these are not valid in animals and should not be used. Reagent strips are adversely affected by moisture and have a limited shelf life. Bottles should be kept tightly capped, and unused strips should be discarded after their expiration date.

pH

Urine pH is typically acidic in dogs and cats and alkaline in horses and ruminants but varies depending on diet, medications, or presence of disease. Reagent strip colorimetric test pads for pH determination are accurate to within ± 0.5 pH units.[11] For example, a reading of 6.5 means the actual pH is likely to be between 6.0 and 7.0. Portable pH meters are more accurate than pH colorimetric test pads. A bacterial urinary tract infection with a urease-producing microbe results in alkaluria. Urine pH affects crystalluria because some crystals, such as struvite, form in alkaline urine, whereas other crystals, such as cystine, form in acidic urine.

Protein

The protein test pad uses a color indicator (tetrabromophenol blue), which detects primarily albumin in urine. Results range from 10 to 1000 mg/dL. Proteinuria can occur from prerenal (fever, strenuous exercise, seizures, extreme environmental temperature, and hyperproteinemia), renal (primarily glomerular and occasionally tubular disease), or postrenal (inflammation, hemorrhage, and infection) causes. A positive reaction must be interpreted in light of USG, pH, and urine sediment examination. For example, a trace amount of protein in concentrated urine is less significant than a trace amount of protein in dilute urine. Alkaluria gives a false-positive reaction. Likewise, presence of other proteins, such as Bence-Jones proteins, gives false-negative results. Proteinuria can be measured using sulfosalicylic acid precipitation, which detects albumin and globulins; however, it is not accurate in dogs and cats. If proteinuria is present with an inactive urine sediment, its significance can be verified and quantitated by dividing the urine protein concentration by the urine creatinine concentration (urine protein to urine creatinine ratio; UP:UC). Interpretation of UP:UC is as follows: less than 0.5:1.0 (dogs) and less than 0.4:1.0 (cats) is normal, 0.4 or 0.5 to 1.0:1.0 is questionable, and greater than 1.0:1.0 is abnormal. With primary renal azotemia, UP:UC greater than 0.4:1.0 in cats and 0.5:1.0 in dogs is considered abnormal.[12] A semiquantitative microalbuminuria test is available to detect urinary albumin in the range of 1 to 30 mg/dL. It uses enzyme-linked immunosorbent assay technology specific for canine or feline albumin. Because of minor species differences to albumin, there are different kits for dogs and cats. The microalbuminuria test detects lower concentrations of albumin than a standard dipstick test pad. Hematuria must be macroscopic to increase the microalbuminuria or UP:UC; however, pyuria increases both.

Glucose

Glucose is detected by a glucose oxidase enzymatic reaction that is specific for glucose. Glucosuria is not present normally because the renal threshold for glucose is greater than 180 mg/dL in most species and greater than 240 mg/dL in cats. With euglycemia, the amount of filtered glucose is less than the renal threshold and all the filtered glucose is reabsorbed in the proximal renal tubules. Glucosuria can result from hyperglycemia (due to diabetes mellitus, excessive endogenous or exogenous glucocorticoids, or stress) or from a proximal renal tubular defect (such as primary renal glucosuria or Fanconi syndrome). If glucosuria is present, blood glucose concentration should be determined. False-negative results can occur with high urinary concentrations of ascorbic acid (vitamin C) or with formaldehyde (a metabolite of the urinary antiseptic, methenamine, which may be used for prevention of bacterial urinary tract infections). False-positive results may occur if the sample is contaminated with hydrogen peroxide, chlorine, or hypochlorite (bleach).

Ketones

Ketones are produced from fatty acid metabolism and include acetoacetic acid, acetone, and β-hydroxybutyrate. The ketone test pad detects acetone and acetoacetic acid but not β-hydroxybutyrate. The test pad contains nitroprusside that reacts with acetoacetic acid and acetone to cause a purple color change; it is more sensitive to acetoacetic acid than acetone. Ketonuria is associated with primary ketosis (ruminants), ketosis secondary to diabetes mellitus (small animals), consumption of low-carbohydrate diets (especially in cats), and occasionally prolonged fasting or starvation. A false-positive reaction can occur with the presence of reducing substances in the urine.

Bilirubin/Urobilinogen

When hemoglobin is degraded, the heme portion is converted to bilirubin, which is conjugated in the liver and excreted in bile. Some conjugated bilirubin is filtered by the glomerulus and excreted in urine. The kidney can metabolize hemoglobin to bilirubin and secrete it in dogs but not in cats. Male dogs have a higher secretory ability than female dogs. Dipstick reagent pads use diazonium salts to create a color change and are more sensitive to conjugated bilirubin than unconjugated bilirubin. Bilirubinuria occurs when the level of conjugated bilirubin exceeds the renal threshold as with liver disease or hemolysis. In dogs with concentrated urine, a small amount of bilirubin can be normal. Pigmenturia and phenothiazine may result in a false-positive reaction; false-negative reactions may occur with large amounts of urinary ascorbic acid (vitamin C).

Urobilinogen, formed from bilirubin by intestinal microflora, is absorbed into the portal circulation and is excreted renally. A small amount of urinary urobilinogen is normal. Increased urinary urobilinogen level occurs with hyperbilirubinemia; a negative test result may be observed with biliary obstruction; however, the test is not specific enough to be clinically useful.

Occult blood

The occult blood test pad uses a pseudoperoxidase method to detect intact RBCs, hemoglobin, and myoglobin. A positive reaction can be due to hemorrhage (hematuria), intravascular hemolysis (hemoglobinuria), or myoglobinuria. The last 2 processes can be distinguished by examination of plasma; plasma appears pink to red after intravascular hemolysis, whereas myoglobin is rapidly cleared from plasma, resulting in clear plasma. As with other colorimetric test pads, discolored urine may yield false-positive results. A positive result should be interpreted with microscopic examination of urine sediment.

URINE SEDIMENT

Microscopic examination of urine sediment should be part of a routine urinalysis. For centrifugation, 3 to 5 mL of urine is transferred to a conical centrifuge tube. Urine is centrifuged at 1000 to 1500 rpm for 5 minutes. The supernatant is decanted, leaving 0.5 to 1.0 mL of urine and sediment in the tip of the conical tube. The sediment is resuspended by tapping the tip of the conical tube against the table several times. A few drops of the sediment are transferred to a glass slide, and a coverslip is applied. Examination of unstained urine is recommended for routine samples. Microscopic examination is performed at 10× objective (for crystals, casts, and cells) and 40× objective (for cells and bacteria) magnifications. Contrast of the sample is enhanced by closing the iris diaphragm and lowering the condenser of the microscope. Stains such as Sedi-Stain and new methylene blue can be used to aid in cell identification but may dilute the specimen and introduce artifacts such as stain precipitate and crystals. Use of a modified Wright stain increases the sensitivity, specificity, and positive and negative predictive values for detection of bacteria.

Red Blood Cells

In an unstained preparation, RBCs are small and round and have a slight orange tint and a smooth appearance (**Fig. 2**). Normal urine should contain less than 5 RBCs per field at 400× magnification (40× objective). Increased RBC count in urine (hematuria) indicates hemorrhage somewhere in the urogenital system; however, sample collection by cystocentesis or catheterization may induce hemorrhage.

White Blood Cells

WBCs are slightly larger than RBCs and have a grainy cytoplasm (see **Fig. 2; Fig. 3**). Normal urine should contain less than 5 WBCs per field at 400× magnification (40× objective). Increased WBC count (pyuria) can occur because of inflammation, infection, trauma, or neoplasia. Catheterization or collection of voided urine may introduce a few WBCs from the urogenital tract.

Epithelial Cells

Transitional epithelial cells, a common urine contaminant derived from the bladder and proximal urethra, resemble WBCs but are larger. They have a greater amount of grainy cytoplasm and a round, centrally located nucleus. In a voided urine sample, squamous epithelial cells may be observed. They are large, oval to cuboidal, and may or may not

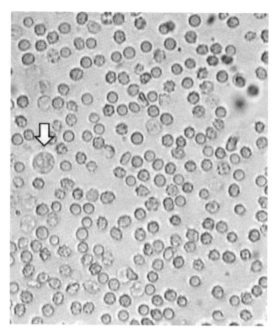

Fig. 2. Red blood cells and 1 white blood cell (*arrow*).

contain a nucleus. Occasionally, neoplastic transitional cells may be observed in an animal with a transitional cell carcinoma. Neoplastic squamous cells may be observed in an animal with a squamous cell carcinoma.

Cylindruria (Casts)

Casts are elongated, cylindrical structures formed by mucoprotein congealing within renal tubules and may contain cells (**Fig. 4**). Hyaline casts are pure protein precipitates, are transparent, have parallel sides and rounded ends, and are composed of mucoprotein. They may occur with fever, exercise, and renal disease. Epithelial cellular casts form from entrapment of sloughed tubular epithelial cells in the

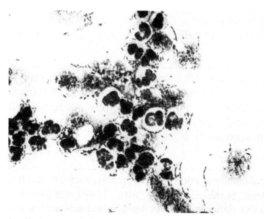

Fig. 3. White blood cells (neutrophils) and bacteria.

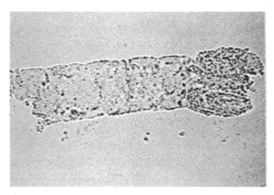

Fig. 4. Granular cast.

mucoprotein; they may be observed with renal tubular disease. Granular casts are thought to represent degenerated epithelial cellular casts. Waxy casts have a granular appearance and are thought to arise from degeneration of long-standing granular casts. They typically have sharp borders with broken ends. Other cellular casts include erythrocyte casts and WBC casts and are always abnormal. Erythrocyte casts form because of renal hemorrhage. WBC casts occur because of renal inflammation, as with pyelonephritis. Fatty casts are not common but can be observed with disorders of lipid metabolism, such as diabetes mellitus. A few hyaline or granular casts are considered normal. However, the presence of cellular casts or other casts in high numbers indicates renal damage and may be one of the earliest abnormalities determined by laboratory tests noted with toxic damage to renal epithelial cells (eg, gentamicin, amphotericin B).

Infectious Organisms

The presence of bacteria in urine collected by cystocentesis indicates infection. Small numbers of bacteria from the lower urogenital tract may contaminate voided samples or samples collected by catheterization and do not indicate infection. Bacterial rods are most easily identified in urine sediment (see **Fig. 3**). Particles of debris may be mistaken for bacteria. Suspected bacteria can be confirmed by staining urine sediment with Gram stain or modified Wright stain; however, aerobic culture is best to confirm a bacterial urinary tract infection. Rarely, yeast and fungi (**Fig. 5**) and parasitic

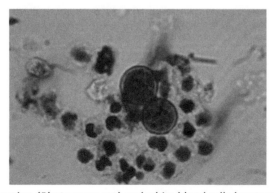

Fig. 5. Fungal organism (*Blastomyces* spp) and white blood cells (neutrophils).

ova may be observed in urine sediment. Their presence is not always associated with clinical disease. Parasitic ova observed include *Stephanus dentatus*, *Capillaria plica*, *Capillaria felis* (**Fig. 6**), and *Dioctophyma renale*. In addition, microfilariae of *Dirofilaria immitis* may be observed in urine sediment.

Crystals

Many urine sediments contain crystals. The type of crystal present depends on urine pH, concentration of crystallogenic materials, urine temperature, and length of time between urine collection and examination. Crystalluria is not synonymous with urolithiasis and is not necessarily pathologic. Furthermore, uroliths may form without observed crystalluria. Struvite crystals (**Fig. 7**) are commonly observed in canine and feline urine. Struvite crystalluria in dogs is not a problem unless there is a concurrent bacterial urinary tract infection with a urease-producing microbe. Without an infection, struvite crystals in dogs are not associated with struvite urolith formation. However, struvite uroliths form in some animals (eg, cats) without a bacterial urinary tract infection. In these animals, struvite crystalluria may be pathologic. Struvite crystals appear typically as coffin lids or prisms; however, they may be amorphous. Calcium oxalate crystalluria occurs less commonly in dogs and cats; if persistent, it may indicate an increased risk for calcium oxalate urolith formation. However, calcium oxalate and calcium carbonate crystalluria is common in healthy horses and cattle. Calcium oxalate dihydrate crystals appear as squares with an X in the middle (**Fig. 8**) or as envelope shaped. Calcium oxalate monohydrate crystals are dumbbell shaped. An unusual form of calcium oxalate crystals is typically seen in association with ethylene glycol toxicity. These crystals occur in neutral to acidic urine. They are small, flat, and colorless and are shaped like picket fence posts. Ammonium acid urate crystals suggest liver disease (eg, portosystemic shunt). These crystals occur in acidic urine and are yellow-brown spheres with irregular, spiny projections (**Fig. 9**); however, they may also be amorphous. Certain species, such as birds and reptiles, and certain breeds of dogs, specifically Dalmatians, can normally have ammonium acid urate crystalluria. Cystine crystals are 6 sided and of variable size

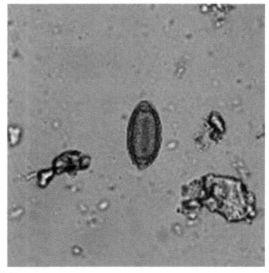

Fig. 6. *Capillaria felis* ovum.

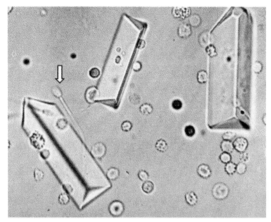

Fig. 7. Struvite crystals, red blood cells, and spermatozoon (*arrow*).

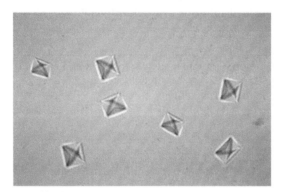

Fig. 8. Calcium oxalate dihydrate crystals.

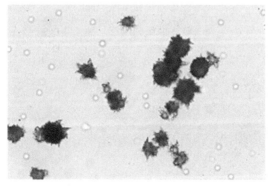

Fig. 9. Ammonium urate crystals.

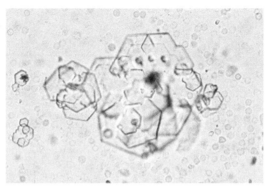

Fig. 10. Cystine crystals.

(**Fig. 10**). They occur in acidic urine. Presence of cystine crystals represents a prox-imal tubular defect in amino acid reabsorption. Cystinuria has been reported to occur in many breeds of dogs and rarely in cats. Dachshunds, Newfoundlands, English bull-dogs, and Scottish terriers have a high incidence of cystine urolithiasis. Bilirubin crys-tals occur with bilirubinuria; however, they may be normal in small numbers in dogs.

Lipids

Fat droplets are commonly present in urine from dogs and cats and may be mistaken for RBC. They often vary in size and tend to float on a different plane of focus than the remainder of the sediment. They are not considered to be pathologic.

Spermatozoa

Spermatozoa may be observed normally in urine collected from male dogs (see **Fig. 7**).

Plant Material

Occasionally, plant material may be observed in urine samples collected by voiding (**Fig. 11**). When present, it indicates contamination of the urine sample and is not pathologic.

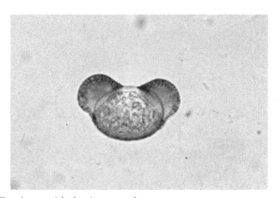

Fig. 11. Plant pollen in a voided urine sample.

REFERENCES

1. Osborne CA, Stevens JB. Urinalysis: a clinical guide to compassionate patient care. Shawnee Mission (KS): Bayer Corporation; 1999.
2. Wamsley H, Alleman R. Complete urinalysis. In: Elliott J, Grauer GF, editors. BSAVA manual of canine and feline nephrology and urology. Gloucester (United kingdom): British Small Animal Veterinary Association; 2007. p. 87–116.
3. Fry MM. Urinalysis. In: Bartges JW, Polzin DJ, editors. Nephrology and urology of small animals. Ames (IA): Blackwell Publishing; 2011. p. 46–57.
4. Defontis M, Bauer N, Failing K, et al. Automated and visual analysis of commercial urinary dipsticks in dogs, cats and cattle. Res Vet Sci 2013;94(3):440–5.
5. Bauer N, Rettig S, Moritz A. Evaluation the Clinitek status automated dipstick analysis device for semiquantitative testing of canine urine. Res Vet Sci 2008; 85(3):467–72.
6. George JW. The usefulness and limitations of hand-held refractometers in veterinary laboratory medicine: an historical and technical review. Vet Clin Pathol 2001;30(4):201–10.
7. O'Neil E, Horney B, Burton S, et al. Comparison of wet-mount, Wright-Giemsa and Gram-stained urine sediment for predicting bacteriuria in dogs and cats. Can Vet J 2013;54(11):1061–6.
8. Swenson CL, Boisvert AM, Gibbons-Burgener SN, et al. Evaluation of modified Wright-staining of dried urinary sediment as a method for accurate detection of bacteriuria in cats. Vet Clin Pathol 2011;40(2):256–64.
9. Swenson CL, Boisvert AM, Kruger JM, et al. Evaluation of modified Wright-staining of urine sediment as a method for accurate detection of bacteriuria in dogs. J Am Vet Med Assoc 2004;224(8):1282–9.
10. Way LI, Sullivan LA, Johnson V, et al. Comparison of routine urinalysis and urine Gram stain for detection of bacteriuria in dogs. J Vet Emerg Crit Care (San Antonio) 2013;23(1):23–8.
11. Heuter KJ, Buffington CA, Chew DJ. Agreement between two methods for measuring urine pH in cats and dogs. J Am Vet Med Assoc 1998;213(7):996–8.
12. Littman MP, Daminet S, Grauer GF, et al. Consensus recommendations for the diagnostic investigation of dogs with suspected glomerular disease. J Vet Intern Med 2013;27(Suppl 1):S19–26.

Diagnostic Imaging of Lower Urinary Tract Disease

Silke Hecht, Dr med vet

KEYWORDS

- Contrast cystography and urethrography • Ultrasonography • CT/MRI
- Urinary bladder • Urethra • Transitional cell carcinoma • Cystitis • Urolithiasis

KEY POINTS

- Diagnostic imaging of the lower urinary tract is commonly performed in small animal patients presented with urinary tract signs such as azotemia, hematuria, dysuria, stranguria, and pollakiuria.
- Ultrasonography is the modality of choice for the diagnosis of most disorders affecting the bladder and intra-abdominal portion of the urethra.
- Survey radiographs of the abdomen are useful in identifying radiopaque bladder or urethral calculi, gas within the urinary tract, and enlarged lymph nodes or bone metastases secondary to lower urinary tract neoplasia.
- Cystography and urethrography are especially useful in the evaluation of bladder or urethral rupture, abnormal communication with other organs, and lesions of the pelvic or penile urethra.
- Advanced diagnostic imaging is useful in assessing the ureterovesical junction, evaluating intrapelvic lesions, improving surgical planning, monitoring the size of known lesions associated with the urinary tract, and evaluating regional lymph nodes and osseous structures for metastases.

INTRODUCTION

Diagnostic imaging of the lower urinary tract is routinely performed in small animal practice. This article reviews the indications, imaging modalities used, and findings to be expected in common lower urinary tract diseases.

INDICATIONS

Indications for diagnostic imaging of the lower urinary tract overlap with indications for general abdominal imaging (eg, nonspecific clinical signs such as anorexia or

The author has nothing to disclose.
Department of Small Animal Clinical Sciences, College of Veterinary Medicine, University of Tennessee, 2407 River Drive, Knoxville, TN 37996, USA
E-mail address: shecht@utk.edu

Vet Clin Small Anim 45 (2015) 639–663
http://dx.doi.org/10.1016/j.cvsm.2015.02.002
0195-5616/15/$ – see front matter © 2015 Elsevier Inc. All rights reserved.

abdominal pain and abnormal findings on abdominal palpation). Specific indications include azotemia, hematuria, dysuria, stranguria, pollakiuria, and abdominal trauma with suspicion of uroabdomen.

IMAGING MODALITIES AND TECHNIQUES USED FOR LOWER URINARY TRACT IMAGING
Survey Radiographs

As radiographic equipment is readily available in small animal practices as well as referral institutions, survey radiographs of the abdomen are commonly the first step used in the evaluation of patients presented with signs referable to the lower urinary tract.[1–4] They are useful in identifying radiopaque bladder or urethral calculi or gas within the urinary tract and in assessing a patient for enlarged lymph nodes or bone metastases secondary to lower urinary tract neoplasia.[5–8] Other disorders of the lower urinary tract usually require additional imaging for diagnosis, although dystrophic mineralization, urethral thickening, or prostatomegaly may on occasion be visible in dogs with urinary tract neoplasia (see later discussion). Standard radiographic projections include lateral and ventrodorsal views. Care should be taken to always include the entire pelvis and perineal area to allow assessment of the pelvic urethra. In addition, ventrodorsal oblique views (**Fig. 1**) and in male dogs lateral views of the pelvis with the legs flexed forward ("lateral perineal views" or "butt shots") may be needed to minimize superimposition of osseous structures, which may obscure urethral calculi (**Fig. 2**).

Normal findings
The normal urinary bladder is of homogenous fluid opacity, is variable in size and shape, and may be partially located within the pelvic canal. Intrapelvic location of the bladder may be noted, the significance of which is controversially discussed.[9,10] The normal urethra is not visible on survey radiographs.[4]

Contrast Cystography and Urethrography

These procedures involve instillation of a positive and/or negative contrast agent into the urinary bladder and/or urethra.[2,3,11–18] They have largely been replaced by abdominal ultrasound but are still indicated for certain conditions (see later discussion).

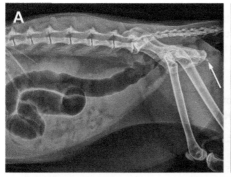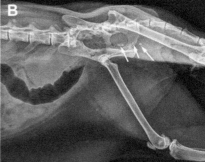

Fig. 1. Urethral calculi in a 13-year-old male castrated domestic shorthair cat. On the lateral view (A), an oblong mineral opacity is partially superimposed over the pelvis and extends into the plane of the perineal soft tissues (arrow). The oblique view of the pelvis (B) allows for identification of additional calculi in the intrapelvic part of the urethra (arrows). Mineralized sediment is present with the urinary bladder. Lumbosacral spondylosis deformans is incidental.

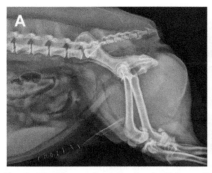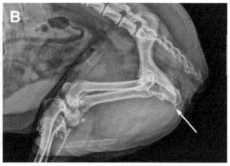

Fig. 2. Bladder and urethral calculi in an 8-year-old male castrated Pembroke Welsh corgi. The routine lateral view of the caudal abdomen (*A*) shows 2 sharply marginated calculi in the plane of the urinary bladder. The lateral perineal view with the legs flexed forward (*B*) shows an additional urethral calculus immediately distal to the ischium (*arrow*). Skin staples associated with the caudal ventral abdominal wall are consistent with recent surgery, and bilateral stifle degenerative joint disease is incidental.

Although these techniques are generally considered safe, adverse effects may occur, including hematuria, infection, (hemorrhagic) cystitis or urethritis, dissection of contrast medium into the bladder wall, iatrogenic bladder or urethral rupture, knotting or breakage of the catheter, and air embolization if using room air as contrast agent.[19–24] Urinalysis and urine culture should be performed before urinary contrast studies because of the risk of contamination during these procedures and because some results may be affected by prior contrast medium administration.[25–27]

Negative contrast cystography
Negative contrast cystography using a gaseous contrast agent is uncommonly performed. CO_2 and N_2O have a higher solubility in blood than room air and therefore pose a lower risk of embolization if absorbed into the vascular system.[2,14,23,24,28] Negative contrast cystography is useful in localizing the bladder if caudal abdominal masses are present or urinary bladder herniation is suspected. The technique is also useful in identification of luminal filling defects (bladder calculi) but is inferior to double-contrast cystography in this regard. It may be used as a complementary technique when performing an intravenous pyelogram because it allows delineation of caudal ureters and ureteral papillae.[29]

Positive contrast cystography
This technique involves instillation of positive contrast medium into the urinary bladder and is the preferred method to diagnose a bladder rupture or abnormal communication with adjacent structures (eg, urethrorectal fistula).[1,2,13,17,28,30–33] It is also useful in distinguishing the urinary bladder from caudal abdominal masses and in evaluating the position of the urinary bladder in the case of abdominal, inguinal, or perineal hernias.

Double-contrast cystography
This technique involves instillation of both positive and negative contrast media into the urinary bladder and is useful in evaluating mural and luminal bladder lesions.[1,2,13,14,16,17,28,33–36] It is the method of choice for the evaluation of the urinary bladder if ultrasonography is not available.

Retrograde urethrography

Because of the at least partially intrapelvic location in dogs and cats and its length in male dogs, urethrography with instillation of a positive contrast medium into the urethra remains the imaging modality of choice to evaluate the entire organ.[11,12,15,18,21]

The materials needed and techniques for these imaging studies are summarized in **Boxes 1–3**.

Box 1
Cystography and retrograde urethrography: materials

- Catheter (type and size dependent on animal size [Foley catheter ideal])
- 3-way valve
- Sterile lubricant
- Syringes
- Sterile gloves
- Sterile saline
- ± Vaginal speculum for female dogs
- ± 2–5 mL of 2% lidocaine without epinephrine
- ± Catheter connectors
- Contrast medium:
  - Positive contrast cystogram:
    - Water-soluble iodinated contrast medium diluted with sterile saline to 15%–20% (150–200 mg iodine [I]/mL)
    - Dogs: 10 (3.5–13.1) mL/kg
    - Cats: 10–50 mL
  - Negative contrast cystogram:
    - Gaseous contrast agent (preferably CO_2 or N_2O)
    - Dose as above
  - Double-contrast cystogram:
    - Water-soluble iodinated contrast medium, undiluted
      - Dogs less than 25 lb: 1–3 mL
      - Dogs greater than 25 lb: 3–6 mL
      - Cats: 0.5–1 mL
    - Gaseous contrast agent (preferably CO_2 or N_2O)
      - Dogs: 10 (3.5–13.1) mL/kg
      - Cats: 10–50 mL
  - Retrograde urethrogram:
    - Water-soluble iodinated contrast medium diluted with sterile saline to 15%–20% (150–200 mg I/mL)
    - Dose highly variable dependent on patient size and lesion location
      - Contrast medium administered in 5–20 mL boluses each
      - Several repetitions may be needed for diagnosis

Box 2
Cystography: technique

- Unless it is an emergency, assure adequate patient preparation
  - Fast patient
  - Administer enema if needed
- Sedation or anesthesia strongly recommended
  - Minimize patient pain/resistance
  - Optimize study quality
  - Reduce radiation exposure of examiner
- Survey lateral and ventrodorsal radiographs of the abdomen
  - Left lateral recumbency recommended by some to minimize risk of gas embolism
- Catheterization
  - Aseptic technique
  - Advance catheter to urinary bladder
  - Inflate cuff and retract catheter until the cuff is lodged within the trigone
  - Connect to 3-way valve
  - Empty bladder and, if needed, flush repeatedly with sterile saline to remove blood clots
- Administration of contrast medium
  - Important: To avoid overdistention of the bladder, injection should be performed under palpation control
  - Positive contrast cystography and negative contrast cystography:
    - Instill contrast agent until the bladder feels firm
  - Double-contrast cystography:
    - Instill negative contrast agent until bladder feels firm
    - Then instill positive contrast agent
    - Gently turn patient to assure even distribution of positive contrast medium along the bladder wall
- Obtain lateral, ventrodorsal, and, if needed, oblique radiographs

---

Other contrast procedures

Catheterization of the urethra in female animals may be challenging. If a catheter cannot be adequately positioned, a *vaginourethrography* can be performed during which the catheter tip is placed in the vaginal vestibule, an atraumatic clamp is placed on the vulva to ovoid leakage, and contrast medium is injected to fill both the vagina and the urethra concurrently.[12,37,38] *Antegrade* and *voiding cystography and urethrography* are technically challenging and not routinely performed. The reader is referred to other publications for further description of these techniques.[4,39–41]

Normal findings

Assuming adequate distention, the normal urinary bladder has a wall thickness of 1 mm (cats) to 2 mm (dogs) and has a smooth mucosal surface and no discernible filling defects associated with wall or lumen.[2,13,15,16] The position varies slightly with degree of distension during the contrast procedure.[42,43] The normal urethra is

---

Box 3
Urethrography: technique

- Unless it is in emergency, assure adequate patient preparation
- Sedation or anesthesia strongly recommended
- Survey lateral and ventrodorsal radiographs of the abdomen
- Catheterization
  - Aseptic technique
  - Initially advance catheter to urinary bladder
  - Connect to 3-way valve
  - Empty bladder and, if needed, flush repeatedly with sterile saline to remove blood clots
  - Distend urinary bladder with positive contrast medium (diluted with saline): this will ensure back pressure during subsequent injection of contrast medium into the urethra and adequate urethral distention, which will optimize evaluation of the wall. (However, normal structures such as the urethral crest may be obscured with this technique.)
  - Position catheter in the urethra
    - In cats and female dogs, the catheter tip should be located as distal in the urethra as possible
    - In male dogs, the evaluation of the entire urethra may require repositioning of the catheter and repeat injections, first from the ischiatic arch, the second from the caudal aspect of the os penis, and the third from the tip of the penis
    - If a balloon-tipped catheter is used, inflate balloon carefully
- Injection and radiographic documentation
  - Initial study most commonly performed in lateral recumbency
  - Fluoroscopy is optimal to monitor injection in real-time
  - If conventional radiographs are used, inject contrast bolus and obtain radiograph toward the end of the injection
  - Several injections may be needed dependent on initial findings
  - In male dogs, successively withdraw catheter and repeat injections from different urethral levels
  - If needed, repeat injections and obtain ventrodorsal and oblique radiographs

---

smoothly marginated and may show longitudinal folds if incompletely distended. It should be of fairly even width with the following exceptions:

- The prostatic urethra in dogs is wider than the membranous urethra.[44]
- In male dogs mild narrowing may be observed at the ischial arch.[18]
- The penile urethra in cats narrows progressively from the ischial arch to the external urethral orifice.[15]
- The colliculus seminalis may appear as a physiologic focal filling defect in male dogs and cats.[4,28]
- In cats a physiologic filling defect is associated with the dorsal urethra representing the urethral crest.[45]

Although an increase in urethral diameter with increased distension of the urinary bladder has been described in the proximal urethra in female dogs and cats and in the prostatic urethra of male dogs, a significant change was not observed in the membranous and penile urethra in male dogs or in male cats.[46] Thin, linear reflux of contrast medium into the prostatic gland may be seen in some normal dogs and is not necessarily an indicator of disease.[47] Similarly, vesicoureteral reflux may be evident in some normal animals.[48]

Ultrasonography

Technique and common artifacts

Patient preparation (clipping of the abdomen and application of alcohol and ultrasound gel) is performed in a routine manner.[49,50] Instillation of a standardized amount of saline solution (5 mL/kg) has been advocated to allow more accurate measurements of bladder wall lesions especially if monitoring a patient's response to treatment of bladder neoplasia.[51]

An extensive discussion of ultrasound physics is beyond the scope of this article and the reader is referred to other references.[52,53] However, a short overview of pertinent ultrasound artifacts is provided because these may be mistaken for lesions or may obscure the area of interest. Artifacts commonly encountered when imaging the urinary tract include acoustic shadowing, reverberation artifact, distal acoustic enhancement, slice thickness artifact, grating or side-lobe artifact, edge shadowing (refraction) artifact, and twinkle artifact.[54–60]

Acoustic shadowing occurs because of mineral or air interfaces causing loss of echo intensity deep to the interface because of absorption and/or reflection. Mineral interfaces such as uroliths typically cause strong distal hypoechoic to anechoic shadows. Air interfaces typically cause echogenic ("dirty") distal shadows because of concurrent reverberation artifact. This artifact is seen when gas is present within the bladder lumen or wall.[57]

Distal acoustic enhancement is due to passage of sound through an area of decreased attenuation resulting in higher echo intensity from tissues deep to the area compared with surrounding tissues at the same depth. This artifact is typically seen with fluid-filled structures such as the urinary bladder.[57]

Slice thickness, side-lobe, and grating-lobe artifacts may cause the appearance of echoic material within anechoic areas. These artifacts can give the false impression of sediment within the urinary bladder.[54]

Edge shadowing artifact is caused by refraction of the ultrasound beam. It occurs at the margin of curved structures and results in a dark line or shadow extending distally. If this artifact involves a curved fluid-filled structure (bladder) surrounded by fluid (abdominal effusion), it will cause the impression of a defect in the bladder wall (**Fig. 3**).[56]

Twinkling artifact is a color Doppler artifact that occurs behind strongly reflective interfaces such as those produced by urinary tract stones or parenchymal calcifications. It appears as a quickly fluctuating mixture of Doppler signals with an associated spectrum of noisy appearance and can be used to differentiate mineral structures from other hyperechoic material.[58]

Normal findings

The urinary bladder is found in the caudoventral abdomen and can vary greatly in normal size because of distention with urine.[59,60] The colon lies dorsally or dorsolaterally and often indents the bladder wall when the bladder is not fully distended. Urinary bladder wall thickness should be measured when the bladder is adequately distended; wall thickness measurements of an empty bladder are significantly thicker and are not reliable.[61] Normal wall thickness should be less than 2 mm in normal dogs, with larger dogs having a slightly thicker wall than smaller dogs. Normal bladder wall thickness varies from 1.3 to 1.7 mm in cats.[62] Lower-frequency transducers show

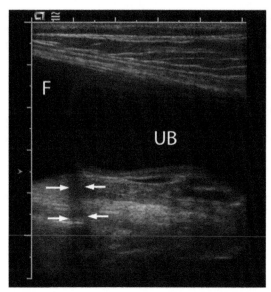

Fig. 3. Edge shadowing artifact in a dog with abdominal effusion (F). There is refraction of the ultrasound beam at the cranial (*curved*) margin of the urinary bladder (UB), resulting in the impression of a bladder wall defect. A dark line extending distally is also noted (*arrows*).

the bladder wall as a single echogenic line; however, high-frequency transducers typically show distinct bladder wall layers.[50] Normal ureteral papillae may be seen in some animals as small focal protrusions of the dorsal wall and should not be confused with abnormal wall thickening or bladder masses.[55] Ureteral "jetting" of urine may on occasion be observed and helps identifying the ureteral openings. Position of the bladder neck within the pelvic canal in some dogs makes complete evaluation difficult because of overlying bone.

Normal dog and cat urine is anechoic. Echogenic debris seen in the urine may be due to crystals, protein, cells, cellular debris, calculi, or fat droplets, and urinalysis is necessary for evaluation of the clinical significance.[49,59,60]

The urethra extends from an ill-defined juncture with the bladder neck into the pelvic canal as a hypoechoic tubular structure. Normally the lumen of the urethra does not contain observable fluid. The intrapelvic urethra is not usually visualized because of overlying pelvic bone but may be observable through the obturator foramen in some cases.[50,59,60] Transrectal imaging of the urethra can be performed but requires expensive specialized transducers.[63] In male dogs part of the prostatic and penile urethra may be evaluated from a perineal and/or ventral approach. Although the mucosal margin of the urethra is best assessed by positive contrast urethrography, ultrasound offers complementary information and can be used to assess urethral thickness and echogenicity.[64]

Advanced Diagnostic Imaging (Computed Tomography, Magnetic Resonance Imaging)

With increasing availability, the use of cross-sectional imaging modalities (computed tomography [CT]; magnetic resonance imaging [MRI]) for diagnostic imaging of the abdomen including the lower urinary tract in small animals is likely to increase. Initial applications described include the use of CT excretory urography to evaluate the ureterovesicular junction in patients with suspected ureteral ectopia and the use of either CT or MRI to evaluate intrapelvic lesions.[65–68] Both CT and MRI allow excellent anatomic delineation and are useful in assessing origin and extent of intrapelvic masses, identifying lesions associated with the pelvic urethra such as wall thickening or calculi, and evaluating surrounding structures including the spine and regional lymph nodes for the presence of additional lesions (eg, metastatic disease). CT has proven superior to ultrasound in accurately measuring the size of bladder wall masses.[51] CT and MRI are useful in planning a surgical approach for intrapelvic lesions and may be needed if radiation therapy planning is to be pursued for pelvic canal neoplasia. Finally, 3-dimensional (3D) volume rendering and virtual endoscopy using CT and MRI datasets are increasingly used in humans and are likely to gain popularity in veterinary medicine with increasing availability of these techniques.[69–74] A detailed discussion of CT and MRI principles, physics, and applications is beyond the scope of this article and readers are referred to specific references.[75] Techniques that have been suggested for evaluation of the ureterovesicular junction[66,68] and volume measurements of bladder masses in dogs,[51] respectively, are shown in **Boxes 4** and **5**.

Normal findings
The urinary bladder is located within the caudal abdomen and is filled with urine of homogenous attenuation/intensity unless contrast medium has been administered, which

---

Box 4
Evaluation of the ureterovesicular junction using CT-excretory urography: technique

- Fast patient for 12 hours and allow to urinate/defecate 2–4 hours before procedure (± enema)

- Place intravenous catheter in peripheral vein

- Sedation or general anesthesia

- (± Place urinary catheter, empty bladder, and distend bladder with negative contrast medium to improve delineation between urinary bladder and ureters)

- Position patient in sternal recumbency

- Precontrast scan from cranial level of kidneys to tuber ischii (± second scan of pelvic canal with smaller field of view)

  o Tube factors: 120 kVp and 120–250 mA

  o Slice thickness: 3–5 mm (thinner if possible dependent on equipment)

- Manual IV injection: Iodinated contrast medium, 400 mg I/kg

- Postcontrast scan (either dynamic or conventional):

  o Dynamic acquisition

    ▪ Slice position stationary and caudal bladder neck

    ▪ 5–10 minutes after injection: Obtain slices at 1-second slice intervals for 30 seconds

  o Standard acquisition:

    ▪ Repeat precontrast scan(s) 3 minutes after injection

    ▪ (± delayed scan [5–10 minutes] if ureters not adequately visualized during first scan)

Modified from Rozear L, Tidwell AS. Evaluation of the ureter and ureterovesicular junction using helical computed tomographic excretory urography in healthy dogs. Vet Radiol Ultrasound 2003;44(2):155–64; and Schwarz T. Urinary system. In: Schwarz T, Saunders J, editors. Veterinary computed tomography. Chichester (United Kingdom): John Wiley & Sons Ltd; 2011. p. 331–8.

Box 5
Urinary bladder CT protocol for tumor volume measurements

- Place IV catheter and induce anesthesia
- Place of an indwelling urinary catheter
- Position patient in dorsal recumbency
- Remove urine from urinary bladder and insufflate CO_2 (5 mL/kg)
- Scan caudal abdomen (1.25-mm slice thickness) from caudal margin of kidneys to pelvic urethra immediately following IV administration of iodinated contrast medium (600 mg I/kg)

From Naughton JE, Widmer WR, Constable PD, et al. Accuracy of three-dimensional and two-dimensional ultrasonography for measurement of tumor volume in dogs with transitional cell carcinoma of the urinary bladder. Am J Vet Res 2012;73(12):1919–24.

---

will result in a layered appearance.[65] Typically, contrast medium accumulates in the dependent portion of the urinary bladder; however, an inverted layering has been reported in CT and has been attributed to increased urine specific gravity.[76] Similar as described for contrast studies and ultrasonography, normal wall thickness of an adequately distended urinary bladder should range from 1 to 2 mm. If intravenous contrast medium has been administered, the ureters are seen entering the urinary bladder at the level of the trigone (**Fig. 4**).[66,68] The normal urethra can be traced caudally from the bladder neck and is clearly delineated within the pelvic canal as a homogenous tubular structure, which should not contain a significant amount of fluid.[65]

IMAGING OF SPECIFIC LOWER URINARY TRACT DISORDERS
Cystitis and Urethritis

Cystitis is common in dogs and cats. Imaging may not show any abnormalities in early or mild cases. In chronic and more severe cases abdominal ultrasound or double-contrast cystography may show diffuse thickening and irregularity of the urinary bladder wall, especially in the cranioventral portion of the bladder (**Fig. 5**, see also **Fig. 10**).[36,77,78] Additional findings might include intraluminal material due to the

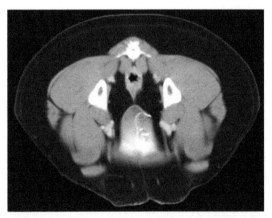

Fig. 4. CT-Excretory urography of the normal ureterovesical junction in a 3-year-old female spayed Swiss mountain dog. The left ureteral opening is associated with the dorsal bladder wall. Positive contrast medium is seen entering the bladder and accumulating ventrally. The right ureteral opening was located slightly more cranially and is not visible on this image.

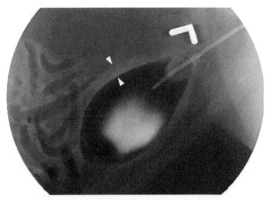

Fig. 5. Double-contrast cystography showing severe generalized bladder wall thickening (between *arrowheads*) in a 5-year-old male castrated domestic shorthair cat with chronic cystitis.

presence of inflammatory products and/or hemorrhage, mineral sediment, or cystic calculi. Mineralization of the bladder wall secondary to severe chronic cystitis has been described but is very rare.[79]

Emphysematous cystitis due to infection with gas-producing bacteria such as *Escherichia coli* or *Clostridium* species is most commonly seen in animals with diabetes mellitus but may affect other patients as well. A diagnosis is usually possible on survey radiographs where variable size gas opacities are associated with the bladder wall (and possibly the lumen) (**Fig. 6**).[6,80,81] Ultrasonographically, these gas inclusions appear as hyperechoic areas with distal reverberation artifacts.[82,83] Care must be taken to distinguish these pathologic gas accumulations from intraluminal gas introduced during cystocentesis, catheterization, or endoscopy, and this can be accomplished by repositioning the dog. While free luminal gas will move with a change in patient position, gas within the wall will remain static.[59]

Polypoid cystitis is a rare disease of the urinary bladder in dogs characterized by inflammation, epithelial proliferation, and development of a polypoid to pedunculated mass or masses without histopathologic evidence of neoplasia.[84,85] Concurrent cystic calculi are common. Most of the masses are located cranioventrally in the bladder (**Fig. 7**) as opposed to transitional cell carcinoma (TCC), which has a predilection for

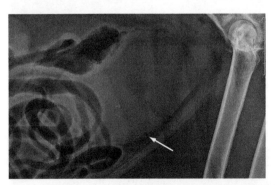

Fig. 6. Emphysematous cystitis in a 12-year-old female spayed Labrador retriever. Linear gas inclusions are associated with the ventral bladder wall (*arrow*). Small bladder calculi are also present.

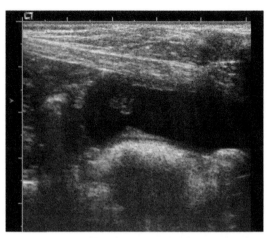

Fig. 7. Polypoid cystitis in a 5-year-old male castrated shih tzu. The ultrasonographic image shows a pedunculated mass attached to the cranial ventral bladder wall by a thin stalk.

the bladder neck or trigone area. However, because bladder neoplasia cannot be excluded based on cystographic or ultrasonographic findings, biopsy may be warranted to establish a definitive diagnosis.

Urethritis is uncommon in small animals and is usually associated with cystitis, prostatitis, or vaginitis.[86] Abdominal ultrasound or a urethrogram shows diffuse and irregular thickening of the urethra, which in the case of granulomatous urethritis may mimic urethral neoplasia.[87]

Urolithiasis

Bladder and urethral calculi are common. In the case of radiopaque calculi (calcium oxalate, calcium phosphate, and struvite) a diagnosis is usually easily possible on survey radiographs where they appear as rounded to spiculated mineral opacities of variable size in the plane of the urinary bladder and/or urethra (**Fig. 8**, see also **Figs. 1** and **2**).[2] Even though contrast resolution of modern digital radiography equipment seems to have improved detectability of less opaque and nonopaque calculi (silica, urate, and cystine calculi) compared with previous film screen radiography (**Fig. 9**),

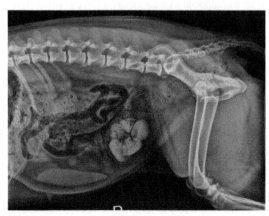

Fig. 8. Lateral survey radiograph of the caudal abdomen showing numerous large well-circumscribed bladder calculi in a 9-year-old female spayed Staffordshire terrier.

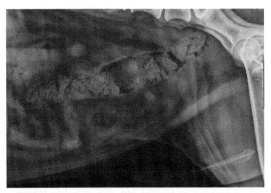

Fig. 9. Lateral radiograph of the caudal abdomen in a 5-year-old male Dalmatian (digital radiograph). Small intestinal segments superimposed over the urinary bladder interfere with evaluation. There are numerous minimally opaque bladder calculi, consistent with urate urolithiasis.

other imaging procedures may be needed to identify calculi, especially if obscured by overlying pelvic bones.[7,88] Using abdominal ultrasound, bladder stones appear as single or multiple strongly hyperechoic structures of variable size and shape (**Fig. 10**).[89] Dependent on size of the calculus and transducer frequency, distal shadowing may be present.[90] Sensitivity of ultrasonographic examination for the detection of cystic calculi is high and similar to double-contrast cystography if using a high-frequency (7.5 MHz or above) transducer. However, if a lower-frequency (5 MHz or lower) transducer is used, false negative results are common especially with small stones.[7] Although size measurements of cystoliths using radiography, double-contrast cystography, and CT are comparable and considered accurate, ultrasonographic measurements may overestimate the true size of calculi and should be interpreted with caution whenever cystolith size may influence patient management.[91] Possible concurrent findings in animals with bladder stones include bladder wall thickening, uroliths

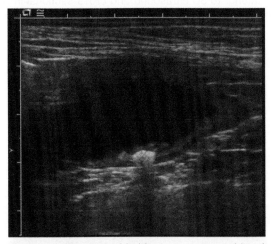

Fig. 10. Ultrasound image of the urinary bladder in an 11-year-old male shih tzu showing bladder calculi with moderate distal acoustic shadowing and mild bladder wall thickening consistent with cystitis.

associated with kidneys, ureters, or urethra, and inflammatory renal changes (pyelectasia, hyperechogenicity of renal cortices, and others).

Urinary calculi may become lodged in the urethra and result in partial or complete urethral obstruction. If the calculus is located in the intra-abdominal portion of the urethra or in the penile urethra in male dogs, it can usually be visualized by means of ultrasonography. Distension of the visible portion of the urethra and failure to visualize an obstructive lesion necessitate further imaging (positive contrast urethrography or possibly CT) (**Fig. 11**).

Neoplasms of the Urinary Bladder and Urethra

Urinary bladder tumors are most commonly identified by means of abdominal ultrasonography; alternatively, double-contrast cystography can be used. Survey radiographs are usually not helpful in identifying the primary lesion, although tumoral dystrophic mineralization may on occasion be visible in the periphery of the urinary bladder.[14] Radiographs are, however, useful in evaluating the patient for metastatic disease to sublumbar lymph nodes, pelvis, and spine. Transitional cell carcinoma (TCC) is the most common tumor type.[92] Other epithelial tumors include transitional cell papillomas, squamous cell carcinomas, adenocarcinomas, and undifferentiated carcinomas. Mesenchymal tumors are less common and include fibromas, fibrosarcomas, leiomyomas, leiomyosarcomas, rhabdomyosarcomas, lymphosarcomas, hemangiomas, and hemangiosarcomas.[93] TCCs are predominantly located at the level of the trigone but may be found in any location. Diffuse infiltration of the bladder wall instead of formation of a distinct mass is also possible.[59] Double-contrast cystography typically demonstrates one or more broad-based irregularly marginated wall–associated filling defects.[1,4,14,34] On abdominal ultrasound bladder TCCs are usually sessile, irregularly shaped masses of variable echogenicity (**Fig. 12**).[59,60,77,94] Concurrent findings may include hydronephrosis/hydroureter secondary to ureteral obstruction and evidence of metastatic disease to the medial iliac lymph nodes or other abdominal organs. Ultrasonographic findings of wall involvement, heterogeneous mass, and trigone location are associated with significantly shorter survival times and may be used as prognostic indicators.[95] Conventional 2-dimensional (2D) ultrasound has proven inferior to 3D ultrasound and cross-sectional imaging in obtaining reliable tumor volume measurements.[51] However, these modalities are currently

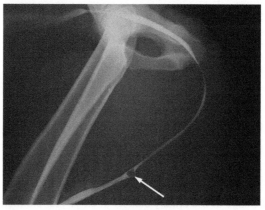

Fig. 11. Urethrogram in a male dog demonstrating a sharply marginated intraluminal filling defect (*arrow*), consistent with a urethral calculus.

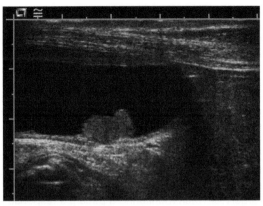

Fig. 12. TCC of the urinary bladder in an 8-year-old female spayed beagle. The sagittal ultrasonographic image demonstrates an approximately 1-cm-length broad-based lobulated mass associated with the dorsal bladder wall. The ventral bladder wall also appears thickened.

limited to specialty institutions. When monitoring a patient's response to treatment using conventional 2D ultrasound, it is important to keep the ultrasound technique and protocol (eg, positioning, degree of bladder filling, radiologist) as consistent as possible between examinations to minimize the chance of measurement errors. Smooth muscle tumors of the urinary bladder appear as smoothly marginated hypoechoic or heterogeneous masses.[59,96] Lymphoma of the urinary bladder wall has been reported to cause masses of variable echogenicity, size, and location.[97] Concurrent ureteral obstruction and lymphadenopathy are common. Differentiation from other tumor types is not possible by means of ultrasonography.

Most urethral tumors are malignant epithelial tumors (TCC or squamous cell carcinoma). A presumptive diagnosis is most commonly established by means of abdominal ultrasound or contrast urethrography. Urethrography demonstrates thickening of the urethra and marked irregularity to the mucosal lining resulting in a moth-eaten appearance (**Fig. 13**).[98] Ultrasound demonstrates hypoechogenicity and irregular thickening of the urethra, with a hyperechoic line along the epithelial surface.[64]

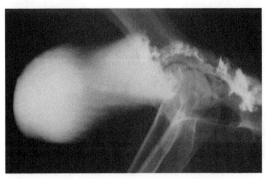

Fig. 13. Urethral TCC in a 10-year-old female spayed German shepherd dog. The urethrogram shows that the urethral wall is severely generally thickened, with marked irregularity of the mucosal surface.

Possible concurrent findings include abnormalities of bladder and/or prostatic gland, hydronephrosis, and medial iliac lymph node enlargement.

Imaging findings in other urinary bladder and urethral tumors are rarely reported and variable.[59,99–101] Neoplasms of structures bordering the urethra, such as prostate, os penis, or vagina/uterus, may involve the urethra, and origin of the disease process may not be obvious in some cases.[102–104]

Advanced diagnostic imaging (CT/MRI) of the bladder is at this point not commonly performed in small animal patients with bladder and urethral neoplasms because of associated cost, need for heavy sedation/general anesthesia, and lack of availability. Both CT and MRI are excellent modalities in evaluating the primary lesion (**Fig. 14**) as well as in the extent of metastatic disease to lymph nodes and osseous structures (**Fig. 15**).[65,68] CT cystography (see **Box 5**) provides an excellent method for accurate tumor volume measurements and should be considered especially if evaluating a patient for possible surgery or when monitoring a patient's response to treatment.[51] In addition, virtual endoscopy using CT or MRI data sets (**Fig. 16**) is increasingly used in human medicine and is likely to gain popularity in veterinary medicine with increasing availability.[70–74]

Because there is overlap in the imaging appearance of various bladder/urethral tumors as well as tumors and inflammatory conditions (eg, polypoid cystitis or granulomatous urethritis), biopsy is necessary for a definitive diagnosis (**Fig. 17**). Samples of

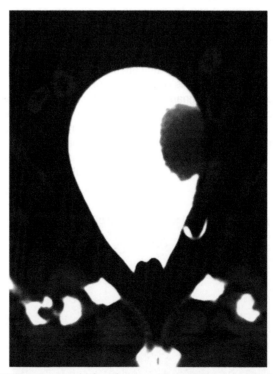

Fig. 14. Bladder TCC in a 6-year-old female spayed West Highland white terrier. Dorsal multiplanar reconstructed CT image obtained after instillation of positive contrast medium into the urinary bladder demonstrates a large broad-based irregularly marginated filling defect (mass) associated with the left bladder wall.

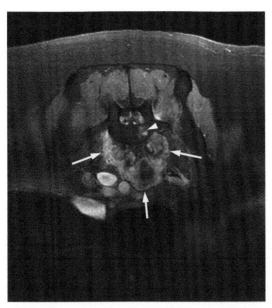

Fig. 15. Metastatic disease from urethral and/or prostatic carcinoma in a 10-year-old male castrated otterhound. The postcontrast T1-weighted fat-saturated image shows a large sublumbar mass abutting the ventral lumbar vertebral bodies (*arrows*), focal contrast enhancement within the left aspect of the vertebral body (*arrowhead*), mild contrast enhancement of the left epaxial muscles, and extradural compressive contrast-enhancing material within the ventral aspect of the vertebral canal.

bladder or urethral masses should be obtained by means of ultrasound-guided traumatic catheterization ("suction biopsy") instead of percutaneous tissue sampling due to the risk of tumor cell implantation along the needle tract[105]; this is especially important for apical tumors in which surgery may be possible.[8]

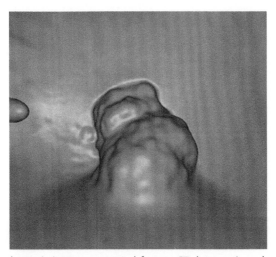

Fig. 16. Virtual endoscopic image generated from a CT data set in a dog with TCC of the urinary bladder (same patient as **Fig. 14**). The 3D display of the mass is comparable to what is seen when performing cystoscopy.

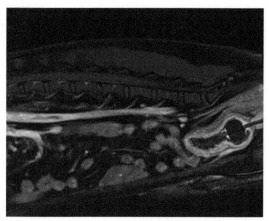

Fig. 17. Severe infiltrative bladder disease in an 8-year-old male castrated bichon frise presented with back pain and urethral obstruction. Prior fine-needle aspiration cytology of the markedly thickened bladder wall yielded a diagnosis of "marked neutrophilic inflammation and possible carcinoma." The postcontrast T1-weighted fat-saturated image shows that the urinary bladder wall is severely thickened and has a markedly irregular mucosal surface. An indwelling Foley catheter is present within the bladder and urethra. There is no evidence of metastatic disease to the spine or sublumbar lymph nodes. Subsequent surgical biopsies yielded the diagnosis of "marked necroulcerative cystitis."

Urinary Bladder and Urethral Rupture

Although the use of contrast cystosonography has been described as a sensitive tool for bladder rupture, positive contrast cystography provides more information on location of the rupture than ultrasound. Similarly, urethrography is considered superior to ultrasonography for the diagnosis of urethral rupture and will show extravasation of contrast medium into surrounding soft tissues and/or peritoneal cavity (**Fig. 18**).[106,107]

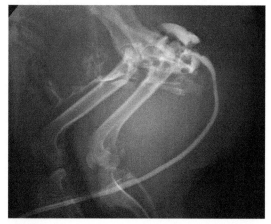

Fig. 18. Urethral rupture in a 1-year-old male miniature dachshund presented after being hit by car. The urethrogram demonstrates extravasation of contrast medium from the urethra into the perineal soft tissues and caudoventral peritoneal cavity.

Other

Abnormal position of the urinary bladder may be observed secondary to displacement by adjacent organs or masses or secondary to an abdominal, inguinal, or perineal hernia. Although ultrasound can be helpful in identifying an abnormally positioned bladder, positive contrast cystography may be given preference especially if the bladder is partially obscured by the pelvis.[13] A focal outpouching from the cranial ventral bladder margin seen on ultrasound or cystogram is consistent with a *persistent urachus/urachal diverticulum*, which is an occasional incidental finding or may be associated with chronic/recurrent cystitis.[2,108,109] An *abnormal communication* (fistula) between the bladder or urethra and other structures (eg, rectum) may be observed as a congenital abnormality or secondary to trauma.[30–32,110–112]; this is best diagnosed by means of positive contrast cystography or urethrography. Although *cystic foreign* bodies in humans are not uncommon and are usually self-inflicted,[113] they are very rare in animals. Potential causes include migration of foreign material from other organs, ballistic fragments, and urinary catheter pieces after catheter failure.[114–116]

SUMMARY

Lower urinary tract disorders are common in small animal patients, and diagnostic imaging is routinely performed as part of the diagnostic workup. Survey radiographs of the abdomen are helpful in identifying radiopaque bladder or urethral calculi, gas within the urinary tract, and enlarged lymph nodes or bone metastases secondary to lower urinary tract neoplasia. Contrast procedures (cystography and urethrography) have largely been replaced with ultrasonography but remain useful in the evaluation of bladder or urethral rupture, abnormal communication with other organs, and lesions of the pelvic or penile urethra. Ultrasonography is the modality of choice for the diagnosis of most disorders affecting the bladder and intra-abdominal portion of the urethra. Advanced diagnostic imaging modalities (CT, MRI) are useful in assessing the ureterovesical junction, evaluating intrapelvic lesions, improving surgical planning, monitoring the size of known lesions associated with the urinary tract, and evaluating regional lymph nodes and osseous structures for metastases.

REFERENCES

1. Johnston GR, Feeney DA. Comparative organ imaging—lower urinary tract. Vet Radiol 1984;25(4):146–53.
2. Marolf AJ, Park RD. The urinary bladder. In: Thrall DE, editor. Textbook of veterinary diagnostic radiology. 6th edition. St Louis (MO): Elsevier Saunders; 2013. p. 726–43.
3. Johnston GR, Feeney DA, Rivers WJ, et al. Diagnostic imaging of the feline lower urinary tract. Vet Clin North Am Small Anim Pract 1996;26(2):401–15.
4. Ackerman N. Radiology and ultrasound of urogenital diseases in dogs and cats. Ames (IA): Iowa State University Press; 1991.
5. Norris AM, Laing EJ, Valli VE, et al. Canine bladder and urethral tumors: a retrospective study of 115 cases (1980–1985). J Vet Intern Med 1992;6(3):145–53.
6. Root CR, Scott RC. Emphysematous cystitis and other radiographic manifestations of diabetes mellitus in dogs and cats. J Am Vet Med Assoc 1971;158(6): 721–8.
7. Weichselbaum RC, Feeney DA, Jessen CR, et al. Urocystolith detection: comparison of survey, contrast radiographic and ultrasonographic techniques in an in vitro bladder phantom. Vet Radiol Ultrasound 1999;40(4):386–400.

8. Allstadt SD, Lee N, Scruggs JL, et al. Clinical rounds—transitional cell carcinoma. Vet Med 2014;109(10):327–33.

9. Adams WM, Dibartola SP. Radiographic and clinical features of pelvic bladder in the dog. J Am Vet Med Assoc 1983;182(11):1212–7.

10. Mahaffey MB, Barsanti JA, Barber DL, et al. Pelvic bladder in dogs without urinary incontinence. J Am Vet Med Assoc 1984;184(12):1477–9.

11. Ackerman N. Positive-contrast retrograde urethrography. Mod Vet Pract 1980; 61(8):684–6.

12. Brown JC. The urethra. In: Thrall DE, editor. Textbook of veterinary diagnostic radiology. 6th edition. St Louis (MO): Elsevier Saunders; 2013. p. 744–56.

13. Essman SC. Contrast cystography. Clin Tech Small Anim Pract 2005;20(1):46–51.

14. Feeney DA, Anderson KL. Radiographic imaging in urinary tract disease. In: Bartges J, Polzin DJ, editors. Nephrology and urology of small animals. Ames (IA): Wiley-Blackwell; 2011. p. 97–127.

15. Johnston GR, Feeney DA, Osborne CA. Urethrography and cystography in cats .1. Techniques, normal radiographic anatomy, and artifacts. Comp Cont Ed Pract Vet 1982;4(10):823–36.

16. Osborne CA, Jessen CR. Double-contrast cystography in the dog. J Am Vet Med Assoc 1971;159(11):1400–4.

17. Pugh CR, Rhodes WH, Biery DN. Contrast studies of the urogenital system. Vet Clin North Am Small Anim Pract 1993;23(2):281–306.

18. Ticer JW, Spencer CP, Ackerman N. Positive contrast retrograde urethrography—a useful procedure for evaluating urethral disorders in the dog. Vet Radiol 1980;21(1):2–11.

19. Barsanti JA, Crowell W, Losonsky J, et al. Complications of bladder distension during retrograde urethrography. Am J Vet Res 1981;42(5):819–21.

20. Farrow CS. Exercise in diagnostic radiology: intimal dissection and luminal involution secondary to double contrast cystography. Can Vet J 1981;22(8):260–1.

21. Johnston GR, Feeney DA, Osborne CA. Urethrography and cystography in cats .2. Abnormal radiographic anatomy and complications. Comp Cont Ed Pract Vet 1982;4(4):931–46.

22. Johnston GR, Stevens JB, Jessen CR, et al. Complications of retrograde contrast urethrography in dogs and cats. Am J Vet Res 1983;44(7):1248–56.

23. Ackerman N, Wingfield WE, Corley EA. Fatal air embolism associated with pneumourethrography and pneumocystography in a dog. J Am Vet Med Assoc 1972; 160(12):1616–8.

24. Zontine WJ, Andrews LK. Fatal air embolization as a complication of pneumocystography in two cats. J Am Vet Rad Soc 1978;19(1):8–11.

25. Breton L, Pennock PW, Valli VE. Effects of hypaque 25-percent and sodium iodide 10-percent in canine urinary bladder. J Am Vet Rad Soc 1978;19(4): 116–24.

26. Feeney DA, Osborne CA, Jessen CR. Effects of radiographic contrast-media on results of urinalysis, with emphasis on alteration in specific gravity. J Am Vet Med Assoc 1980;176(12):1378–81.

27. Ruby AL, Ling GV, Ackerman N. Effect of sodium diatrizoate on the in vitro growth of three common canine urinary bacterial species. Vet Radiol 1983; 24(5):222–5.

28. Feeney DA, Johnston GR. Urogenital imaging: a practical update. Semin Vet Med Surg (Small Anim) 1986;1(2):144–64.

29. Silverman S, Long CD. The diagnosis of urinary incontinence and abnormal urination in dogs and cats. Vet Clin North Am Small Anim Pract 2000;30(2):427–48.

30. Silverstone AM, Adams WM. Radiographic diagnosis of a rectourethral fistula in a dog. J Am Anim Hosp Assoc 2001;37(6):573–6.
31. Osuna DJ, Stone EA, Metcalf MR. A urethrorectal fistula with concurrent urolithiasis in a dog. J Am Anim Hosp Assoc 1989;25(1):35–9.
32. Waknitz D, Greer DH. Urethrorectal fistula in a cat. Vet Med Small Anim Clinician 1983;78(1):1551–3.
33. Bischoff MG. Radiographic techniques and interpretation of the acute abdomen. Clin Tech Small Anim Pract 2003;18(1):7–19.
34. Scrivani PV, Léveillé R, Collins RL. The effect of patient positioning on mural filling defects during double contrast cystography. Vet Radiol Ultrasound 1997;38(5):355–9.
35. Mahaffey MB, Barber DL, Barsanti JA, et al. Simultaneous double-contrast cystography and cystometry in dogs. Vet Radiol 1984;25(6):254–9.
36. Mahaffey MB, Barsanti JA, Crowell WA, et al. Cystography—effect of technique on diagnosis of cystitis in dogs. Vet Radiol 1989;30(6):261–7.
37. Léveillé R, Atilola MA. Retrograde vaginocystography—a contrast study for evaluation of bitches with urinary incontinence. Compend Contin Educ Vet 1991;13(6):934–41.
38. Rivers B, Johnston GR. Diagnostic imaging of the reproductive organs of the bitch—methods and limitations. Vet Clin North Am Small Anim Pract 1991; 21(3):437–66.
39. Moreau PM, Lees GE, Gross DR. Simultaneous cystometry and uroflowmetry (micturition study) for evaluation of the caudal part of the urinary tract in dogs—studies of the technique. Am J Vet Res 1983;44(9):1769–73.
40. Moreau PM, Lees GE, Gross DR. Simultaneous cystometry and uroflowmetry (micturition study) for evaluation of the caudal part of the urinary tract in dogs: reference values for healthy animals sedated with xylazine. Am J Vet Res 1983;44(9):1774–81.
41. Poogird W, Wood AK. Radiologic study of the canine urethra. Am J Vet Res 1986;47(12):2491–7.
42. Johnston GR, Osborne CA, Jessen CR. Effects of urinary bladder distension on the length of the dog and cat urethra. Am J Vet Res 1985;46(2):509–12.
43. Johnston GR, Osborne CA, Jessen CR, et al. Effects of urinary bladder distension on location of the urinary bladder and urethra of healthy dogs and cats. Am J Vet Res 1986;47(2):404–15.
44. Feeney DA, Johnston GR, Osborne CA, et al. Dimensions of the prostatic and membranous urethra in normal male dogs during maximum distension retrograde urethrocystography. Vet Radiol 1984;25(6):249–53.
45. Scrivani PV, Chew DJ, Buffington CA, et al. Results of retrograde urethrography in cats with idiopathic, nonobstructive lower urinary tract disease and their association with pathogenesis: 53 cases (1993–1995). J Am Vet Med Assoc 1997;211(6):741–8.
46. Johnston GR, Jessen CR, Osborne CA. Effects of bladder distension on canine and feline retrograde urethrography. Vet Radiol 1983;24(6):271–7.
47. Ackerman N. Prostatic reflux during positive contrast retrograde urethrography in the dog. Vet Radiol 1983;24(6):251–9.
48. Christie BA. Vesicoureteral reflux in dogs. J Am Vet Med Assoc 1973;162(9): 772–6.
49. Hecht S. Applications of ultrasound in diagnosis and management of urinary disease. In: Bonagura J, Twedt D, editors. Kirk's current veterinary therapy XV. St Louis (MO): Elsevier Saunders; 2014. p. 840–5.

50. Hecht S, Henry GA. Ultrasonography of the urinary tract. In: Bartges J, Polzin DJ, editors. Nephrology and urology of small animals. Ames (IA): Wiley-Blackwell; 2011. p. 128–45.
51. Naughton JE, Widmer WR, Constable PD, et al. Accuracy of three-dimensional and two-dimensional ultrasonography for measurement of tumor volume in dogs with transitional cell carcinoma of the urinary bladder. Am J Vet Res 2012;73(12): 1919–24.
52. Kremkau FW. Doppler ultrasound—principles and instruments. 2nd edition. Philadelphia: W. B. Saunders Company; 1995.
53. Kremkau FW. Diagnostic ultrasound. 6th edition. Philadelphia: W. B. Saunders Company; 2002.
54. Barthez PY, Léveillé R, Scrivani PV. Side lobes and grating lobes artifacts in ultrasound imaging. Vet Radiol Ultrasound 1997;38(5):387–93.
55. Douglass JP. Bladder wall mass effect caused by the intramural portion of the canine ureter. Vet Radiol Ultrasound 1993;34(2):107.
56. Douglass JP, Kremkau FW. Ultrasound corner—the urinary bladder wall hypoechoic pseudolesion. Vet Radiol Ultrasound 1993;34(1):45–6.
57. Kirberger RM. Imaging artifacts in diagnostic ultrasound—a review. Vet Radiol Ultrasound 1995;36(4):297–306.
58. Louvet A. Twinkling artifact in small animal color-Doppler sonography. Vet Radiol Ultrasound 2006;47(4):384–90.
59. Sutherland-Smith J. Bladder and urethra. In: Penninck D, d'Anjou MA, editors. Atlas of small animal ultrasonography. Ames (IA): Blackwell Publishing; 2008. p. 365–83.
60. Barrett E. Bladder and urethra. In: Barr F, Gaschen L, editors. BSAVA manual of canine and feline ultrasonography. Gloucester (United Kingdom): British Small Animal Veterinary Association; 2011. p. 155–64.
61. Geisse AL, Lowry JE, Schaeffer DJ, et al. Sonographic evaluation of urinary bladder wall thickness in normal dogs. Vet Radiol Ultrasound 1997;38(2):132–7.
62. Finn-Bodner ST. The urinary bladder. In: Cartee RE, Selcer BA, Hudson JA, et al, editors. Practical veterinary ultrasound. Philadelphia: Lea and Febiger; 1995. p. 210–35.
63. Levy DA, Cromeens DM, Evans R, et al. Transrectal ultrasound-guided intraprostatic injection of absolute ethanol with and without carmustine: a feasibility study in the canine model. Urology 1999;53(6):1245–51.
64. Hanson JA, Tidwell AS. Ultrasonographic appearance of urethral transitional cell carcinoma in ten dogs. Vet Radiol Ultrasound 1996;37(4):293–9.
65. MacLeod AG, Wisner ER. Computed tomography and magnetic resonance imaging of the urinary tract. In: Bartges J, Polzin DJ, editors. Nephrology and urology of small animals. Ames (IA): Wiley-Blackwell; 2011. p. 146–60.
66. Rozear L, Tidwell AS. Evaluation of the ureter and ureterovesicular junction using helical computed tomographic excretory urography in healthy dogs. Vet Radiol Ultrasound 2003;44(2):155–64.
67. Samii VF, McLoughlin MA, Mattoon JS, et al. Digital fluoroscopic excretory urography, digital fluoroscopic urethrography, helical computed tomography, and cystoscopy in 24 dogs with suspected ureteral ectopia. J Vet Intern Med 2004;18(3):271–81.
68. Schwarz T. Urinary system. In: Schwarz T, Saunders J, editors. Veterinary computed tomography. Chichester (United Kingdom): John Wiley & Sons ltd; 2011. p. 331–8.
69. Orabi H, Aboushwareb T, Tan J, et al. Can computed tomography-assisted virtual endoscopy be an innovative tool for detecting urethral tissue pathologies? Urology 2014;83(4):930–8.

70. Behrens A, Heisterklaus I, Muller Y, et al. 2-D and 3-D visualization methods of endoscopic panoramic bladder images. Medical imaging 2011: visualization, image-guided procedures, and modeling. In: Proceedings of SPIE, vol. 7964. 2011. http://proceedings.spiedigitallibrary.org/volume.aspx?volumeid=163#1599SessionName.
71. Heinz-Peer G, Happel B, Memarsadeghi M, et al. Virtual multislice computed tomography cystoscopy for evaluation of urinary bladder lesions. Radiologe 2005; 45(10):897–904.
72. Russell ST, Kawashima A, Vrtiska TJ, et al. Three-dimensional CT virtual endoscopy in the detection of simulated tumors in a novel phantom bladder and ureter model. J Endourol 2005;19(2):188–92.
73. Stenzl A, Frank R, Eder R, et al. 3-dimensional computerized tomography and virtual reality endoscopy of the reconstructed lower urinary tract. J Urol 1998; 159(3):741–6.
74. Suleyman E, Yekeler E, Dursun M, et al. Bladder tumors: virtual MR cystoscopy. Abdom Imaging 2006;31(4):483–9.
75. Tidwell AS. Principles of computed tomography and magnetic resonance imaging. In: Thrall DE, editor. Textbook of veterinary diagnostic radiology. 5th edition. St Louis (MO): Saunders Elsevier; 2007. p. 50–77.
76. Samii VF. Inverted contrast medium-urine layering in the canine urinary bladder on computed tomography. Vet Radiol Ultrasound 2005;46(6):502–5.
77. Léveillé R. Ultrasonography of urinary bladder disorders. Vet Clin North Am Small Anim Pract 1998;28(4):799–821.
78. Scrivani PV, Chew DJ, Buffington CA, et al. Results of double-contrast cystography in cats with idiopathic cystitis: 45 cases (1993–1995). J Am Vet Med Assoc 1998;212(12):1907–9.
79. Zotti A, Fant P, De Zan G, et al. Chronic cystitis with ossification of the bladder wall in a 6-month-old German shepherd dog. Can Vet J 2007;48(9):935–8.
80. Aizenberg I, Aroch I. Emphysematous cystitis due to Escherichia coli associated with prolonged chemotherapy in a non-diabetic dog. J Vet Med B Infect Dis Vet Public Health 2003;50(8):396–8.
81. Middleton DJ, Lomas GR. Emphysematous cystitis due to Clostridium perfringens in a non-diabetic dog. J Small Anim Pract 1979;20(7):433–8.
82. Moon R, Biller DS, Smee NM. Emphysematous cystitis and pyelonephritis in a nondiabetic dog and a diabetic cat. J Am Anim Hosp Assoc 2014;50(2):124–9.
83. Petite A, Busoni V, Heinen MP, et al. Radiographic and ultrasonographic findings of emphysematous cystitis in four nondiabetic female dogs. Vet Radiol Ultrasound 2006;47(1):90–3.
84. Martinez I, Mattoon JS, Eaton KA, et al. Polypoid cystitis in 17 dogs (1978–2001). J Vet Intern Med 2003;17(4):499–509.
85. Takiguchi M, Inaba M. Diagnostic ultrasound of polypoid cystitis in dogs. J Vet Med Sci 2005;67(1):57–61.
86. Polzin DJ, Jeraj K. Urethritis, cystitis, and ureteritis. Vet Clin North Am Small Anim Pract 1979;9(4):661–78.
87. Moroff SD, Brown BA, Matthiesen DT, et al. Infiltrative urethral disease in female dogs: 41 cases (1980–1987). J Am Vet Med Assoc 1991;199(2):247–51.
88. Langston C, Gisselman K, Palma D, et al. Diagnosis of urolithiasis. Compend Contin Educ Vet 2008;30(8):447–50, 452–4; [quiz: 455].
89. Voros K, Wladar S, Vrabely T, et al. Ultrasonographic diagnosis of urinary bladder calculi in dogs. Canine Pract 1993;18(1):29–33.

90. Weichselbaum RC, Feeney DA, Jessen CR, et al. Relevance of sonographic artifacts observed during in vitro characterization of urocystolith mineral composition. Vet Radiol Ultrasound 2000;41(5):438–46.
91. Byl KM, Kruger JM, Kinns J, et al. In vitro comparison of plain radiography, double-contrast cystography, ultrasonography, and computed tomography for estimation of cystolith size. Am J Vet Res 2010;71(3):374–80.
92. Knapp DW. Tumors of the urinary system. In: Withrow SJ, Vail DM, editors. Small animal clinical oncology. 4th edition. St Louis (MO): Saunders Elsevier; 2007. p. 649–58.
93. Confer AW, Panciera RJ. The urinary system. In: McGavin MD, Carlton WW, Zachary JF, editors. Thomson's special veterinary pathology. 3rd edition. St Louis (MO): Mosby; 2001. p. 235–77.
94. Léveillé R, Biller DS, Partington BP, et al. Sonographic investigation of transitional cell carcinoma of the urinary bladder in small animals. Vet Radiol Ultrasound 1992;33(2):103–7.
95. Hanazono K, Fukumoto S, Endo Y, et al. Ultrasonographic findings related to prognosis in canine transitional cell carcinoma. Vet Radiol Ultrasound 2014; 55(1):79–84.
96. Heng HG, Lowry JE, Boston S, et al. Smooth muscle neoplasia of the urinary bladder wall in three dogs. Vet Radiol Ultrasound 2006;47(1):83–6.
97. Benigni L, Lamb CR, Corzo-Menendez N, et al. Lymphoma affecting the urinary bladder in three dogs and a cat. Vet Radiol Ultrasound 2006;47(6):592–6.
98. Ticer JW, Spencer CP, Ackerman N. Transitional cell carcinoma of the urethra in 4 female dogs: its urethrographic appearance. Vet Radiol 1980;21(1):12–7.
99. Liptak J, Dernell WS, Withrow SJ. Haemangiosarcoma of the urinary bladder in a dog. Aust Vet J 2004;82(4):215–7.
100. Mellanby RJ, Chantrey JC, Baines EA, et al. Urethral haemangiosarcoma in a boxer. J Small Anim Pract 2004;45(3):154–6.
101. Olausson A, Stieger SM, Loefgren S, et al. A urinary bladder fibrosarcoma in a young dog. Vet Radiol Ultrasound 2005;46(2):135–8.
102. Mirkovic TK, Shmon CL, Allen AL. Urinary obstruction secondary to an ossifying fibroma of the os penis in a dog. J Am Anim Hosp Assoc 2004;40(2):152–6.
103. Suzuki K, Nakatani K, Shibuya H, et al. Vaginal rhabdomyosarcoma in a dog. Vet Pathol 2006;43(2):186–8.
104. Winter MD, Locke JE, Penninck DG. Imaging diagnosis—urinary obstruction secondary to prostatic lymphoma in a young dog. Vet Radiol Ultrasound 2006;47(6): 597–601.
105. Nyland TG, Wallack ST, Wisner ER. Needle-tract implantation following US-guided fine-needle aspiration biopsy of transitional cell carcinoma of the bladder, urethra, and prostate. Vet Radiol Ultrasound 2002;43(1):50–3.
106. Côté E, Carroll MC, Beck KA, et al. Diagnosis of urinary bladder rupture using ultrasound contrast cystography: in vitro model and two case-history reports. Vet Radiol Ultrasound 2002;43(3):281–6.
107. Stafford JR, Bartges JW. A clinical review of pathophysiology, diagnosis, and treatment of uroabdomen in the dog and cat. J Vet Emerg Crit Care 2013; 23(2):216–29.
108. Groesslinger K, Tham T, Egerbacher M, et al. Prevalence and radiologic and histologic appearance of vesicourachal diverticula in dogs without clinical signs of urinary tract disease. J Am Vet Med Assoc 2005;226(3):383–6.
109. Rahal SC. What is your diagnosis? J Am Vet Med Assoc 2004;225(7): 1041–2.

110. Agut A, Lucas X, Castro A, et al. A urethrorectal fistula due to prostatic abscess associated with urolithiasis in a dog. Reprod Domest Anim 2006;41(3):247–50.
111. Hage MC, Duarte TS, Tavares TR, et al. Radiographic diagnosis of traumatic urethrorectal fistula in dog. Ciencia Rural 2011;41(5):848–51.
112. Miller CF. Urethrorectal fistula with concurrent urolithiasis in a dog. Vet Med Small Anim Clinician 1980;75(1):73–6.
113. Kochakarn W, Pummanagura W. Foreign bodies in the female urinary bladder: 20-year experience in Ramathibodi Hospital. Asian J Surg 2008;31(3):130–3.
114. Henninger W. Air-gun pellet forming the nucleus of a cystic calculus in a dog. Wien Tierarztl Monatsschr 1998;85(11):395–8.
115. Houston DM, Eaglesome H. Unusual case of foreign body-induced struvite urolithiasis in a dog. Can Vet J 1999;40(2):125–6.
116. Wyatt KM, Marchevsky AM, Kelly A. An enterovesical foreign body in a dog. Aust Vet J 1999;77(1):27–9.

Cystoscopy in Dogs and Cats

Megan Morgan, VMD, Marnin Forman, DVM*

KEYWORDS

- Cystoscopy • Urethroscopy • Urinary incontinence • Ectopic ureter • Hematuria
- Pollakiuria • Urinary obstruction • Urinary cancer

KEY POINTS

- For experienced, well trained clinicians, cystoscopy is a minimally invasive tool that has advanced urology in veterinary medicine.
- Cystoscopy provides the ability to diagnose conditions that cannot easily be diagnosed using other modalities.
- Cystoscopy enables thorough and minimally invasive assessment and treatment of conditions diagnosed using other modalities.
- As technology advances, a wider range of patients will be able to be assessed via cystoscopy, and more cystoscopic guided treatment options will become available.
- Advanced training and a wide range of specialized equipment are necessary to perform cystoscopy appropriately.

INTRODUCTION: NATURE OF THE PROBLEM

Cystourethroscopy is a technique used to gain access to the lower genitourinary tract (urethra, urinary bladder, ureteral orifices, vagina). In most cases, cystourethroscopy is used as a diagnostic tool to visually assess the lower urinary tract if routine diagnostic evaluation (blood work, urinalysis, urine culture, radiography, ultrasonography) does not yield a definitive diagnosis for the cause of a patient's lower urinary tract disease. In addition, some treatment modalities can be administered with cystoscopic guidance. Cystourethroscopy is considered a minimally invasive procedure but does require general anesthesia in order to minimize patient movement and secondary iatrogenic injury to the lower urinary tract.

INDICATIONS FOR CYSTOURETHROSCOPY
Persistent/Recurrent Lower Urinary Tract Signs

Common lower urinary tract signs in dogs and cats include dysuria, pollakiuria, stranguria, hematuria, and inappropriate urination (**Boxes 1** and **2**). The most common

Internal Medicine Department, Cornell University Veterinary Specialists, 880 Canal Street, Stamford, CT 06902, USA
* Corresponding author.
E-mail address: mforman@cuvs.org

Vet Clin Small Anim 45 (2015) 665–701
http://dx.doi.org/10.1016/j.cvsm.2015.02.010
0195-5616/15/$ – see front matter © 2015 Elsevier Inc. All rights reserved.

vetsmall.theclinics.com

differentials for these signs in dogs are urinary tract infection (**Fig. 1**), urolithiasis (**Fig. 2**), and lower urinary tract neoplasia (**Fig. 3**), whereas in cats feline idiopathic cystitis (also known as feline lower urinary tract disease, **Fig. 4**) is also a common differential for lower urinary tract signs.[1] Cystoscopy is indicated when routine diagnostic evaluation (blood work, urinalysis, urine culture, radiography, ultrasonography) does not yield an obvious cause for a patient's lower urinary tract signs. It is also indicated when there has been an apparent therapeutic failure for a diagnosed cause of lower urinary tract signs. An example of this is a patient with lower urinary tract signs that do not abate after appropriate antibiotic therapy is instituted for a urinary tract

---

Box 1
Indications for cystoscopy

Assessment of persistent or recurrent lower urinary tract signs of unknown origin

    Urethral or bladder masses

    Urethral strictures

    Occult uroliths

Assessment of persistent or recurrent urinary tract infections

    Investigate for anatomic abnormalities that may predispose the patient to development of infections

    Identify urethral or bladder masses

    Identify uroliths

    Identify vestibulovaginal stenosis

    Identify and resect (via laser) vestibulovaginal septal remnants

Assessment of chronic hematuria

    Identify bladder or urethral masses

    Identify occult uroliths

    Identify primary renal hematuria (hematuria seen exiting ureteral orifices)

Assessment of bladder or urethral masses

    Assess extent of mass

    Cystoscopic guided biopsy

    Cystoscopic guided laser resection of cystic polyps

Treatment of cystic or urethral calculi

    Cystoscopic guided stone basketing

    Laser lithotripsy

    Electrohydraulic lithotripsy

    Laparoscopic assisted cystoscopic urolith removal

    Percutaneous cystolithotomy

Assessment and treatment of urinary incontinence

    Assess for the presence of ectopic ureters

    Cystoscopic guided laser ablation of ectopic ureters

    Cystoscopic guided submucosal injection of urethral bulking agents

Box 2
Cystoscopic guided treatment options for various urinary tract disease processes

Disease Processes Diagnosed via Cystoscopy and Treatable with Cystoscopic Guided Procedures

Disease Process	Cystoscopic Guided Treatment Options
Cystic or urethral calculi	1. Retrograde cystoscopic guided stone basketing 2. Retrograde cystoscopic guided laser lithotripsy 3. Antegrade percutaneous cystolithotomy
Cystic polypoid masses	Cystoscopic guided laser resection
Idiopathic renal hematuria	Cystoscopic guided sclerotherapy
Ureteral ectopia (intramural)	Cystoscopic guided laser ablation of ectopic ureters
Urethral sphincter mechanism incompetence (presumptively diagnosed when other causes of urinary incontinence are ruled out)	1. Cystoscopic guided submucosal bulking agent injections 2. Cystoscopic guided botulinum toxin injections

infection diagnosed via urine culture and sensitivity testing. It is possible that such a patient may have a concurrent condition, such as occult urolithiasis or urinary tract neoplasia. Similarly, a patient that has previously undergone a cystotomy for urolith extraction but continues to have lower urinary tract signs may have suture remnants present in the urinary bladder (**Fig. 5**).[2]

Evaluation of Hematuria

Hematuria can be caused by bleeding from any portion of the urinary or genital tract. Cystoscopy is a useful tool for the diagnosis of the source and cause of hematuria in dogs and cats. It is particularly useful in patients for which thorough diagnostic

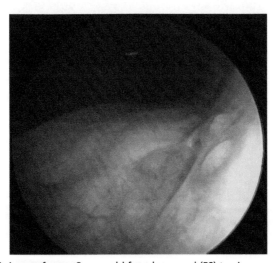

Fig. 1. Cystoscopic image from a 2-year-old female spayed (FS) terrier cross dog with urinary tract infection and urinary bladder wall pustules.

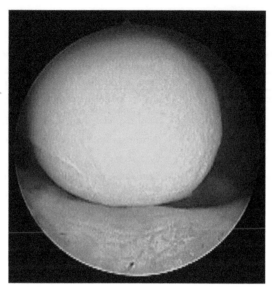

Fig. 2. Cystoscopic image from a 7-year-old female spayed bichon frise with struvite and calcium phosphate carbonate uroliths.

evaluation, including coagulation testing, does not diagnose a definitive cause of hematuria. In patients that do not have obvious inflammatory lesions (**Fig. 6**) within the lower urinary tract, primary renal hematuria (**Fig. 7**) becomes a likely differential. This condition can be diagnosed definitively by monitoring the urine jets (**Fig. 8**) from each ureteral orifice for obvious bleeding.[3,4] Cystoscopic guided sclerotherapy can be performed in select patients with primary renal hematuria.

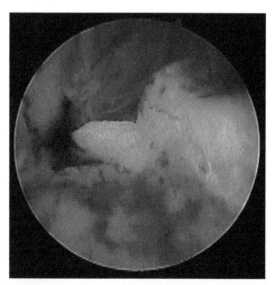

Fig. 3. Cystoscopic image from a 12-year-old female spayed mixed breed dog with a transitional cell carcinoma at the trigone.

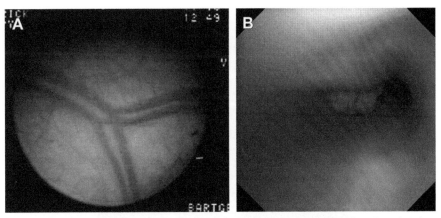

Fig. 4. (*A*) Cystoscopic image from a 3-year-old spayed female domestic short hair (DSH) cat with vascular congestion secondary to feline lower urinary tract disease. (*B*) Cystoscopic image from a male dog of unknown age with a urethrolith at the base of the os penis.

Urinary Tract Masses

Cystoscopy can be helpful in the diagnosis of lower urinary tract masses. In many cases, these masses are diagnosed using other modalities (most commonly transabdominal ultrasonography). Occasionally, cystoscopy reveals masses not visualized using other diagnostic tools, particularly when they are located only in the urethra, vagina, or vestibular vault. Transitional cell carcinoma and prostatic carcinoma are the most common malignant neoplasms of the lower urinary tract, but other types of neoplasia (rhabdomyosarcoma, leiomyosarcoma, lymphosarcoma, hemangiosarcoma, fibrosarcoma, metastatic neoplasia) have also been reported.[5–20] Cystoscopic guided mass biopsy can be performed via introduction of a flexible biopsy instrument

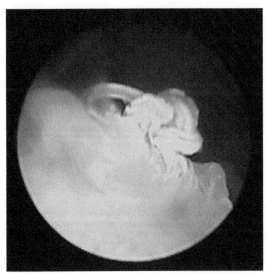

Fig. 5. Cystoscopic image from a 9-year-old female spayed Lhasa apso with a suture knot in the urinary bladder.

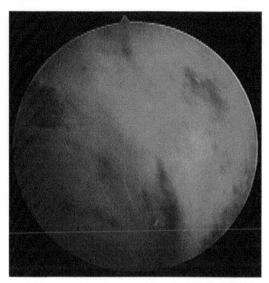

Fig. 6. Cystoscopic image from a 5-year-old female spayed Labrador dog with hemorrhagic cystitis secondary to recurrent UTIs.

through the cystoscopy sheath's instrument port.[21–23] Inflammatory polyps are common benign masses of the urinary bladder. Inflammatory polyps can appear similar to transitional cell carcinoma based on visual inspection (**Fig. 9**), and cystoscopic guided biopsy must be performed to definitively differentiate the two. Inflammatory polyps often have a stalklike base (**Fig. 10**), and are most commonly located at the apex of

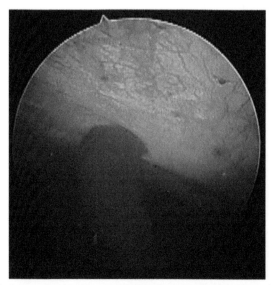

Fig. 7. Cystoscopic image from a 5-year-old female spayed mixed breed dog with bloody urine passing from the right ureteral orifice secondary to primary renal hematuria.

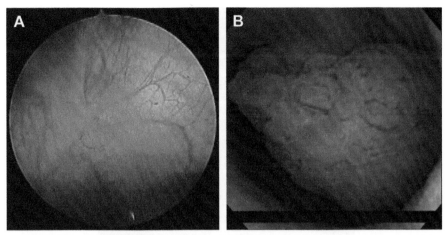

Fig. 8. (*A*) Cystoscopic image from a 7-year-old female spayed Yorkshire terrier dog with a normal left ureter passing yellow urine. (*B*) Cystoscopic image from a male dog of unknown age with urinary bladder transitional cell carcinoma.

the urinary bladder, whereas transitional cell carcinoma masses are most commonly located at the bladder trigone.[24,25] Holmium yttrium aluminum garnet lasers or diode lasers can be used to ablate the stalks of inflammatory polyps with cystoscopic guidance.[26] A cystoscopic stone basket or cystoscopic biopsy instrument can then be used to grasp the polyp and remove it from the urinary tract through the urethra. Care must be taken to ensure that the polyp is of an appropriate size to be removed through the urethra, because an inability to remove the polyp after detachment could result in a risk of urinary obstruction. Proliferative urethritis (also known as granulomatous urethritis) is a severe, proliferative, inflammatory process that occurs in the urethra and which, on gross examination, can appear identical (**Fig. 11**) to urethral neoplasia.[27]

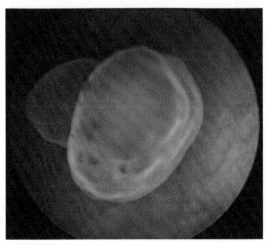

Fig. 9. Cystoscopic image from a male dog of unknown age with polypoid cystitis secondary to stones.

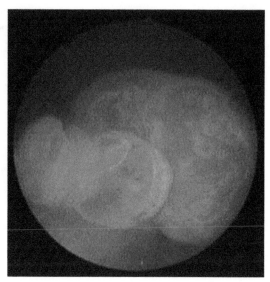

Fig. 10. Cystoscopic image from a 10-year-old female spayed Lhasa apso with polypoid cystitis.

Urolithiasis

Cystoscopy can be helpful in the diagnosis of uroliths not visualized with other common diagnostic tools, such as radiolucent calculi that are located in areas not able to be visualized by ultrasonography (eg, distal urethra). In patients previously diagnosed with urolithiasis via other modalities, cystoscopy can be used to gain access to the calculi (**Fig. 12**) and then cystoscopic assisted removal can be performed. For small

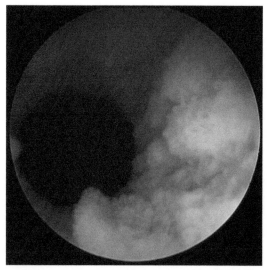

Fig. 11. Cystoscopic image from a 9-year-old female spayed retriever cross dog with lymphoplasmacytic urethritis.

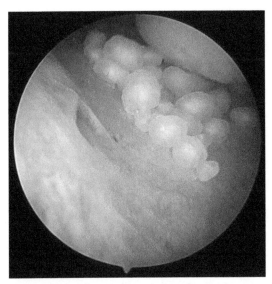

Fig. 12. Cystoscopic image from a female spayed dog of unknown age with uroliths in the urinary bladder. Note the normal right ureteral orifice.

calculi that can pass easily through the urethra, a stone basket (**Figs. 13** and **14**) can be passed through the cystoscope instrument port and used to grasp the calculi and remove them from the urinary bladder. Previous literature on voiding urohydropulsion provides information about the largest uroliths that were able to pass through the urethras of patients of varying sizes, sexes, and species (**Box 3**).[28] This information can be used to help determine the likelihood that cystoscopic guided stone basketing would be a viable option for urolith removal in a patient. For larger calculi, a lithotripsy fiber

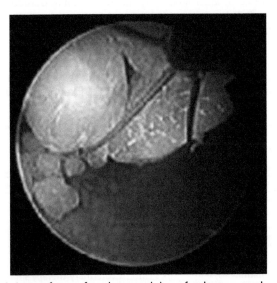

Fig. 13. Cystoscopic image from a female spayed dog of unknown age having multiple uroliths retrieved by a stone basket forceps.

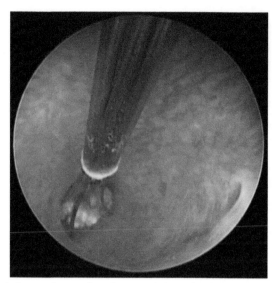

Fig. 14. Cystoscopic image from a female spayed dog of unknown age having urethrolith retrieved by graspers.

(**Fig. 15**) can be passed through the cystoscope instrument port and used to fragment the calculi into smaller pieces that can then be removed through the urethra via stone basketing or voiding urohydropulsion.[29–32] Because of the small size of the urethras of male dogs, and the resultant need to use a flexible cystoscope (**Figs. 16** and **17**), laser lithotripsy procedure times can be prolonged and there is a higher risk of incomplete urolith removal in male dogs than in female dogs.[29,31] For these reasons, antegrade approaches to the lower urinary tract have been described as a minimally invasive alternative to laser lithotripsy or cystotomy in male dogs.[33–35] An antegrade approach may also be preferable to laser lithotripsy for female cats, particularly those with a large stone burden.[36] This approach also provides a minimally invasive option for stone removal in male cats.

Recurrent Urinary Tract Infections

Cystoscopic evaluation of the lower urinary tract can reveal anatomic abnormalities that may predispose the patient to recurrence of UTIs. Examples of such abnormalities

---

Box 3
Maximum diameter of uroliths passed through the urethra via voiding urohydropulsion

Maximum Urolith Size Passed During Voiding Urohydropulsion			
Species	Sex	Body Weight (kg)	Maximum Urolith Size (mm)
Canine	Female	7.4	7
	Male	9	5
Feline	Female	4.6	5
	Male	6.6	1

From Lulich JP, Osborne CA. Voiding urohydropulsion: a nonsurgical technique for removal of urocystoliths. In: Bonagura JD, editor. Kirk's current veterinary therapy small animal practice. 12th edition. Philadelphia: WB Saunders; 1995:1006; with permission.

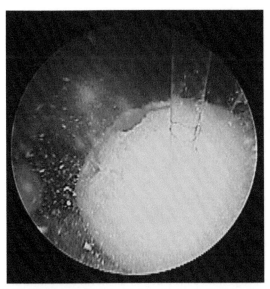

Fig. 15. Cystoscopic image from a 7-year-old female spayed bichon frise with struvite and calcium phosphate carbonate uroliths managed with lithotripsy.

include ectopic ureters (**Figs. 18** and **19**), urinary masses (**Figs. 20** and **21**), uroliths, vestibulovaginal stenosis, urachal diverticulum (**Fig. 22**), persistent paramesonephric remnant (hymen), vaginourethral fistula, and urethrorectal fistula.[37–42] In some cases, these abnormalities can be corrected cystoscopically (intramural ectopic ureters, uroliths, inflammatory polyps, persistent paramesonephric remnants).[29,31,37,43–46]

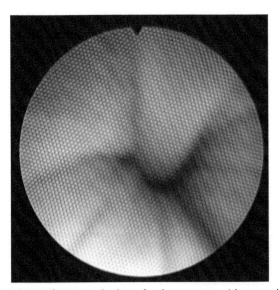

Fig. 16. Cystoscopic image from a male dog of unknown age with normal urethra. The image was obtained from a fiberoptic cystoscope.

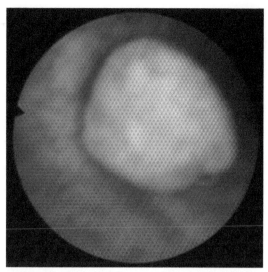

Fig. 17. Cystoscopic image from a male dog of unknown age with a urethrolith.

Urinary Incontinence

Cystoscopic evaluation of the lower urinary tract can reveal anatomic abnormalities resulting in urinary incontinence. Examples include ectopic ureters, intrapelvic bladder (short urethra), urethral hypoplasia (**Fig. 23**), vaginourethral fistula, and persistent vestibulovaginal septae.[37,38,45–48] Intramural ectopic ureters can be ablated via cystoscopic laser ablation.[43,44,46] Patients with no obvious anatomic or neurologic causes for urinary incontinence are typically presumed to have urethral sphincter

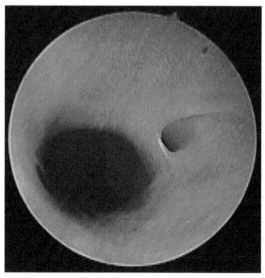

Fig. 18. Cystoscopic image from a 4-year-old female spayed Labrador dog with ectopic ureter (tear-shaped opening on the right).

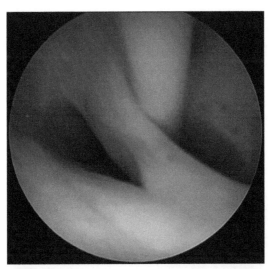

Fig. 19. Cystoscopic image from an 8-month-old female spayed rottweiler with an ectopic ureter (catheter in ectopic ureter).

mechanism incompetence. Urodynamics, including urethral pressure profilometry and cystometrography can be performed in patients with refractory incontinence to confirm abnormalities in urethral and/or urinary bladder tone, but have limited availability. Patients with urethral sphincter mechanism incompetence can be treated with cystoscopic guided submucosal bulking agent injections (**Fig. 24**) or possibly botulinum toxin injections.[49–52]

CONTRAINDICATIONS
Thrombocytopenia or Other Coagulopathy

Cystoscopy is minimally invasive and induces minimal trauma to the urinary tract when performed correctly (**Box 4**). However, in patients with defective primary or secondary

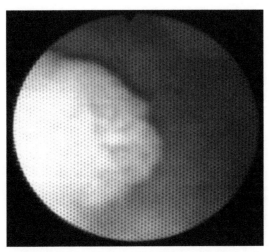

Fig. 20. Cystoscopic image from a male dog of unknown age with polypoid cystitis.

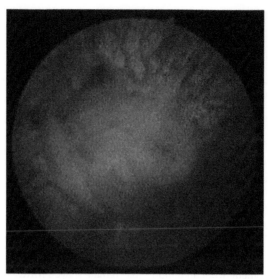

Fig. 21. Cystoscopic image from a 10-year-old female spayed miniature poodle with a sterile suture–induced urinary bladder granuloma.

hemostasis, even mild trauma could result in significant hemorrhage, potentially placing the patient at risk of blood loss as well as the formation of obstructive urethral blood clots. In addition, intraprocedural hemorrhage can cause deterioration of the cystoscopic image quality, thus decreasing the diagnostic utility of the procedure.

Anesthetic Intolerance

In dogs and cats, cystoscopy should be performed under general anesthesia because of the risk of iatrogenic injury to the urinary tract if the patient is excessively mobile during the procedure. Alterations to the anesthetic protocol can be made based on an individual patient's needs.

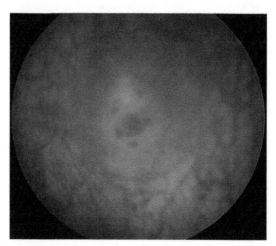

Fig. 22. Cystoscopic image from a male dog of unknown age with a urachal diverticulum.

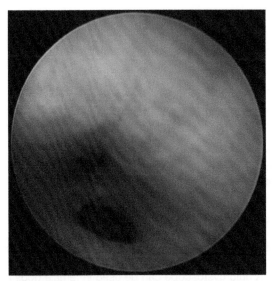

Fig. 23. Cystoscopic image from a 9-month-old female intact (FI) rottweiler with urethral hypoplasia.

Ruptured Urinary Bladder or Urethra, Recent (<7 Days) Urinary Tract Surgery

Cystoscopy on patients with rupture of any portion of the urinary tract can be challenging because of a loss of normal anatomic markers and difficulty distending the bladder or urethral lumen.[22,26] In addition, the vestibular vault, vagina, and distal urethra are not sterile environments, leading to a risk of introducing bacteria to the abdominal cavity (bladder and proximal urethral rupture) or the perineal region (distal urethral rupture).[53]

Complete Urethral Obstruction

Obstruction of the urethra could be considered a contraindication to cystourethroscopy in that complete urinary obstruction may render thorough assessment of the

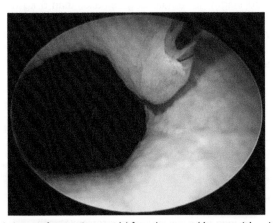

Fig. 24. Cystoscopic image from a 6-year-old female spayed boxer with urinary incontinence treated with urethral bulking polydimethylsiloxane.

Box 4
Contraindications to cystoscopy
Coagulopathy
Anesthetic intolerance
Bladder/urethral rupture
Recent cystotomy or urethrotomy (<7 days before procedure)

entire lower urinary tract impossible. However, urethroscopy can be used to determine the cause of the obstruction and can potentially be part of the treatment of the problem (eg, laser lithotripsy of urethroliths).[26]

TECHNIQUE
Equipment

A variety of cystoscopes is needed to perform transurethral cystoscopy in both male and female dogs and cats because of anatomic variations and marked variability in urethral diameter. A rigid cystoscope can be used in female dogs and cats. Flexible cystoscopes are required in male dogs and cats for complete evaluation of the urethra and urinary bladder. Most rigid cystoscopes are composed of 2 parts (**Fig. 25**): the inner telescope, which permits the conduction of light and the image; and the outer sheath, which protects the telescope and has ports and channels for the instillation of sterile liquid (or gas); drainage of urine; and passage of biopsy forceps, stone removal baskets, or lithotripsy fibers. The sheath also provides a smooth edge to protect the urethral and bladder mucosa. The sheath has a locking device to connect it to the telescope. Some cystoscopes have been developed that contain both the sheath and telescope in 1 unit. This design provides a slightly smaller outer diameter.[2,26] Telescopes are available in a wide range of sizes and lengths. The most commonly used cystoscope is a 2.7-mm diameter, 18-cm-long cystoscope with a 14.5-Fr sheath. This cystoscope is appropriate for female dogs greater than 5 kg and less than 20 kg. In dogs larger than 15 to 20 kg, the 2.7-mm cystoscope typically permits visualization of the urethra and bladder trigone, but not a complete bladder examination. In these larger female dogs, a 3.5-mm diameter, 30-cm-long cystoscope with a 17-Fr sheath provides the needed length. In female dogs smaller than 5 kg and female cats, a 1.9-mm diameter, 18-cm-long cystoscope with a 10-Fr sheath is required. Image quality is typically better with the larger telescopes. Telescopes are available with a

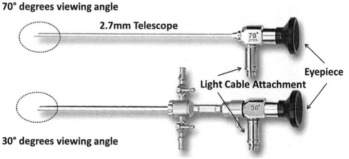

Fig. 25. Labeled 2.7-mm telescope cystoscope with and without a sheath.

variety of viewing angles, but a 30° angle of view is most commonly used in veterinary medicine.[2,26] Cystoscopy in male dogs requires a flexible cystoscope because of the anatomy of the urethra. These endoscopes are classified as ureteroscopes or ureterorenoscopes by most companies that sell cystoscopic equipment, because these endoscopes are used to visualize the ureters and renal pelvis in humans. Multiple flexible cystoscopes are available, with the most commonly used endoscope being 7.5 Fr and 55 to 100 cm long (**Fig. 26**). When selecting a flexible cystoscope it is important to consider the degree of deflection of the distal tip (ideal is 270° dual deflection), particularly if interventional procedures are to be performed. Cystoscopy in male cats is limited by the small luminal diameter of the male cat urethra but is possible with a flexible 1.2-mm diameter or semirigid 1.0-mm cystourethroscope. Both endoscopes provide visualization only. They have no biopsy channels and have poor image and light transmission quality because of the limited numbers of fiber optic bundles. Alternative techniques that could be used to image the urinary bladder and proximal urethra in male cats are rigid retrograde cystourethroscopy using a 1.9-mm, 18-cm-long rigid cystoscope following perineal urethrostomy, or antegrade cystourethroscopy after obtaining access to the urinary bladder surgically or laparoscopically.[2,26,34,35] Additional equipment needed to perform cystoscopy includes a light source (xenon light sources provide the best light quality), light-transmitting cable, sterile infusion fluid (typically 0.9% NaCl [saline] or lactated Ringer solution [LRS]), and irrigation lines. A suction device is also needed for flexible cystoscopy. Many endoscopists also use a high-definition camera (with connector) that attaches to the eyepiece of the telescope and transfers the image to an image processor. The image processor projects the image on a video monitor. This equipment can be stored on an endoscopy tower. A separate camera is also frequently used for flexible cystoscopy performed with a fiber optic endoscope but is not needed with a video endoscope. An image capturing device permits storage of images and/or videos for documentation in the patient medical record, future comparisons, and client education. Biopsy forceps, stone removal baskets or nets, electrocautery, or lithotripsy instruments are needed if these interventions are to be performed. After being cleaned and air dried, rigid telescopes and flexible cystoscopes should be stored in storage bins designed to avoid compression damage.[2,26]

Preparation

Cystoscopy should be performed under general anesthesia.

Female dogs or cats

The perivulvar region is clipped and cleaned with surgical scrub. An antiseptic vaginal flush (0.05% chlorhexidine acetate solution [12.5 mL of chlorhexidine added to 500 mL

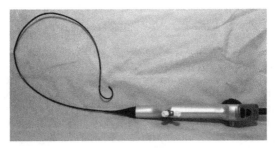

Fig. 26. Flexible cystoscope.

of sterile LRS or a 0.9% NaCl bag makes a 0.05% solution]) should be used before cystoscopy, particularly in patients with excessive vaginal discharge.

Male dogs
Preputial and peripreputial hair is clipped and the preputial and peripreputial region is cleaned with surgical scrub. The prepuce is then flushed with 0.05% chlorhexidine acetate solution for 2 minutes.[54]

Male cats
Preputial and peripreputial hair is clipped and the preputial and peripreputial region is cleaned with surgical scrub. Stay sutures are placed through the reflection of the prepuce at the base of the penis in order to facilitate penile extrusion.[22]

Patient Positioning

Female dogs or cats
The authors prefer to perform rigid cystoscopy in dorsal recumbency because of an improved ability to access the ureteral orifices for procedures such as ureteral stent placement or cystoscopic guided laser ablation of ectopic ureters, and decreased chance of fecal contamination of the vulva in dorsal recumbency.[55] Lateral recumbency and sternal recumbency have also been described.[2,56] If dorsal recumbency is used, the patient is placed in a radiology positioning trough located at the end of the examination table. The tail base is positioned at the edge of the trough. The hind limbs are tied in a frog-legged position. A sterile patient drape is placed over the patient and a hole is made to expose the vulva.

Male dogs
Lateral recumbency is used most commonly, but male dogs may also be positioned in dorsal recumbency, which offers some benefits with regard to complete visualization of the ureteral orifices.[56] A sterile patient drape is placed over the patient, and a hole is made to expose the prepuce. Care is taken to ensure that the cranial aspect of the drape is sufficiently long to reduce the risk of contamination of the flexible cystourethroscope.

Male cats
The patient is placed in dorsal recumbency. A patient drape is placed over the patient, and a hole is made to expose the prepuce.

Approach and Procedure

Female dogs: rigid retrograde cystourethroscopy
The rigid cystoscope should be fully assembled (telescope, sheath, camera, light source, light transmitting cable, irrigation lines connected) before introduction into the lower urinary tract. The rigid cystoscope should be liberally lubricated with sterile lubricating jelly before passage into the vestibular vault. The vulva is grasped and gently retracted caudally using the thumb and index finger of the endoscopist's nondominant hand. The cystoscope is then passed using the dominant hand between the fingers that are retracting the vulva, thus creating a seal around the cystoscope with the vulvar folds. Care is taken not to introduce the cystoscope into the clitoral fossa (**Fig. 27**). Irrigation is introduced to allow filling and complete assessment of the anatomy of the vestibular vault. In dorsal recumbency, the vaginal vault is located at the bottom of the image, and the urethral os is located at the top of the image (**Fig. 28**). The cystoscope is not initially advanced into the vagina, which has a larger number of bacteria than the urethra.[53] The cystoscope is slowly passed into the

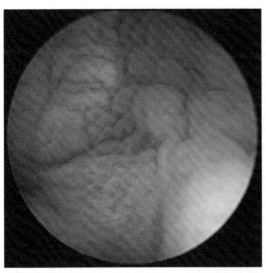

Fig. 27. A female spayed dog of unknown age with a normal clitoral fossa.

urethral os and irrigation is used to distend the urethra in order to enable visualization before cystoscope advancement. In order to prevent iatrogenic urethral trauma, care must be taken to keep the lumen of the urethra toward the bottom of the field of view because of the 30° angle of the rigid cystourethroscope. The cystoscope is gently advanced through the urethra and into the urinary bladder. If resistance is met at any point during cystoscope advancement through the urethra, the endoscopist stops advancing the cystoscope and withdraws the cystoscope slightly to visualize the

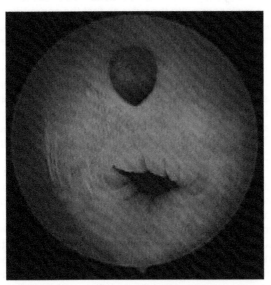

Fig. 28. Cystoscopic image from a 10-year-old female spayed miniature poodle with a normal vaginal vestibule distended with fluid (the vagina is the lower opening; the external urethral opening is at the top).

urethra and determine the reason for resistance. If there is no obvious reason for resistance, then it is most likely that the endoscopist is not appropriately centering the cystoscope in the lumen of the urethra (ie, the lumen is not being kept at the bottom of the screen) and therefore the cystoscope tip is encountering the dorsal wall of the urethra. The best way to correct this problem is for the endoscopist to lower the wrist slightly, such that the urethral lumen drops to the bottom of the screen. Once the cystoscope enters the urinary bladder, it is centered within the bladder lumen and the egress port is opened to allow the urinary bladder to be emptied. A urine sample should be obtained for analysis and bacterial culture if not already performed. Once the bladder is empty, it is filled with sterile saline. If the view of the bladder wall is still cloudy because of the presence of turbid urine, the bladder is again emptied of fluid and refilled with saline until the bladder wall is able to be visualized clearly. The entire bladder wall is carefully assessed (**Fig. 29**). The cystoscope sheath is moved counterclockwise while the camera is held stable such that the light source connection to the cystoscope is pointing upward. By doing this, the 30°angle of the cystoscope tip is pointing downward, which enables excellent visualization of both ureteral orifices. The ureteral orifices are C-shaped structures that face each other on the dorsal wall of the urinary bladder's trigone. The orifices are assessed with regard to their positioning within the urinary bladder, their anatomy, and the production of a jet of normal urine from each ureteral orifice (see **Fig. 6**). The cystoscope is then gradually withdrawn from the urethra. Following cystourethroscopy, vaginoscopy (see **Fig. 29**A) should be performed to assess for vestibulovaginal septal remnants (see **Fig. 29**B, C), vaginal masses (see **Fig. 29**D, E), vaginitis (see **Fig. 29**F), or vaginourethral fistulae.

Female cats: rigid retrograde cystourethroscopy

The rigid cystourethroscope should be fully assembled (telescope, sheath, camera, light source, light transmitting cable, irrigation lines connected) before introduction into the lower urinary tract. The cystoscope should be liberally lubricated with sterile lubricating jelly before passage into the vestibular vault. Saline irrigation is started before inserting the cystoscope into the vulva so that the appropriate rate of irrigation can be determined. Aggressive irrigation can result in overdistension of the urinary bladder and potential bladder rupture. The vulva is gently grasped and retracted caudally using the thumb and index finger of the endoscopist's nondominant hand. The cystoscope is then passed using the dominant hand between the fingers that are retracting the vulva, thus creating a seal around the cystoscope with the vulvar folds. The cystoscope is pointed downward so that the vestibular vault can be accessed. The urethral opening appears as a vertical slit at the top of the field of view, whereas the vaginal opening is a small circular opening at the bottom of the field of view (**Fig. 30**).[21,22,36] The cystoscope is gently passed into the urethral orifice and is gently advanced through the urethra, which is longer and narrower in female cats than in female dogs.[21,22,36] The urethra of female cats is often most narrow at its distal aspect, so entering the urethral orifice can be challenging in some female cats.[36] Care must be taken to keep the lumen of the urethra toward the bottom of the field of view because of the 30°angle of the rigid cystourethroscope in order to prevent iatrogenic urethral trauma. The cystoscope is gently advanced through the urethra and into the urinary bladder. Starting in the midurethra, there is a smooth ridge of tissue that arises from the dorsal wall of the urethra. This ridge is present along the remaining length of the urethra, up to the urethrovesicular junction. If resistance is met at any point during cystoscope advancement through the urethra, the endoscopist stops advancing the cystoscope and withdraws the cystoscope slightly to visualize the urethra and determine the reason for resistance. If there is no obvious reason for

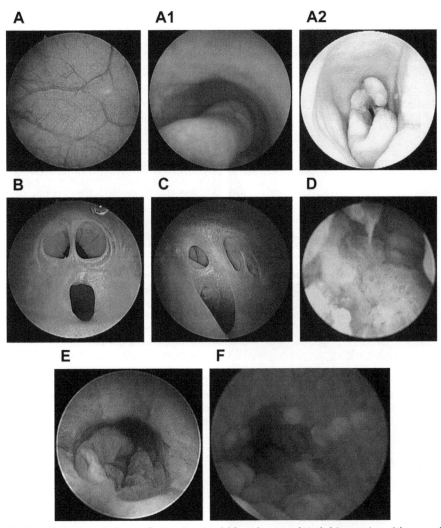

Fig. 29. (*A*) Cystoscopic image from a 7-year-old female spayed Yorkshire terrier with normal urinary bladder mucosa. (*A1*) Vaginoscopy image from a female spayed anestrous dog of unknown age with close cervical os. (*A2*) Vaginoscopy image from a 4-year-old female intact (FI) beagle with open cervical os in estrous. (*B*) A 7-year-old female spayed Yorkshire terrier with a thin frenulum in the vaginal vestibule. (*C*) Cystoscopic image from a 4-year-old Labrador with complex wide band frenulum (the patient also had bilateral ectopic ureters, which are not visible in this image). (*D*) A 9-year-old female spayed Norwegian elkhound with vaginal squamous cell carcinoma mass extending to the level of the external urethral papilla. (*E*) Vaginoscopy from a female spayed dog of unknown age with a vaginal transitional cell carcinoma. (*F*) Vaginoscopy from a female intact dog of unknown age with vaginitis (the patient also had urethritis, which is not visible in this image).

resistance, one possibility is that the endoscopist is not appropriately centering the cystoscope in the lumen of the urethra (ie, the lumen is not being kept at the bottom of the screen), and therefore the cystoscope tip is encountering the dorsal wall of the urethra. As is the case in female dogs, the best way to correct this problem is for the

A

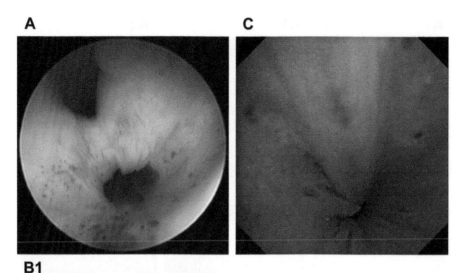

C

B1

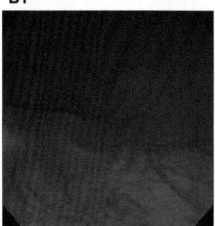

B2

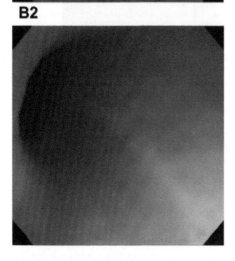

Fig. 30. (*A*) Cystoscopic image from a feline of unknown age with a normal urethral orifice and vagina (petechial hemorrhage is iatrogenic). (*B1*) Cystoscopic image from a male dog of unknown age with a normal-appearing perineal urethra. (*B2*) Cystoscopic image from a male dog of unknown age with a normal-appearing right ureteral orifice. (*C*) Cystoscopic image from a male dog of unknown age with a normal-appearing prostatic urethra with openings of ducts.

operator to lower the wrist slightly, such that the urethral lumen drops to the bottom of the screen. If resistance is still met, then it is most likely that the urethra is too narrow for cystoscopy. Retrograde cystourethroscopy should be aborted, and antegrade cystourethroscopy should be performed instead.[36] Once the cystoscope enters the urinary bladder, it is centered within the bladder lumen and the egress port is opened to allow the urinary bladder to be emptied. A urine sample should be obtained for analysis and bacterial culture at this time if not already performed. Once the bladder is empty, it is filled with saline. If the view of the bladder wall is still cloudy because of the presence of turbid urine, the bladder is again emptied of fluid and refilled with saline until the bladder wall is able to be visualized clearly. The entire bladder wall is carefully assessed. The cystoscope sheath is then moved counterclockwise while the camera is held stable such that the light source connection to the cystoscope is pointing upward. By doing this, the 30°angle of the cystoscope tip is pointing downward, which enables visualization of both ureteral orifices. Unlike female dogs, the ureteral orifices of female cats are located in the most proximal urethra.[22,36] The ureteral papillae arise from the previously described ridge of tissue on the dorsal urethral wall, and each ureteral orifice appears as a small slit on the top of each ureteral papilla.[36] The orifices are assessed with regard to their positioning, their anatomy, and the production of a jet of normal urine from each ureteral orifice (**Fig. 31**). The cystoscope is then gradually withdrawn from the urethra.

Male dogs: flexible retrograde cystourethroscopy
The authors typically empty the urinary bladder using a red rubber catheter attached to a 60-mL syringe before the procedure. The penis is extruded from the prepuce by an assistant. The penis is then gently grasped and the flexible cystourethroscope is passed into the urethral orifice. Care is taken not to enter the prepuce instead of the urethra, because the prepuce is a nonsterile environment. An assistant facilitates the infusion of saline through the cystoscope into the urethra. Because the working channel of flexible cystourethroscopes is narrow, using only a hanging bag of saline for infusion does not typically provide an adequate stream of saline to distend the urethra. The authors typically use a system in which the

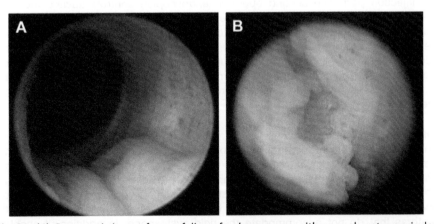

Fig. 31. (A) Cystoscopic image from a feline of unknown age with normal ureterovesicular junctions at the urinary bladder neck. (B) Cystoscopic image from an 8-year-old female spayed Labrador with small distal urethral perforation (noted at the 5 o'clock position) and urethral transitional cell carcinoma.

primary infusion line connected to the hanging bag of saline is attached to a 3-way stopcock. The other 2 ports of the stopcock are connected to an extension line that enters the ingress/egress port of the flexible cystourethroscope, and a 60-mL syringe. Saline is drawn into the 60-mL syringe from the saline bag, and is then infused into the cystoscope. Using this system, a higher pressure stream of saline can be used to dilate the urethral lumen, which drastically improves visualization of the urethra. Unlike female dog and cat cystourethroscopy, the urethral lumen should be kept in the center of the image as the cystourethroscope is advanced through the urethra, because the flexible cystourethroscope has a 0° angle tip. Once the prostatic urethra is entered, the prostatic ductules can be seen opening into the urethra. These ductules should not be mistaken for ectopic ureteral orifices. The bladder is then entered. The bladder is mostly empty and saline is infused to distend the bladder's lumen and the bladder's wall is thoroughly assessed. One major downside of flexible cystourethroscopy is that complete assessment of the bladder wall can be challenging because of the limitations of using a fiber optic scope with a narrow field of view. As the cystourethroscope is backed out of the urinary bladder, the cystoscope tip is deflected dorsally so that the ureteral orifices can be visualized. Assessment of the ureteral orifices using flexible cystoureteroscopy can be challenging, and the authors typically wait to see a jet of urine in order to guide the cystourethroscope to the appropriate location to assess the orifices. Following assessment of the urinary bladder and ureteral orifices, the cystourethroscope is gradually backed out of the urethra and the urethra is assessed a second time. Following assessment of the urethra and urinary bladder, the preputial fossa is examined with the cystourethroscope.

Male cats: semiflexible retrograde urethroscopy
This technique can only be used to assess the urethra of male cats.[22] If evaluation of the urinary bladder is necessary, antegrade cystourethroscopy is recommended (discussed later). Two operators are required for this procedure. The penis is kept extruded from the prepuce by preplaced stay sutures in the reflection of the prepuce. The penis is gently grasped and the semirigid cystoscope is passed into the urethral orifice. One operator (assistant) controls the infusion of saline through the injection port. The second operator (endoscopist) controls advancement of the cystourethroscope. The urethral lumen must be kept in the center of the image. Because the tip of the semirigid cystourethroscope cannot be deflected, this depends on tension exerted on the penis, saline infusion into the cystourethroscope, and torque placed on the cystourethroscope.[22] The normal bulbocavernosus glands and prostate appear as narrowings in the urethra. The entire urethra is carefully assessed as the cystourethroscope is advanced and withdrawn from the urethra.

Antegrade cystourethroscopy
This approach is appropriate for male dogs, male cats, and small female cats. The benefit of this approach is that it allows use of the rigid cystoscope to assess the urinary bladder and the proximal urethra, thus providing superior image quality compared with the flexible fiber optic cystoscope in male dogs and semirigid cystoscope in male cats. It allows access to the urinary tract in small female cats with urethras that do not accommodate the rigid cystoscope. In addition, it enables more rapid stone removal in male patients compared with laser lithotripsy and stone basketing via flexible cystourethroscopy.[35] A 1-cm skin incision is made over the apex of the urinary bladder. The urinary bladder is isolated and a stay suture is

placed into the apex of the bladder. The bladder is then gently retracted toward the body wall and the stay suture at the bladder's apex is tacked to the patient drape. Two stay sutures are then placed on each lateral aspect of the bladder and tacked to the patient drape, thus positioning the apex of the urinary bladder at the body wall. A stab incision is made into the apex of the urinary bladder and a screw trocar with diaphragm is inserted into the stab incision. The rigid cystourethroscope is passed through the trocar into the urinary bladder to assess the wall of the urinary bladder and the ureteral orifices, as well as the proximal urethra. The flexible cystourethroscope is then passed through the trocar and into the urethra to assess the urethral lumen. The penile urethra of male cats cannot be assessed with this technique because it is too small to accommodate the 7.5-Fr flexible cystourethroscope.[36]

Percutaneous perineal approach for rigid retrograde cystourethroscopy in male dogs
This approach is appropriate for large male dogs when rigid retrograde cystourethroscopy is desirable; for example, when interventional endoscopic procedures are required (eg, cystoscopic laser ablation of ectopic ureters).[57] Although cystoscopic laser ablation of ectopic ureters has been described in male dogs using flexible cystourethroscopy, it is not possible to have a ureteral catheter in place to protect the lateral wall of the ectopic ureter when using this approach.[43] In addition, it is significantly more technically challenging to perform cystoscopic laser ablation of ectopic ureters using a flexible cystourethroscope than it is to perform the procedure with a rigid cystourethroscope. This difficulty is primarily caused by limitations in image quality resulting from many flexible cystourethroscopes being fiber optic scopes rather that videoscopes, as well as from limitations in the maneuverability of flexible cystourethroscopes. The patient is placed in dorsal recumbency and the perineal region and preputial region are clipped and aseptically prepared with surgical scrub. The prepuce is flushed using 0.05% chlorhexidine acetate solution. A sterile drape is placed over the patient and holes are made in the drape over the midischial region and preputial region. A red rubber catheter is passed into the urethra and is palpated in the urethra in the midischial region. It is gradually backed out of the urethra until the tip of the catheter can be felt just distal to the midischial urethra. Saline is introduced through the catheter to distend the urethra. The urethra is stabilized between the finger and thumb of the endoscopist's nondominant hand, and an 18-gauge intravenous catheter is inserted into the urethra through the skin, making sure to orient the catheter dorsally toward the urinary bladder. Once saline is seen entering the hub of the cannula, the cannula is removed and the catheter is left in place. A 0.89-mm (0.035-inch) hydrophilic guide wire (Weasel Wire, Infiniti Medical) is passed through the catheter and into the urethra, and is allowed to curl within the urinary bladder. The catheter is then removed over the wire, and serial fascial dilators are passed over the guide wire, starting at 4 to 5 Fr and ending at 16 Fr. A 16-Fr vascular access sheath with dilator is then passed into the urethra and the hydrophilic guide wire is removed. The dilator is removed, and the rigid cystoscope is then introduced into the urethra through the vascular access sheath. The proximal urethra and urinary bladder are then assessed as described for female dogs. Because the vascular access sheath is within the urethral lumen, assessment of the entire accessible portion of the urethra requires the sheath and cystoscope to be concurrently withdrawn from the urethra. Following the procedure, a standard urinary catheter is passed and attached to a closed collection system. An indwelling urinary catheter is kept in place for at least 24 hours after the procedure.

COMPLICATIONS AND MANAGEMENT
Mild Trauma of the Urethra and Urinary Bladder

Low-grade urethral and bladder mucosal injury is common during cystourethroscopy and typically does not require any form of treatment (**Box 5**). Hematuria may be present for 2 to 3 days after cystoscopy.[22]

Stranguria, Pollakiuria, and Inappropriate Urination

Patients occasionally have lower urinary tract clinical signs of varying severity following cystourethroscopy.[22] These signs typically persist for 2 to 5 days after cystoscopy. Lower urinary tract signs seem to be particularly common in females following lithotripsy. The authors typically preemptively treat these patients with tramadol (2–3 mg/kg orally every 6–8 hours) or oral buprenorphine (0.01 mg/kg orally every 6–8 hours). If the urethra appears hyperemic and inflamed at the end of a cystoscopy procedure, topical bupivacaine (2 mg/kg diluted 50:50 with saline) can be administered through the cystourethroscope as it is withdrawn. Steroidal or nonsteroidal antiinflammatories can be used to reduce urethritis in patients that have significant

---

Box 5
Complications associated with cystourethroscopy and their management

Complications Associated with Cystourethroscopy

Complication	Management Options
Mild trauma to urethral wall or urinary bladder wall	No treatment necessary (self-limiting)
Urethritis (resulting in stranguria, pollakiuria, or inappropriate urination)	1. Pain control: tramadol (2–3 mg/kg every 6–8 hours) or buprenorphine (0.01 mg/kg orally every 6–8 hours)
	2. Topical analgesia (2 mg/kg diluted 50:50 with saline administered through cystoscope or urinary catheter into urethral lumen)
	3. Antiinflammatory therapy (nonsteroidal antiinflammatory drug vs weaning course of prednisone)
	4. Urethral antispasmodic therapy (prazosin 1 mg/15 kg orally every 8 hours in dogs; 0.5 mg total dose orally every 8–12 hours in cats)
Urinary incontinence	No treatment necessary (self-limiting)
Urethral perforation	Indwelling urinary catheter with closed collection system for 7–10 days
Bladder rupture	1. Indwelling urinary catheter with closed collection system for 7–10 days (only for small rents)
	2. Surgical bladder wall closure
Urine passage through perineal access site (applies only to rigid cystoscopy in male dogs using the percutaneous perineal approach)	Indwelling urinary catheter for 24–72 hours postprocedure

clinical signs.[26] In addition, a urethral antispasmodic, such as prazosin (1 mg/15 kg every 8 hours in dogs; 0.25–0.5 mg [total dose] orally every 8–12 hours in cats) can be prescribed.

Incontinence

Following cystoscopy, continent female patients rarely have incontinence, which is potentially caused by excessive distension of the urethra.[22] This condition is self-limiting and does not require treatment, but may persist for 3 to 5 days after cystoscopy.

Urethral Perforation

This is a rare complication of cystourethroscopy and is typically caused by the use of excessive force and operator inexperience.[2,22,58] Perforation can also be caused by inadvertent damage to the urethral wall during laser lithotripsy or urethral biopsy acquisition (see **Fig. 31**B). In most cases, urethral perforations can be treated with the placement of an indwelling urinary catheter. Most sources recommend mainte-nance of the catheter for 7 to 10 days to allow complete healing of the tear.[59–61] However, some sources suggest that shorter periods of urinary catheterization (24–48 hours) should suffice.[22,60] Rarely, surgical correction of the urethral perforation may be required if the defect is very large or circumferential.[1,59–61]

Bladder Rupture

This is a very rare complication of cystourethroscopy and is typically caused by over-distension of the bladder with saline during the procedure. It can also occur if the pro-cedure is performed soon after a cystotomy (<7 days) and care is not taken to avoid overdistending the bladder. This complication may potentially be managed with an indwelling urinary catheter for a minimum of 7 days. However, if the rent is large, sur-gical closure is recommended.[1]

Urine Passage Through Perineal Access Site

The owners of male patients for which the percutaneous perineal approach for rigid retrograde cystourethroscopy is used should be warned that urine may pass through both the penis and the perineal access site for a few days following the proce-dure.[21,57] In addition, minor bleeding and occasional blood clot passage may occur through both sites. These complications typically resolve within 7 days of the proce-dure (usually by day 3).[57] They are worst immediately following the procedure and gradually resolve over the next several days. For this reason, an indwelling urinary catheter should be placed and maintained with a closed collection for at least 24 hours after the procedure in order to decompress the bladder and bypass the ure-thral access site.

POSTPROCEDURAL CARE

The patient is monitored carefully for complete anesthetic recovery, and is kept in the hospital until the patient is observed urinating with a subjectively good urine stream. Patients with significant stranguria or that are unable to form a urine stream should be kept in the hospital. The patient is provided with pain control, antispasmodic ther-apy, and/or antiinflammatory therapies as needed, and is closely monitored for urine retention. If these interventions do not improve the patient's urinary patterns, then an indwelling urinary catheter is placed and maintained with a closed collection system to allow the urethra to be bypassed for a brief period of time as the urethritis subsides.

Most patients are discharged from the hospital within a few hours of an uncomplicated diagnostic cystourethroscopy, but are usually hospitalized overnight following procedures such as laser lithotripsy or cystoscopic guided laser ablation of ectopic ureters. For pets with sterile urine before cystoscopy, some investigators prescribe a 3-day course of amoxicillin (10–20 mg/kg orally every 12 hours) to treat inadvertent urinary tract bacterial contamination during the procedure; however, this practice has not been critically evaluated.[21,22,26,55]

OUTCOMES

The outcomes of cystoscopy depend on the goals set before performing the procedure. Cystoscopy can be purely a diagnostic procedure or it may be combined with therapeutic procedures. Cystoscopy can be used to diagnose problems that can then be treated using other modalities such as surgery or interventional radiology. For example, urethral strictures (**Fig. 32**) diagnosed via cystoscopy can be treated via urethral balloon dilation or urethral stent placement, both of which typically require fluoroscopic guidance. Patients with urethral obstruction caused by urethral masses may be treated with urethral stent placement (**Fig. 33**). Vaginourethral fistulae require surgical intervention to be corrected. In contrast, there are disease processes that can be treated via cystoscopic guided procedures. Examples include cystoscopic laser ablation of intramural ectopic ureters, removal of cystic or urethral calculi via lithotripsy, percutaneous cystolithotomy, cystoscopic guided laser resection of cystic polyps, laser ablation of vestibulovaginal septal remnants, extraction of remnant suture material, sclerotherapy for idiopathic renal hematuria, and injection of submucosal bulking agents or botulinum toxin for urethral sphincter mechanism incompetence.[3,26,29–35,37,43,44,46,49–52]

Reporting, Follow-up, and Clinical Implications

A standardized cystoscopy reporting form is valuable to ensure that all anatomic structures are evaluated and abnormalities are recorded. The combination of a

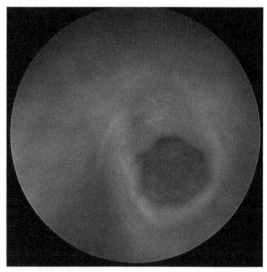

Fig. 32. Cystoscopic image from a female spayed dog of unknown age with a urethral stricture.

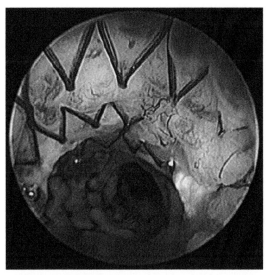

Fig. 33. Cystoscopic image from a female spayed dog of unknown age with a urethral transitional cell carcinoma after stent placement.

standardized cystoscopy report and images (still images and/or video) provides documentation for the medical record and facilitates communication with the owner and consulting veterinarians. Standardized reports have been published for female and male cystoscopy that also permit collection of data for prospective or retrospective research data, including grading urinary bladder mucosal abnormalities at low and high pressures and the volume of fluid to distend the urinary bladder to 80 cm of pressure. The authors recognize the benefits of these reports, but propose a simplified report (**Boxes 6** and **7**). Minimal follow-up is required immediately following diagnostic cystoscopy without therapeutic procedures. Because the procedure is performed under general anesthesia, standard postanesthesia recommendations are made for monitoring the pet until completely awake from anesthesia and for the reintroduction of food and water. Long-term follow-up depends on the cystoscopic diagnosis, results of histopathology, stone analysis results, culture results, and outcome following therapeutic interventions.[2]

CURRENT CONTROVERSIES/FUTURE CONSIDERATIONS

One of the limiting issues that have delayed the advancement of cystoscopy and urinary tract interventional endoscopy in dogs and cats is the lack of equipment that is of an appropriate size for these patients. There are gradual advancements being made in this regard, and the hope is that, as technology advances, the ability of veterinarians to treat urinary tract disease in a noninvasive fashion will progress. A current source of controversy in veterinary medicine is how best to treat urolithiasis. Advocates of traditional cystotomy cite its lower cost, more rapid procedure times, and universal availability as benefits.[62] However, as is the case in human medicine, many veterinary clinicians are currently attempting to advance veterinary urology with the use of less invasive modalities that may reduce length of hospital stay and postprocedural complications. In addition, given that up to 20% of dogs treated with traditional cystotomy have incomplete urolith extraction, there is evidence that there is significant room to

Box 6
Female cystoscopy report

Procedure length:

Anesthesia used:

Patient position

  Dorsal [ ]

  Right lateral [ ]

  Sternal [ ]

Miscellaneous:

  Emergency procedure [ ]

  Fluoroscopy [ ]

  Computed tomography [ ]

  Procedural radiography [ ]

  Other [ ]

Equipment used:

  Cystoscope: 1.9-mm diameter, 18 cm long with a 10-Fr sheath [ ]

  Cystoscope: 2.7-mm diameter, 18 cm long with a 14.5-Fr sheath [ ]

  Cystoscope: 3.5-mm diameter, 30 cm long with a 17-Fr sheath [ ]

  Flexible biopsy forceps [ ]

  Stone basket [ ]

  Other [ ]

Findings

  Grades

    Normal/absent = 0

    If abnormal: mild = 1, moderate = 2, severe = 3; and describe

  Urethra

    Quality of examination:

    External urethral meatus [ ]

    Vascularity [ ]

    Calculi/crystals [ ]

    Erosions [ ]

    Diverticulum [ ]

    Mass lesions [ ]

    Ectopic ureteral opening [ ]

  Urinary bladder

    Quality of examination:

    Left ureter opening [ ]

    Right ureter opening [ ]

    Trigone [ ]

    Vascularity [ ]

Calculi/crystals [ ]

Erosions [ ]

Diverticulum [ ]

Mass lesions [ ]

Ectopic ureteral opening [ ]

Vessel tortuosity [ ]

Mucous/amorphous debris [ ]

Hemorrhage [ ]

Glomerulations [ ]

Edema [ ]

Granularity [ ]

Inadequate insufflation [ ]

Vagina

Quality of examination:

Frenula (remnants of paramesonephric septae) [ ]

Vascularity [ ]

Erosions [ ]

Mass lesions [ ]

Ectopic ureteral opening [ ]

Mucous/amorphous debris [ ]

Hemorrhage [ ]

Granularity [ ]

Therapeutic procedures:

Biopsies [ ], number taken [ ]

Basket retrieval [ ]

Lithotripsy [ ]

Voiding urohydropulsion [ ]

Stent placement [ ]

Collagen implants [ ]

Image storage:

Electronic [ ]

Printed [ ]

Complications:

During procedure [ ]

Postprocedure [ ]

Cystoscopic diagnosis:

Clinician performing procedure:

Box 7
Male cystoscopy report

Procedure length:

Anesthesia used:

Patient position

  Right lateral [ ]

  Sternal [ ]

Miscellaneous:

  Percutaneous perineal approach [ ]

  Emergency procedure [ ]

  Fluoroscopy [ ]

  Computed tomography [ ]

  Procedural radiography [ ]

  Other [ ]

Equipment used:

  Cystoscope: 1.2 mm, flexible [ ]

  Cystourethroscope: 1.0 mm, semirigid [ ]

  Cystoscope: 7.5 Fr, 100 cm long, flexible [ ]

  Flexible biopsy forceps [ ]

  Stone basket [ ]

  Other [ ]

Findings

  Grades

    Normal/absent = 0

    If abnormal: mild = 1, moderate = 2, severe = 3; and describe

  Urethra

    Note location of abnormalities (preprostatic or postprostatic)

    Quality of examination:

    Quality of urine stream [ ]

    External urethral meatus [ ]

    Vascularity [ ]

    Calculi/crystals/plug [ ]

    Erosions [ ]

    Diverticulum [ ]

    Mass lesions [ ]

    Ectopic ureteral opening [ ]

    Prostatic openings [ ]

  Urinary bladder

    Quality of examination:

    Left ureter opening [ ]

Right ureter opening [ ]

Trigone [ ]

Vascularity [ ]

Calculi/crystals [ ]

Erosions [ ]

Diverticulum [ ]

Mass lesions [ ]

Ectopic ureteral opening [ ]

Vessel tortuosity [ ]

Mucous/amorphous debris [ ]

Hemorrhage [ ]

Glomerulations [ ]

Edema [ ]

Granularity [ ]

Inadequate insufflation [ ]

Therapeutic procedures:

Biopsies [ ], number taken [ ]

Basket retrieval [ ]

Lithotripsy [ ]

Voiding urohydropulsion [ ]

Stent placement [ ]

Collagen implants [ ]

Image storage:

Electronic [ ]

Printed [ ]

Complications:

During procedure [ ]

Postprocedure [ ]

Cystoscopic diagnosis:

Clinician performing procedure:

improve the success of urolith extraction in veterinary medicine.[63] It is the opinion of the authors that the specifics of an individual case (such as stone size, number of stones, stone composition [if known], sex, and size of patient) should always dictate the procedure used for stone removal, and that cystotomy, percutaneous cystolithotomy/laparoscopic assisted cystoscopy, laser lithotripsy, and voiding urohydropulsion are all techniques that are appropriate under certain circumstances. Another common source of controversy in veterinary medicine is the best approach for the treatment of ureteral ectopia. There should be no argument that extramural ectopic ureters are best treated surgically. However, in the case of intramural ectopic ureters, particularly in female dogs, surgical correction is more costly and invasive than cystoscopic laser ablation, and there is a higher postoperative complication rate.[43,44,46] In addition, cystoscopic laser ablation offers the benefit of concurrent diagnosis and treatment of ureteral ectopia. Therefore, the authors support the use of cystoscopic guided laser ablation of intramural ectopic ureters in dogs.

SUMMARY

For experienced, well-trained clinicians, cystoscopy is a minimally invasive tool that has advanced urology in veterinary medicine. Cystoscopy provides the ability to diagnose conditions that cannot easily be diagnosed using other modalities. It also enables more thorough assessment and potentially treatment of conditions diagnosed using other modalities. As technology advances, a wider range of patients will be able to be assessed via cystoscopy, and more treatment modalities will become available. Advanced training and a wide range of specialized equipment are necessary to perform cystoscopy appropriately.

REFERENCES

1. Adams LG, Syme HM. Canine ureteral and lower urinary tract diseases. In: Ettinger SJ, Feldman EC, editors. Textbook of veterinary internal medicine. 7th edition. St Louis (MO): Saunders Elsevier; 2010. p. 2086–115.
2. Messer JS, Chew DJ, McLoughlin MA. Cystoscopy: techniques and clinical applications. Clin Tech Small Anim Pract 2005;20:52–64.
3. Berent AC, Weisse CW, Branter E, et al. Endoscopic-guided sclerotherapy for renal-sparing treatment of idiopathic renal hematuria in dogs: 6 cases (2010–2012). J Am Vet Med Assoc 2013;242:1556–63.
4. Di Cicco MF, Fetzer T, Secoura PL, et al. Management of bilateral idiopathic renal hematuria in a dog with silver nitrate. Can Vet J 2013;54:761–4.
5. Amores-Fuster I, Elliott JW, Freeman AI, et al. Histiocytic sarcoma of the urinary bladder in a dog. J Small Anim Pract 2011;52:665.
6. Benigni L, Lamb CR, Corzo-Menendez N, et al. Lymphoma affecting the urinary bladder in three dogs and a cat. Vet Radiol Ultrasound 2006;47:592–6.
7. Blackwood L, Sullivan M, Thompson H. Urethral leiomyoma causing post renal failure in a bitch. Vet Rec 1992;131:416–7.
8. Davis GJ, Holt D. Two chondrosarcomas in the urethra of a German shepherd dog. J Small Anim Pract 2003;44:169–71.
9. Gerber K, Rees P. Urinary bladder botryoid rhabdomyosarcoma with widespread metastases in an 8-month-old Labrador cross dog. J S Afr Vet Assoc 2009;80: 199–203.
10. Heng HG, Lowry JE, Boston S, et al. Smooth muscle neoplasia of the urinary bladder wall in three dogs. Vet Radiol Ultrasound 2006;47:83–6.
11. Kessler M, Kandel-Tschiederer B, Pfleghaar S, et al. Primary malignant lymphoma of the urinary bladder in a dog: longterm remission following treatment with radiation and chemotherapy. Schweiz Arch Tierheilkd 2008;150:565–9.
12. Liptak JM, Dernell WS, Withrow SJ. Haemangiosarcoma of the urinary bladder in a dog. Aust Vet J 2004;82:215–7.
13. Mellanby RJ, Chantrey JC, Baines EA, et al. Urethral haemangiosarcoma in a boxer. J Small Anim Pract 2004;45:154–6.
14. Mutsaers AJ, Widmer WR, Knapp DW. Canine transitional cell carcinoma. J Vet Intern Med 2003;17:136–44.
15. Norris AM, Laing EJ, Valli VE, et al. Canine bladder and urethral tumors: a retrospective study of 115 cases (1980–1985). J Vet Intern Med 1992;6:145–53.

16. Olausson A, Stieger SM, Loefgren S, et al. A urinary bladder fibrosarcoma in a young dog. Vet Radiol Ultrasound 2005;46:135–8.
17. Santos M, Dias Pereira P, Montenegro L, et al. Recurrent and metastatic canine urethral transitional cell carcinoma without bladder involvement. Vet Rec 2007; 160:557–8.
18. Sapierzynski R, Malicka E, Bielecki W, et al. Tumors of the urogenital system in dogs and cats. Retrospective review of 138 cases. Pol J Vet Sci 2007;10:97–103.
19. Takiguchi M, Watanabe T, Okada H, et al. Rhabdomyosarcoma (botryoid sarcoma) of the urinary bladder in a Maltese. J Small Anim Pract 2002;43:269–71.
20. Wilson HM, Chun R, Larson VS, et al. Clinical signs, treatments, and outcome in cats with transitional cell carcinoma of the urinary bladder: 20 cases (1990–2004). J Am Vet Med Assoc 2007;231:101–6.
21. McCarthy TC. Cystoscopy and biopsy of the feline lower urinary tract. Vet Clin North Am Small Anim Pract 1996;26:463–82.
22. Chew DJ, Buffington T, Kendall MS, et al. Urethroscopy, cystoscopy, and biopsy of the feline lower urinary tract. Vet Clin North Am Small Anim Pract 1996;26:441–62.
23. Childress MO, Adams LG, Ramos-Vara JA, et al. Results of biopsy via transurethral cystoscopy and cystotomy for diagnosis of transitional cell carcinoma of the urinary bladder and urethra in dogs: 92 cases (2003–2008). J Am Vet Med Assoc 2011;239:350–6.
24. Bohme B, Ngendahayo P, Hamaide A, et al. Inflammatory pseudotumours of the urinary bladder in dogs resembling human myofibroblastic tumours: a report of eight cases and comparative pathology. Vet J 2010;183:89–94.
25. Martinez I, Mattoon JS, Eaton KA, et al. Polypoid cystitis in 17 dogs (1978–2001). J Vet Intern Med 2003;17:499–509.
26. Rawlings CA. Diagnostic rigid endoscopy: otoscopy, rhinoscopy, and cystoscopy. Vet Clin North Am Small Anim Pract 2009;39:849–68.
27. Hostutler RA, Chew DJ, Eaton KA, et al. Cystoscopic appearance of proliferative urethritis in 2 dogs before and after treatment. J Vet Intern Med 2004;18:113–6.
28. Lulich JP, Osborne CA. Voiding urohydropulsion: a nonsurgical technique for removal of urocystoliths. In: Bonagura JD, editor. Kirk's current veterinary therapy small animal practice. 12th edition. Philadelphia: WB Saunders; 1995. p. 1008–10.
29. Adams LG, Berent AC, Moore GE, et al. Use of laser lithotripsy for fragmentation of uroliths in dogs: 73 cases (2005–2006). J Am Vet Med Assoc 2008;232: 1680–7.
30. Defarges A, Dunn M. Use of electrohydraulic lithotripsy in 28 dogs with bladder and urethral calculi. J Vet Intern Med 2008;22:1267–73.
31. Lulich JP, Osborne CA, Albasan H, et al. Efficacy and safety of laser lithotripsy in fragmentation of urocystoliths and urethroliths for removal in dogs. J Am Vet Med Assoc 2009;234:1279–85.
32. Rawlings C. Endoscopic removal of urinary calculi. Compend Contin Educ Vet 2009;31:476–84.
33. Libermann SV, Doran IC, Bille CR, et al. Extraction of urethral calculi by transabdominal cystoscopy and urethroscopy in nine dogs. J Small Anim Pract 2011;52: 190–4.
34. Rawlings CA, Mahaffey MB, Barsanti JA, et al. Use of laparoscopic-assisted cystoscopy for removal of urinary calculi in dogs. J Am Vet Med Assoc 2003; 222:759–61, 737.
35. Runge JJ, Berent AC, Mayhew PD, et al. Transvesicular percutaneous cystolithotomy for the retrieval of cystic and urethral calculi in dogs and cats: 27 cases (2006–2008). J Am Vet Med Assoc 2011;239:344–9.

36. Berent A. Cystourethroscopy in the cat: what do you need? When do you need it? How do you do it? J Feline Med Surg 2014;16:34–41.
37. Burdick S, Berent AC, Weisse C, et al. Endoscopic-guided laser ablation of vestibulovaginal septal remnants in dogs: 36 cases (2007–2011). J Am Vet Med Assoc 2014;244:944–9.
38. Crawford JT, Adams WM. Influence of vestibulovaginal stenosis, pelvic bladder, and recessed vulva on response to treatment for clinical signs of lower urinary tract disease in dogs: 38 cases (1990–1999). J Am Vet Med Assoc 2002;221: 995–9.
39. Kieves NR, Novo RE, Martin RB. Vaginal resection and anastomosis for treatment of vestibulovaginal stenosis in 4 dogs with recurrent urinary tract infections. J Am Vet Med Assoc 2011;239:972–80.
40. Kyles AE, Vaden S, Hardie EM, et al. Vestibulovaginal stenosis in dogs: 18 cases (1987–1995). J Am Vet Med Assoc 1996;209:1889–93.
41. Wang KY, Samii VF, Chew DJ, et al. Vestibular, vaginal, and urethral relations in spayed dogs with and without lower urinary tract signs. J Vet Intern Med 2006; 20:1065–73.
42. Bailiff NL, Westropp JL, Jang SS, et al. Corynebacterium urealyticum urinary tract infection in dogs and cats: 7 cases (1996–2003). J Am Vet Med Assoc 2005;226: 1676–80.
43. Berent AC, Mayhew PD, Porat-Mosenco Y. Use of cystoscopic-guided laser ablation for treatment of intramural ureteral ectopia in male dogs: four cases (2006–2007). J Am Vet Med Assoc 2008;232:1026–34.
44. Berent AC, Weisse C, Mayhew PD, et al. Evaluation of cystoscopic-guided laser ablation of intramural ectopic ureters in female dogs. J Am Vet Med Assoc 2012; 240:716–25.
45. Davidson AP, Westropp JL. Diagnosis and management of urinary ectopia. Vet Clin North Am Small Anim Pract 2014;44:343–53.
46. Smith AL, Radlinsky MG, Rawlings CA. Cystoscopic diagnosis and treatment of ectopic ureters in female dogs: 16 cases (2005–2008). J Am Vet Med Assoc 2010;237:191–5.
47. Samii VF, McLoughlin MA, Mattoon JS, et al. Digital fluoroscopic excretory urography, digital fluoroscopic urethrography, helical computed tomography, and cystoscopy in 24 dogs with suspected ureteral ectopia. J Vet Intern Med 2004; 18:271–81.
48. Holt PE. Importance of urethral length, bladder neck position and vestibulovaginal stenosis in sphincter mechanism incompetence in the incontinent bitch. Res Vet Sci 1985;39:364–72.
49. Barth A, Reichler IM, Hubler M, et al. Evaluation of long-term effects of endoscopic injection of collagen into the urethral submucosa for treatment of urethral sphincter incompetence in female dogs: 40 cases (1993–2000). J Am Vet Med Assoc 2005;226:73–6.
50. Byron JK, Chew DJ, McLoughlin ML. Retrospective evaluation of urethral bovine cross-linked collagen implantation for treatment of urinary incontinence in female dogs. J Vet Intern Med 2011;25:980–4.
51. Lew S, Majewski M, Radziszewski P, et al. Therapeutic efficacy of botulinum toxin in the treatment of urinary incontinence in female dogs. Acta Vet Hung 2010;58: 157–65.
52. Sumner JP, Hardie RJ, Henningson JN, et al. Evaluation of submucosally injected polyethylene glycol-based hydrogel and bovine cross-linked collagen in the

canine urethra using cystoscopy, magnetic resonance imaging and histopathology. Vet Surg 2012;41:655–63.
53. Pressler B, Bartges JW. Urinary tract infections. In: Ettinger SJ, Feldman EC, editors. Textbook of veterinary internal medicine. 7th edition. St Louis (MO): Saunders Elsevier; 2010. p. 2036–47.
54. Neihaus SA, Hathcock TL, Boothe DM, et al. Presurgical antiseptic efficacy of chlorhexidine diacetate and providone-iodine in the canine preputial cavity. J Am Anim Hosp Assoc 2011;47:406–12.
55. Lulich JP. Endoscopic vaginoscopy in the dog. Theriogenology 2006;66:588–91.
56. Senior DF. Cystoscopy. In: Tams TR, editor. Small animal endoscopy. 2nd edition. St Louis (MO): Mosby; 1999. p. 447–53.
57. Brearley MJ, Milroy EJ, Rickards D. A percutaneous perineal approach for cystoscopy in male dogs. Res Vet Sci 1988;44:380–2.
58. McCarthy TC, McDermaid SL. Cystoscopy. Vet Clin North Am Small Anim Pract 1990;20:1315–39.
59. Addison ES, Halfacree Z, Moore AH, et al. A retrospective analysis of urethral rupture in 63 cats. J Feline Med Surg 2014;16:300–7.
60. Anderson RB, Aronson LR, Drobatz KJ, et al. Prognostic factors for successful outcome following urethral rupture in dogs and cats. J Am Anim Hosp Assoc 2006;42:136–46.
61. Meige F, Sarrau S, Autefage A. Management of traumatic urethral rupture in 11 cats using primary alignment with a urethral catheter. Vet Comp Orthop Traumatol 2008;21:76–84.
62. Arulpragasam SP, Case JB, Ellison GW. Evaluation of costs and time required for laparoscopic-assisted versus open cystotomy for urinary cystolith removal in dogs: 43 cases (2009–2012). J Am Vet Med Assoc 2013;243:703–8.
63. Grant DC, Harper TA, Werre SR. Frequency of incomplete urolith removal, complications, and diagnostic imaging following cystotomy for removal of uroliths from the lower urinary tract in dogs: 128 cases (1994–2006). J Am Vet Med Assoc 2010;236:763–6.

Congenital Diseases of the Lower Urinary Tract

Joseph W. Bartges, DVM, PhD*, Amanda J. Callens, BS, LVT

KEYWORDS

- Congenital • Urinary bladder • Urethra • Lower urinary tract

KEY POINTS

- Congenital lower urinary tract disorders occur uncommonly in dogs and cats.
- Many congenital disorders are associated with congenital urinary incontinence.
- Treatment depends on the underlying congenital anomaly and if the anomaly is associated with clinical signs.

Genetic or acquired diseases may affect differentiation and development of the lower urinary tract. More than 400 regulatory genes seem to be involved in embryogenesis of the urinary system, which depends on a coordinated and orderly interaction of multiple embryonic tissues.[1–3] An alteration in one or more of these genes or disruption of normal development may result in an anomaly.

URINARY BLADDER

Urinary Bladder Agenesis and Hypoplasia

Agenesis or hypoplasia of the urinary bladder results in diminished capacity for urine storage and presents as urinary incontinence.[4–7] Embryonic maldevelopment may result in a hypoplastic bladder but is more commonly associated with ectopic ureters.[7] Ectopic ureters may result in diminished bladder capacity, which may contribute to urinary incontinence even with surgical correction; however, bladder capacity may increase over time.[8,9]

Pelvic Bladder

A pelvic bladder is one that has a blunt trigone, which is located in an intrapelvic location associated with a shortened urethra (**Fig. 1**).[10] The role of pelvic bladder with urinary incontinence is controversial, and dogs with pelvic bladder may be continent.[10–12] Normally, the trigone tapers and connects to the urethra in an

The authors have nothing to disclose.
Cornell University Veterinary Specialists, 880 Canal Street, Stamford, CT 06902, USA
* Corresponding author.
E-mail address: joe.bartges@cuvs.org

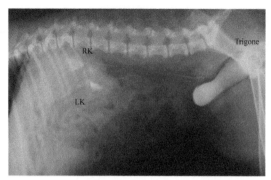

Fig. 1. Lateral abdominal radiograph of an excretory urogram in a dog with a pelvic bladder and pyelonephritis. Pyelectasia is present bilaterally. The dog had urinary incontinence and recurrent bacterial urinary tract infections. LK, left kidney; RK, right kidney; Trigone, trigone of bladder located in pelvic canal.

intra-abdominal location. The degree of distention of the bladder affects location of the trigone; therefore, the bladder should be adequately distended during contrast urethrocystography before diagnosing pelvic bladder.[12] Pelvic bladder has also been associated with urinary tract infection.[10] Although some dogs with pelvic bladders are continent, other dogs with pelvic bladders have refractory urinary incontinence without any other identifiable cause.[10,13] A diagnosis of pelvic bladder is established by contrast radiography. If pelvic bladder is associated with urinary incontinence, pharmacologic management with estrogens and/or α-adrenergic agonists should be tried before more invasive interventions. If urinary incontinence is refractory to medical therapy, urethral bulking with collagen or surgery (urethropexy or colposuspension) may be attempted.[14–16]

Exstrophy and Herniation

Exstrophy refers to eversion of the urinary bladder, and often the intestines and external genitalia, due to absence of a portion of the ventral abdominal wall.[17] This disorder is rare, being reported in an 8-month-old female English bulldog with urinary incontinence and pyelonephritis.[18] Treatment involves managing associated conditions and reconstructive surgery.[19]

Urinary Bladder Herniation

Exteriorization of the urinary bladder through an inguinal hernia has been described in a 2-year-old cat.[20] Clinical signs included chronic lower urinary tract signs, and a soft mass was palpated in the region. Radiography revealed the urinary bladder to be extra-abdominal. Treatment consisted of repositioning of the urinary bladder in the abdominal cavity with an incisional cystopexy and partial closure of the enlarged inguinal canals.

Urachal Anomalies

Urachal anomalies occur commonly in dogs and cats. The urachus is a fetal connection allowing urine to pass between the developing urinary bladder and the placenta. It undergoes complete atrophy and is nonfunctional at birth. If it fails to completely atrophy, macroscopic or microscopic remnants may remain and result in persistent urachal patency or formation of urachal cysts or diverticula.[21,22]

A persistent urachus occurs when the urachal canal remains functionally patent between the urinary bladder and the umbilicus (**Fig. 2**). It is characterized by

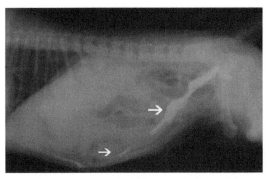

Fig. 2. Lateral contrast cystogram in an immature dog with a patent urachus (*arrows*).

inappropriate urine loss through the umbilicus.[23–27] A patent urachus is often accompanied by omphalitis, ventral dermatitis, and urinary tract infections. Rarely, uroabdomen may occur when a persistent urachus terminates in the abdominal cavity.[28] A urachal cyst may develop if the urachal epithelium in an isolated segment of a persistent urachus continues to secrete fluid (**Fig. 3**).[21,29]

A vesicourachal diverticulum occurs when a portion of the urachus located at the bladder vertex fails to close, resulting in a blind diverticulum that protrudes from the bladder apex (**Fig. 4**). Vesicourachal diverticula may be microscopic or macroscopic. Microscopic vesicourachal diverticula are microscopic lumens lined by transitional epithelium that may persist at the bladder vertex from the level of the submucosa to the subserosa.[21] Approximately 40% of bladders from 80 cats had microscopic

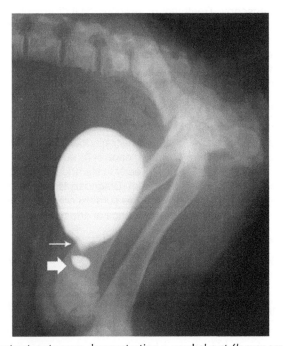

Fig. 3. Lateral contrast cystogram demonstrating a urachal cyst (*larger arrow*) and urachal diverticulum (*smaller arrow*).

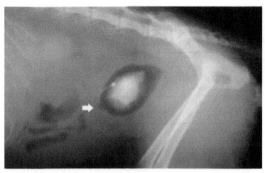

Fig. 4. Lateral double-contrast cystogram showing a urachal diverticulum (*arrow*) in a 3-year-old castrated male domestic shorthair cat with idiopathic cystitis.

diverticula in one study.[30] Usually microscopic diverticula are insignificant clinically; however, they may become macroscopic when acquired bladder and/or urethral diseases develop (eg, urinary tract infections, urolithiasis, or idiopathic cystitis).[31–33] A microscopic diverticulum may open because of inflammation and/or increased intraluminal pressure from an acquired disease. Many of these macroscopic diverticula disappear within 2 to 3 weeks following treatment of the acquired disease and resolution of clinical signs.[21,32] Congenital macroscopic vesicourachal diverticula are thought to be caused by urine outflow obstruction and develop before or shortly after birth. These diverticula increase the risk of bacterial urinary tract infection and associated clinical signs of lower urinary tract disease.[34]

Vesicourachal diverticula may be visualized by contrast urethrocystography, ultrasonography, or cystoscopy. Treatment of vesicourachal diverticula depends on their size and association with clinical disease. Many macroscopic diverticula associated with active lower urinary tract disease regress with successful treatment of the acquired disease; therefore, documentation of regression of diverticulum following treatment is important.[31,32] If the diverticulum does not resolve and recurrent disease occurs, then diverticulectomy may be warranted.[33,35]

Urinary Bladder Duplication

Complete and partial urinary bladder duplication with and without concurrent urethral duplication has been reported in dogs.[36] Urinary bladder duplication may result from any alteration of normal development of the cloaca or its subdivision into the urogenital sinus and rectum.[37] Clinical signs develop early in life and include lower urinary tract signs, incontinence, and distended abdomen. Diagnosis is made by physical examination and imaging studies. Treatment involves surgical correction; however, success depends on degree of malformation and presence of additional congenital anomalies.

Colovesical Fistula and Uterine-Bladder Communication

Rarely, the urinary bladder may communicate with the colon or uterine horn.[21,38,39] Clinical signs included urinary incontinence, lower urinary tract signs, and urinary tract infection. Treatment is limited to surgical correction.

Primary Urinary Bladder Neoplasia

Urinary bladder neoplasia of immature dogs and cats is rare.[40] Botryoid rhabdomyosarcoma has been observed to occur in large breed dogs younger than 18 months but can occur in other dogs.[41–50] Botryoid rhabdomyosarcomas are embryonic mesenchymal tumors arising from pleuripotent stem cells originating from primitive urogenital ridge remnants. They are infiltrating tumors arising from the trigone and projecting into the bladder lumen as botryoid (resembling a cluster of grapes) masses.[44] Clinical signs are consistent with lower urinary tract disease, and the tumor may result in urinary outflow obstruction and hypertrophic osteoarthropathy.[44,45] Treatment includes surgery with or without additional chemotherapy (doxorubicin, cyclophosphamide, and vincristine sulfate).[51,52] Metastases to local tissues (lymph nodes, mesentery, omentum, prostate) and distant organs (lung, liver, kidney, spleen) have been described with this tumor.[42,48,50]

Urocystolithiasis

Urocystolithiasis has been described in immature dogs and cats. Most commonly, struvite secondary to infection with a urease-producing microbial organism and urate secondary to congenital hepatic disease occur (**Figs. 5** and **6**).[53–55] Although certain breeds of dogs are prone to formation of metabolic uroliths, for example, Dalmatians and urate and English bulldogs and urate or cystine, uroliths do not typically form in immature animals despite the metabolic abnormality relative to other breeds.

URETHRA
Urethral Aplasia and Hypoplasia

Urethral aplasia is a rare congenital anomaly characterized by complete absence of a patent urethra. Incontinence occurs associated with ectopic location of the ureters.[25,56] Urethral hypoplasia described in immature female cats is associated with juvenile-onset urinary incontinence.[5,57,58] Diagnosis is based on clinical signs and imaging studies. Radiographic features include urethral shortening and vaginal aplasia. Urethral hypoplasia may be associated with other congenital anomalies and bacterial urinary tract infection. Some affected animals respond to sympathomimetic treatment,[58] whereas in others, surgical reconstruction of the bladder neck may improve or resolve clinical signs.[57]

Ectopic Ureters

Normally, the ureter enters the dorsolateral caudal surface of the bladder and empties into the trigone after a short intramural course. Ectopic ureter results from termination of one or both ureters at a site other than the trigone as a result of an embryologic abnormality of the ureteral bud of the mesonephric duct. The degree of deviation of the ureteral bud from the normal position determines the location of the ectopic opening.

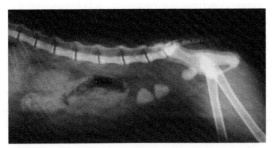

Fig. 5. Lateral abdominal radiograph of a kitten showing 3 radiodense uroliths. The uroliths were composed of struvite that formed secondary to an infection with a urease-producing microbial organism (*Staphylococcus* spp).

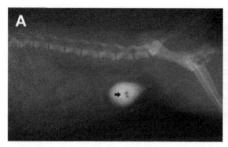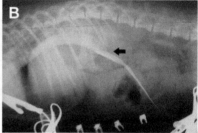

Fig. 6. (A) Lateral double-contrast cystogram of a 1-year-old castrated male Pomeranian showing urocystoliths (*arrow*) composed of ammonium urate that formed secondary to a congenital extrahepatic portovascular anomaly. (B) Lateral contrast portography of the dog described in (A) showing a single extrahepatic portovascular anomaly (*arrow*).

Ectopic ureters may be unilateral or bilateral and intramural or extramural. An extramural ectopic ureter bypasses insertion at the trigone and inserts distally in the urethra, vagina or vestibule in females, or ductus deferens in males. An intramural ectopic ureter inserts at the trigone but tunnels in the urethral wall to open distally. Variations of the intramural ectopic ureter include ureteral troughs, double ureteral openings, multiple fenestrated openings, and 2 intramural ureters opening in a single orifice.[59] Ectopic ureters may be associated with other congenital defects of the urogenital tract, including agenesis, hypoplasia, or irregular shape of the kidneys; hydroureter; ureterocele; urachal remnants, pelvic bladder; vulvovaginal strictures; and persistent hymen.[60,61]

Young female dogs (median age of 10 months) are most commonly diagnosed with ectopic ureter; bilateral intramural ectopic ureters occur most commonly.[6,61] Males with ectopic ureter present later, with a median age of 24 months,[6] or they may be undiagnosed because they remain continent presumably because of the urethral length and external urethral sphincter. Breeds reported to be at greater risk for ectopic ureter include the Siberian husky, Labrador retriever, golden retriever, Newfoundland, English bulldog, West Highland white terrier, fox terrier, Skye terrier, and miniature and toy poodles.[61] A genetic basis may exist but is unproven in most cases. Cats are rarely diagnosed with ectopic ureter.

Intermittent or continuous urinary incontinence since birth or weaning is the most frequently reported clinical sign in patients with ectopic ureter; however, most dogs void normally. Physical examination findings are often unremarkable, with the exception of moist or urine-stained hair in the perivulvar or preputial region. Urine scalding may cause secondary dermatitis, and owners may report frequent licking of the vulval or preputial area. Some dogs have vulvovaginitis, a vulvovaginal stricture, or a persistent hymen that can be detected digitally or with vaginoscopy. Dogs often have a history of bacterial urinary tract infections, and bacterial urinary tract infections have been reported to occur in 64% of patients.[59] Some animals may respond partially or completely to pharmacologic management of urethral sphincter mechanism incompetence.

Survey radiography should be performed to assess size, shape, and location of kidneys and bladder. Excretory urography combined with pneumocystography (**Fig. 7**),[61] abdominal ultrasonography,[62] contrast urethrocystography with vesicoureteral reflux, fluoroscopy, or contrast-enhanced computerized tomography may be used to diagnose ectopic ureter; however, urethrocystoscopy (**Fig. 8**) is more reliable especially when combined with other imaging modalities.[61] Dilation of the ectopic ureter is often but not always present.

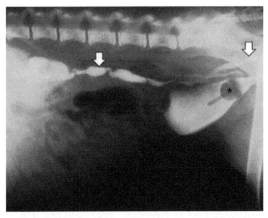

Fig. 7. Excretory urogram demonstrating a dilated extramural ectopic ureter (*arrows*) in a 10-month old intact female Setter. Air in the balloon of the Foley catheter (*asterisk*) is visible at the trigone of the urinary bladder.

Although medical management may help control urinary incontinence, surgical correction or laser ablation is the preferred treatment. An extramural ectopic ureter is ligated at the distal end of the ureter at its attachment and reimplanted into the urinary bladder between the apex and the trigone (neoureterocystostomy). The bladder wall or urine from the renal pelvis should be collected at the time of surgery and cultured because of the common occurrence of bacterial urinary tract infections.

Traditionally, intramural ectopic ureter is treated by ligating the distal submucosal ureteral segment and creating a new ureteral opening in the trigone of the urinary bladder (neoureterostomy and urethral-trigonal reconstruction); however, incontinence persists commonly (44%–67%)[61,63,64] because the intramural segment of the ureter disrupts the functional anatomy of the internal urethral sphincter mechanism. Transurethral laser ablation may also be used to correct intramural ectopic ureter. A rigid (in females) or flexible (in males) endoscope is inserted retrograde into the urethra; diagnostic urethrocystosopy is performed. A catheter is inserted into the lumen of the ectopic ureter to protect the urethral wall. A laser fiber, diode[65] or preferably Holmium:YAG,[66–68] is inserted through the operating channel of the cystoscope and

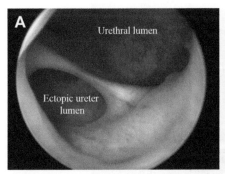
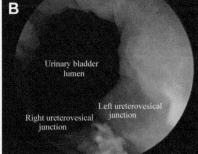

Fig. 8. (*A*) Cystoscopic image of a right intramural ectopic ureter in a 9-month old, intact female, Standard poodle positioned in dorsal recumbency. (*B*) Cystoscopic image of the right intramural ectopic ureter following laser ablation of the medial wall of the ectopic ureter to the level of the normally positioned left ureterovesical junction.

used to transect the free wall of the ectopic ureter until the opening is as close as possible to the normal anatomic location at the trigone. Incontinence may persist if the ectopic ureter is located intramurally because of disruption of the proximal urethra and internal urethral sphincter mechanism.[69] It seems that dogs are more likely to be continent with this procedure than with surgical correction. In patients in which the kidney cannot be spared because of hydronephrosis or pyelonephritis, nephroureterectomy can be performed.

Epispadias and Hypospadias

Epispadias refers to congenital defects in the dorsal aspect of the distal urethra, and hypospadias refers to anomalous ventral malposition of the urethral meatus.[70] Epispadias has been associated with exstrophy of the urinary bladder in an 8-month-old female English bulldog.[18]

Hypospadias occurs more commonly and usually in male dogs; Boston terriers and dalmatians have been described as having an increased risk (**Fig. 9**).[70,71] It has been described in a Himalayan cat.[72] It has been described in an East Greenland male sledge dog associated with potential in utero exposure to organochlorine, which was estimated to be 320 μg/d, corresponding to 128 pg toxic equivalents (TEQ)/kg/d. This value is 32- to 128-fold more than the World Health Organization guidelines and threshold levels for teratogen and reproductive effects.[73]

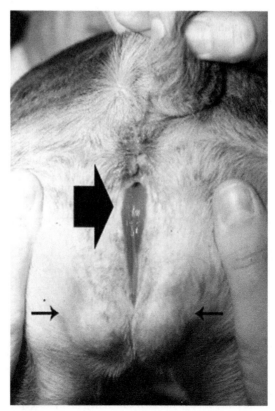

Fig. 9. Perineal hypospadias (*larger arrow*) in a 6-month-old male English bulldog. Smaller arrows designate position of the testicles.

In affected male dogs, an abnormal ventral urethral meatus may be located anywhere along the shaft of the penis, scrotum, or perineum. It is usually associated with malformation of the prepuce and penis.[74,75] Hypospadias has been described in female dogs in association with concurrent disorders of intersexuality. Embryonically, hypospadias results from incomplete fusion of the urogenital fold. Affected dogs present at various ages and may be asymptomatic or have clinical signs of urinary incontinence, periurethral dermatitis, or bacterial urinary tract infection.[74,76] Diagnosis is often based on physical examination. The presence of an os penis in male dogs precludes surgical reconstruction in most cases. Scrotal or perineal urethrostomy combined with castration and removal of vestigial prepucial and penile tissues may be of cosmetic value. Shortening of the penis, amputation, and urethral reconstruction have also been described.[77–80] One technique described creating an advancement flap from the dorsal mucosa of the incompletely formed prepuce and suturing it circumferentially to construct a longer distal preputial mucosa. V- to Y-plasty of the ventral abdominal skin was used to create the preputial skin overlying the mucosal flap. Urethrostomy and partial penile amputation were also performed. This technique may be considered for glandular or penile hypospadias or after resection of the ventral aspect of the distal prepuce when inadequate tissue is present for a simple 2-layer closure of the preputial mucosa and skin.[81]

Urethrogenital Malformations

Urethrogenital malformations associated with diseases of intersexuality, especially pseudohermaphroditism, are often associated with urinary incontinence.[82] Pseudohermaphrodites have gonads of one sex and external genitalia resembling those of the opposite sex.[83] It occurs in both sexes as a result of simultaneous development of Mullerian duct derivatives (oviduct, uterus, and portions of the vagina) and masculinization of the urogenital sinus. The phenotypic appearance of the animal depends on the degree of masculinization of the urogenital sinus. Incontinence develops early in life and may be accompanied by signs of lower urinary tract disease due to a bacterial urinary tract infection. Urinary incontinence likely results from retention of urine in anomalous communications between the urethra and the genital tract and subsequent passive leakage.[84] Diagnosis is based on clinical signs and imaging studies. Urinary incontinence may resolve with surgical correction.[82]

Prostatic urethral diverticulae have been observed in male dogs (**Fig. 10**).[85] It has been associated with a shortened and wide intrapelvic urethra, widened urinary bladder neck, and ureteral anomalies. This condition seems to be similar to a condition described in an infant with congenital obstructive posterior urethral membrane whereby a membrane extended proximally from the verumontanum toward the bladder neck. Although this often results in chronic renal disease, a milder degree of obstruction and protective pressure pop-off mechanisms have been reported resulting in dilation of the prostatic utricle.[86]

Urethral Duplication

Urethral duplication is an uncommon congenital anomaly described only in immature dogs.[87–91] Because of the close association between embryonic development of the urogenital and gastrointestinal systems, urethral duplication is almost always accompanied by other duplication anomalies. These anomalies result from abnormal sagittal midline division and subsequent parallel development of the embryonic hindgut, cloaca, rectum, or urogenital sinus.[37] Associated anomalies accompanying urethral duplication depends on the stage at which dysmorphogenesis occurs. Examination of affected animals may reveal anatomic abnormalities, urinary incontinence, or

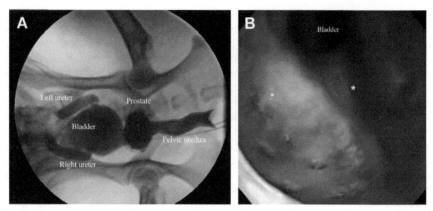

Fig. 10. Prostatic urethral diverticulae with ureteral and urethral anomalies in a 10-month-old castrated male Labrador. (*A*) Ventrodorsal contrast urethrocystogram with ureteral reflux of contrast using fluoroscopy. Bilateral hydroureter is present, and the ureters enter the urinary bladder through one vesicoureteral junction. The urinary bladder neck is nonexistent, and there is posprostatic urethral dilation. (*B*) Cystoscopic image of prostatic urethral diverticulae. The prostatic median raphe is visible (*asterisk*).

clinical signs associated with secondary bacterial urinary tract infection. Diagnosis is based on physical examination, imaging studies, and exploratory surgery. Urethral duplication may in some cases be amenable to surgical extirpation of the duplicated structure; however, surgical reconstruction has rarely been attempted with extensive duplication.

Ectopic Urethra

Ectopic urethra is characterized by abnormal position of the external urethral orifice. Embryonically, urethral ectopia results from anomalous morphogenesis of the urogenital sinus, paramesonephric ducts (Mullerian ducts), or mesonephric ducts.[1] Clinical signs depend on the site of the termination of the abnormal urethra and other concurrent urogenital anomalies. Lifelong urinary incontinence was the predominant clinical feature in a 21-month-old female English bulldog with unilateral ureteral ectopia and an ectopic urethra terminating in the distal vagina.[92] In contrast, a 2-month-old female domestic shorthair cat with ectopic urethra terminating in the ventral rectum did not have urinary incontinence but did void urine through the anus.[93]

Urethrorectal, Urethrovaginal, and Urethroperineal Fistula and Urethral Diverticula

Fistulas connecting the urethral lumen with the large bowel, vagina, and perineal region have been described in dogs and cats.[90,94–101] Fistula may be congenital or may be acquired because of traumatic, inflammatory, or neoplastic processes.[102] Male dogs seem to be affected more frequently, and English bulldogs seem to have a predilection for urethrorectal fistula.[102] Clinical signs are due to abnormal passage of urine from the fistula during urination. Additional signs may include diarrhea, perineal dermatitis, and signs associated with secondary bacterial urinary tract infections. Fistulas have been associated with infection-induced struvite urolithiasis.[95,97,99] Diagnosis is based on clinical signs and imaging studies (**Fig. 11**). Treatment involves surgical correction or surgical urinary diversion. In one dog with a urethrorectal fistula secondary to a prostatic abscess, conservative therapy using an indwelling urinary catheter, low-residue diet, and antibiotics was successful.[97] Micropenis and midline

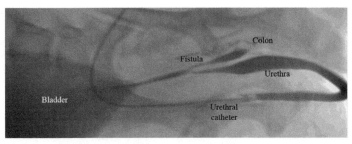

Fig. 11. Contrast urethrogram using fluoroscopy demonstrating a urethral-colonic fistula in a 1-year-old intact male English bulldog.

vestibuloperineal fistula were described in 2 dogs with urinary incontinence considered to be intersexes having 78XX karyotype.[103]

Urethral Prolapse

Prolapse of the urethral mucosal lining through the external urethral orifice occurs primarily in male dogs younger than 5 years **(Fig. 12)**[104]; English bulldogs and Boston terriers seem to have a predilection.[105–107] Urethral prolapse may not be associated with clinical signs, or owners may only notice a red to purple mass at the tip of the penis during urination; however, it may be associated with dripping of blood, licking of the prepuce or penis, or signs of lower urinary tract disease. Diagnosis is based on physical examination. If urethral prolapse is associated with no to minimal clinical signs, treatment may not be necessary.[108] If associated with clinical signs, manual reduction if small or surgical correction if large may be done.[105,107]

Urethral Stricture and Hypoplasia

Presumed congenital urethral strictures and hypoplasia have been described in young dogs and cats.[57,109] Clinical signs relate to partial or complete urethral obstruction with stricture or urinary incontinence with hypoplasia. Systemic signs, bladder

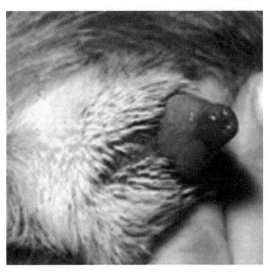

Fig. 12. Urethral prolapse in a 2-year-old intact male English bulldog.

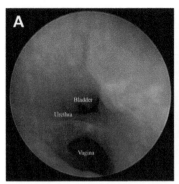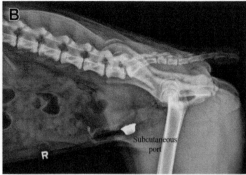

Fig. 13. Urethral hypoplasia in a 9-month-old spayed female rottweiler presented for urinary incontinence. (*A*) Cystoscopic image in dorsal recumbency of the urethral orifice and hypoplastic urethra with the lumen of the urinary bladder visible. The urethra measured approximately 2 cm long. (*B*) Immediate postoperative lateral survey abdominal radiograph demonstrating the placement of a hydraulic urethral occlude attached by tubing to the metallic subcutaneous port.

distention or rupture, overflow incontinence, secondary bacterial urinary tract infection, and hydronephrosis occur secondary to the urinary outflow obstruction or urinary incontinence with urethral hypoplasia. Urinary incontinence and bilateral hydroureter and hydronephrosis were observed in an 8-month-old male German shepherd with congenital midurethral stricture.[109] Treatment involves surgery. If the stricture occurs in the extrapelvic urethra, urethrostomy may be performed; if it occurs in the intrapelvic or intra-abdominal urethra, then urethral resection and anastomosis or prepubic urethrostomy may be indicated.[110,111] Dilation of the urethral stricture may also be attempted with balloon or bougienage catheters. Urinary incontinence secondary to urethral hypoplasia may be treated surgically or with a hydraulic urethral occluder with variable success (**Fig. 13**).[57]

Congenital Urinary Incontinence

Many congenital disorders are associated with congenital urinary incontinence. In addition to those described in the preceding sections, spinal dysraphism is associated with urinary and fecal incontinence. Spinal dysraphism refers to cleftlike malformations of the spine and spinal cord resulting from incomplete closure of the neural tube. Congenital urethral sphincter mechanism incompetency has been described in dogs and cats associated with urethral hypoplasia[57] or due to neurogenic causes associated with pseudohermaphrodism[84]; however, ectopic ureter is most commonly associated with juvenile urinary incontinence.[61,66,112]

REFERENCES

1. Noden DA, deLahunta A. The embryology of domestic animals. Baltimore (MA): Willilams & Wilkins; 1985.
2. Kruger JM, Osborne CA, Lulich JP. Inherited and congenital disease of the lower urinary tract. In: Osborne CA, Finco DR, editors. Canine and feline nephrology and urology. Baltimore (MA): Williams & Wilkins; 1995. p. 681–92.
3. Haraguchi R, Motoyama J, Sasaki H, et al. Molecular analysis of coordinated bladder and urogenital organ formation by Hedgehog signaling. Development 2007;134:525–33.

4. Pearson H, Gibbs C, Hillson JM. Some abnormalities of the canine urinary tract. Vet Rec 1965;77:775–80.
5. Holt PE, Gibbs C. Congenital urinary incontinence in cats: a review of 19 cases. Vet Rec 1992;130:437–42.
6. Holt PE, Moore AH. Canine ureteral ectopia: an analysis of 175 cases and comparison of surgical treatments. Vet Rec 1995;136:345–9.
7. Agut A, Fernandez del Palacio MJ, Laredo FG, et al. Unilateral renal agenesis associated with additional congenital abnormalities of the urinary tract in a Pekingese bitch. J Small Anim Pract 2002;43:32–5.
8. Schmaelzle JF, Cass AS, Hinman F Jr. Effect of disuse and restoration of function on vesical capacity. J Urol 1969;101:700–5.
9. Sutherland-Smith J, Jerram RM, Walker AM, et al. Ectopic ureters and ureteroceles in dogs: treatment. Compend Contin Educ Vet 2004;26:311–5.
10. Adams WM, DiBartola SP. Radiographic and clinical features of pelvic bladder in the dog. J Am Vet Med Assoc 1983;182:1212–7.
11. Mahaffey MB, Barsanti JA, Barber DL, et al. Pelvic bladder in dogs without urinary incontinence. J Am Vet Med Assoc 1984;184:1477–9.
12. Johnston GR, Osborne CA, Jessen CR, et al. Effects of urinary bladder distention on location of the urinary bladder and urethra of healthy dogs and cats. Am J Vet Res 1986;47:404–15.
13. Lane IF, Lappin MR. Urinary incontinence and congenital urogenital anomalies in small animals. In: Bonagura JD, Kirk RW, editors. Current veterinary therapy XII. Philadelphia: WB Saunders; 1995. p. 1022–6.
14. Rawlings C, Barsanti JA, Mahaffey MB, et al. Evaluation of colposuspension for treatment of incontinence in spayed female dogs. J Am Vet Med Assoc 2001; 219:770–5.
15. White RN. Urethropexy for the management of urethral sphincter mechanism incompetence in the bitch. J Small Anim Pract 2001;42:481–6.
16. Barth A, Reichler IM, Hubler M, et al. Evaluation of long-term effects of endoscopic injection of collagen into the urethral submucosa for treatment of urethral sphincter incompetence in female dogs: 40 cases (1993–2000). J Am Vet Med Assoc 2005;226:73–6.
17. Caione P, Capozza N, Zavaglia D, et al. Anterior perineal reconstruction in exstrophy-epispadias complex. Eur Urol 2005;47:872–7 [discussion: 877–8].
18. Hobson HP, Ader PL. Exstrophy of the bladder in a dog. J Am Anim Hosp Assoc 1979;15:103–7.
19. Shimada K, Matsumoto F, Tohda A, et al. Surgical management of urinary incontinence in children with anatomical bladder-outlet anomalies. Int J Urol 2002;9:561–6.
20. Zulauf D, Voss K, Reichler IM. Herniation of the urinary bladder through a congenitally enlarged inguinal canal in a cat. Schweiz Arch Tierheilkd 2007; 149:559–62.
21. Osborne CA, Johnston GR, Kruger JM, et al. Etiopathogenesis and biological behavior of feline vesicourachal diverticula. Don't just do something–stand there. Vet Clin North Am Small Anim Pract 1987;17:697–733.
22. Bartges JW. Diseases of the urinary bladder. In: Birchard SJ, Sherding RG, editors. Saunders manual of small animal practice. 2nd edition. Philadelphia: WB Saunders; 2000. p. 943–57.
23. Osborne CA, Rhoades JD, Hanlon GR. Patent urachus in the dog. J Am Anim Hosp Assoc 1966;2:245–50.
24. Greene RW, Bohning RH Jr. Patent persistent urachus associated with urolithiasis in a cat. J Am Vet Med Assoc 1971;158:489–91.

25. Pearson H, Gibbs C. Urinary tract abnormalities in the dog. J Small Anim Pract 1971;12:67–84.
26. Cornell KK. Cystotomy, partial cystectomy, and tube cystostomy. Clin Tech Small Anim Pract 2000;15:11–6.
27. Laverty PH, Salisbury SK. Surgical management of true patent urachus in a cat. J Small Anim Pract 2002;43:227–9.
28. Hanson JS. Patent urachus in a cat. Vet Med Small Anim Clin 1972;67: 379–81.
29. Archibald J, Owen RR. Urinary system. In: Archibald J, editor. Canine surgery. Santa Barbara (CA): American Veterinary Publications; 1974. p. 627–701.
30. Wilson GP, Dill LS, Goodman RZ. The relationship of urachal defects in the feline urinary bladder to feline urological syndrome. In: 7th Kal Kan Symp. Columbus (OH); 1983;125–29.
31. Lulich JP, Osborne CA, Johnston GR. Non-surgical correction of infection-induced struvite uroliths and a vesicourachal diverticulum in an immature dog. J Small Anim Pract 1989;30:613–7.
32. Osborne CA, Kroll RA, Lulich JP, et al. Medical management of vesicourachal diverticula in 15 cats with lower urinary tract disease. J Small Anim Pract 1989;30:608–12.
33. Scheepens ET, L'Eplattenier H. Acquired urinary bladder diverticulum in a dog. J Small Anim Pract 2005;46:578–81.
34. Gotthelf LN. Persistent urinary tract infection and urolithiasis in a cat with a urachal diverticulum. Vet Med Small Anim Clin 1981;76:1745–7.
35. Lobetti RG, Goldin JP. Emphysematous cystitis and bladder trigone diverticulum in a dog. J Small Anim Pract 1998;39:144–7.
36. Hoskins JD, Abdelbaki YZ, Root CR. Urinary bladder duplication in a dog. J Am Vet Med Assoc 1982;181:603–4.
37. Abrahamson J. Double bladder and related anomalies: clinical and embryological aspects and a case report. Br J Urol 1961;33:195–214.
38. van Schouwenburg SJ, Louw GJ. A case of dysuria as a result of a communication between the urinary bladder and corpus uteri in a cairn terrier. J S Afr Vet Assoc 1982;53:65–6.
39. Lawler DV, Monti KL. Morbidity and mortality in neonatal kittens. Am J Vet Res 1984;45:1455–9.
40. Caywood DD, Osborne CA, Johnston GR. Neoplasia of the canine and feline urinary tracts. In: Kirk RW, editor. Current veterinary therapy VII. Philadelphia: WB Saunders; 1980. p. 1203–12.
41. Osborne CA, Low DG, Perman V, et al. Neoplasms of the canine and feline urinary bladder: incidence, etiologic factors, occurrence and pathologic features. Am J Vet Res 1968;29:2041–55.
42. Stamps P, Harris DL. Botryoid rhabdomyosarcoma of the urinary bladder of a dog. J Am Vet Med Assoc 1968;153:1064–8.
43. Roszel JF. Cytology of urine from dogs with botryoid sarcoma of the bladder. Acta Cytol 1972;16:443–6.
44. Kelly DF. Rhabdomyosarcoma of the urianry bladder in dogs. Vet Pathol 1973; 10:375–84.
45. Halliwell WH, Ackerman N. Botryoid rhabdomyosarcoma of the urinary bladder and hypertrophic osteoarthropathy in a young dog. J Am Vet Med Assoc 1974; 165:911–3.
46. Pletcher JM, Dalton L. Botryoid rhabdomyosarcoma in the urinary bladder of a dog. Vet Pathol 1981;18:695–7.

47. Stone EA, George TF, Gilson SD, et al. Partial cystectomy for urinary bladder neoplasia: surgical technique and outcome in 11 dogs. J Small Anim Pract 1996;37:480–5.
48. Takiguchi M, Watanabe T, Okada H, et al. Rhabdomyosarcoma (botryoid sarcoma) of the urinary bladder in a Maltese. J Small Anim Pract 2002;43:269–71.
49. Madarame H, Ito A, Tanaka R. Urinary bladder rhabdomyosarcoma (botryoid rhabdomyosarcoma) in a labrador retriever dog. J Toxicol Pathol 2003;16: 279–81.
50. Bae IH, Kim Y, Pakhrin B, et al. Genitourinary rhabdomyosarcoma with systemic metastasis in a young dog. Vet Pathol 2007;44:518–20.
51. Van Vechten M, Goldschmidt MH, Wortman JA. Embryonal rhabdomyosarcoma of the urinary bladder in dogs. Compend Contin Educ Vet 1990;12:783–93.
52. Senior DF, Lawrence DT, Gunson C. Successful treatment of boytroid rhabdomyosarcoma in the bladder of a dog. J Am Anim Hosp Assoc 1993; 29:386–90.
53. Bartges JW, Cornelius LM, Osborne CA. Ammonium urate uroliths in dogs with portosystemic shunts. In: Bonagura JD, editor. Current veterinary therapy XIII. Philadelphia: WB Saunders; 1999. p. 872–4.
54. Bartges JW, Osborne CA, Lulich JP, et al. Canine urate urolithiasis. Etiopathogenesis, diagnosis, and management. Vet Clin North Am Small Anim Pract 1999;29:161–91, xii–xiii.
55. Osborne CA, Bartges JW, Lulich JP, et al. Canine urolithiasis. In: Hand MS, Thatcher CD, Remillard RL, et al, editors. Small animal clinical nutrition. 4th edition. Marceline (MO): Wadsworth Publishing Co; 2000. p. 605–88.
56. Bargai U, Bark H. Multiple congenital urinary tract abnormalities in a bitch: a case history report. Vet Radiol Ultrasound 1982;23:10–2.
57. Holt PE. Surgical management of congenital urethral sphincter mechanism incompetence in eight female cats and a bitch. Vet Surg 1993;22:98–104.
58. Baines SJ, Speakman AJ, Williams JM, et al. Genitourinary dysplasia in a cat. J Small Anim Pract 1999;40:286–90.
59. Stone EA, Mason LK. Surgery of ectopic ureters: types, method of correction, and postoperative results. J Am Anim Hosp Assoc 1990;26:81–8.
60. Mason LK, Stone EA, Biery DN, et al. Surgery of ectopic ureters - preoperative and postoperative radiographic morphology. J Am Anim Hosp Assoc 1990;26: 73–9.
61. McLoughlin MA, Chew DJ. Diagnosis and surgical management of ectopic ureters. Clin Tech Small Anim Pract 2000;15:17–24.
62. Lamb CR. Ultrasonography of the ureters. Vet Clin North Am Small Anim Pract 1998;28:823–48.
63. McLaughlin R Jr, Miller CW. Urinary incontinence after surgical repair of ureteral ectopia in dogs. Vet Surg 1991;20:100–3.
64. Anders KJ, McLoughlin MA, Samii VF, et al. Ectopic ureters in male dogs: review of 16 clinical cases (1999-2007). J Am Anim Hosp Assoc 2012;48:390–8.
65. McCarthy TC. Endoscopy brief: transurethal cystoscopy and diode laser incision to correct an ectopic ureter. Vet Med 2006;101:558–9.
66. Berent AC, Mayhew PD, Porat-Mosenco Y. Use of cystoscopic-guided laser ablation for treatment of intramural ureteral ectopia in male dogs: four cases (2006-2007). J Am Vet Med Assoc 2008;232:1026–34.
67. Bartges JW. Laser ablation of ectopic ureter. In: Bartges JW, Polzin DJ, editors. Nephrology and urology of small animals. Ames (IA): Wiley-Blackwell; 2011. p. 383–5.

68. Berent AC, Weisse C, Mayhew PD, et al. Evaluation of cystoscopic-guided laser ablation of intramural ectopic ureters in female dogs. J Am Vet Med Assoc 2012; 240:716–25.

69. Ho LK, Troy GC, Waldron DR. Clinical outcomes of surgically managed ectopic ureters in 33 dogs. J Am Anim Hosp Assoc 2011;47:196–202.

70. Hayes HM Jr, Wilson GP. Hospital incidence of hypospadias in dogs in North America. Vet Rec 1986;118:605–7.

71. Cassata R, Iannuzzi A, Parma P, et al. Clinical, cytogenetic and molecular evaluation in a dog with bilateral cryptorchidism and hypospadias. Cytogenet Genome Res 2008;120:140–3.

72. King GJ, Johnson EH. Hypospadias in a Himalayan cat. J Small Anim Pract 2000;41:508–10.

73. Sonne C, Dietz R, Born EW, et al. Is there a link between hypospadias and organochlorine exposure in East Greenland sledge dogs (Canis familiaris)? Ecotoxicol Environ Saf 2008;69:391–5.

74. Ader L, Hobson HP. Hypospadias: a review of the veterinary literature and a report of three cases in the dog. J Am Anim Hosp Assoc 1978;14:721–7.

75. Grieco V, Riccardi E, Veronesi MC, et al. Evidence of testicular dysgenesis syndrome in the dog. Theriogenology 2008;70:53–60.

76. Jurka P, Galanty M, Zielinska P, et al. Hypospadias in six dogs. Vet Rec 2009; 164:331–3.

77. Rawlings CA. Correction of congenital defects of the urogenital system. Vet Clin North Am Small Anim Pract 1984;14:49–60.

78. Lefebvre R, Lussier B. A clinical case of hypospodias in a dog. Can Vet J 2005; 46:1022–5 [in French].

79. Pavletic MM. Reconstruction of the urethra by use of an inverse tubed bipedicled flap in a dog with hypospadias. J Am Vet Med Assoc 2007;231: 71–3.

80. Galanty M, Jurka P, Zielinska P. Surgical treatment of hypospadias. Techniques and results in six dogs. Pol J Vet Sci 2008;11:235–43.

81. Grossman J, Baltzer W. Use of a preputial circumferential mucosal flap for hypospadias management in a Boston terrier. J Small Anim Pract 2012;53:292–6.

82. Holt PE, Long SE, Gibbs C. Disorders of urination associated with canine intersexuality. J Small Anim Pract 1983;24:475–87.

83. Jackson DA. Pseudohermaphroditism. In: Kirk RW, editor. Current veterinary therapy VII. Philadelphia: WB Saunders; 1980. p. 1241–3.

84. Jackson DA, Osborne CA, Brasmer TH, et al. Nonneurogenic urinary incontinence in a canine female pseudohermaphrodite. J Am Vet Med Assoc 1978; 172:926–30.

85. Holt PE. Urinary incontinence. In: Holt PE, editor. Urological disorders of the dog and cat. London: Manson Publishing; 2008. p. 134–59.

86. Siomou E, Papadopoulou F, Salakos C, et al. Rare combination of unilateral renal agenesis, congenital obstructive posterior urethral membrane, and enlarged prostatic utricle, with absence of hydroureteronephrosis. Urology 2007;70: 1008.e1001–3.

87. Wolff A, Radecky M. Anomaly in a poodle puppy. Vet Med Small Anim Clin 1973; 68:732–3.

88. Johnston SD, Bailie NC, Hayden DW. Diphallia in a mixed-breed dog with multiple anomalies. Theriogenology 1989;31:1253–60.

89. Longhofer SL, Jackson RK, Cooley AJ. Hindgut and bladder duplication in a dog. J Am Vet Med Assoc 1991;64:520–3.

90. Tobias KS, Barbee D. Abnormal micturition and recurrent cystitis associated with multiple congenital anomalies of the urinary tract in a dog. J Am Vet Med Assoc 1995;207:191–3.
91. Duffey MH, Barnhart MD, Barthez PY, et al. Incomplete urethral duplication with cyst formation in a dog. J Am Vet Med Assoc 1998;213:1287–9, 1279.
92. Osborne CA, Hanlon GF. Canine congenital ureteral ectopia: Case report and review of literature. J Am Anim Hosp Assoc 1967;3:111–22.
93. Lulich JP, Osborne CA, Lawler DF, et al. Urologic disorders of immature cats. Vet Clin North Am Small Anim Pract 1987;17:663–96.
94. Osborne CA, Engen MH, Yano BL, et al. Congenital urethrorectal fistula in two dogs. J Am Vet Med Assoc 1975;166:999–1002.
95. Miller CF. Urethrorectal fistula with concurrent urolithiasis in a dog. Vet Med Small Anim Clin 1980;75:73–6.
96. Whitney WO, Schrader LA. Urethrorectal fistulectomy in a dog, using a perineal approach. J Am Vet Med Assoc 1988;193:568–9.
97. Agut A, Lucas X, Castro A, et al. A urethrorectal fistula due to prostatic abscess associated with urolithiasis in a dog. Reprod Domest Anim 2006;41:247–50.
98. Gray LA. Urethrovaginal fistulas. Am J Obstet Gynecol 1968;101:28–36.
99. Osuna DJ, Stone EA, Metcalf MR. A urethrorectal fistula with concurrent urolithiasis in a dog. J Am Anim Hosp Assoc 1989;25:35–9.
100. Foster SF, Hunt GB, Malik R. Congenital urethral anomaly in a kitten. J Feline Med Surg 1999;1:61–4.
101. Lautzenhiser SJ, Bjorling DE. Urinary incontinence in a dog with an ectopic ureterocele. J Am Anim Hosp Assoc 2002;38:29–32.
102. Osborne CA. Urethrorectal fistulas. In: Kirk RW, editor. Current veterinary therapy VI. Philadelphia: WB Saunders; 1977. p. 985–6.
103. Gregory SP, Trower ND. Surgical treatment of urinary incontinence resulting from a complex congenital abnormality in two dogs. J Small Anim Pract 1997;38:25–8.
104. Ragni RA. Urethral prolapse in three male Yorkshire terriers. J Small Anim Pract 2007;48:180.
105. Sinibaldi KR, Green RW. Surgical correction of prolapse of the male urethra in three English bulldogs. J Am Anim Hosp Assoc 1973;9:450–3.
106. Osborne CA, Sanderson SL. Medical management of urethral prolapse in male dogs. In: Bonagura JD, Kirk RW, editors. Current veterinary therapy XII. Philadelphia: WB Saunders; 1995. p. 1027–9.
107. Kirsch JA, Hauptman JG, Walshaw R. A urethropexy technique for surgical treatment of urethral prolapse in the male dog. J Am Anim Hosp Assoc 2002;38:381–4.
108. Osborne CA, Sanderson SL, Lulich JP, et al. Medical management of iatrogenic rents in the wall of the feline urinary bladder. Vet Clin North Am Small Anim Pract 1996;26:551–62.
109. Breitschwerdt EB, Olivier NB, King GK, et al. Bilateral hydronephrosis and hydroureter in a dog associated with congenital urethral stricture. J Am Anim Hosp Assoc 1982;18:799–803.
110. Baines SJ, Rennie S, White RS. Prepubic urethrostomy: a long-term study in 16 cats. Vet Surg 2001;30:107–13.
111. Bernarde A, Viguier E. Transpelvic urethrostomy in 11 cats using an ischial ostectomy. Vet Surg 2004;33:246–52.
112. Silverman S, Long CD. The diagnosis of urinary incontinence and abnormal urination in dogs and cats. Vet Clin North Am Small Anim Pract 2000;30:427–48.

Urinary Tract Infections
Treatment/Comparative Therapeutics

Shelly J. Olin, DVM[a],*, Joseph W. Bartges, DVM, PhD[b]

KEYWORDS

- Veterinary medicine • Canine • Feline • Cystitis • Pyelonephritis • Prostatitis
- Urinary tract infection

KEY POINTS

- Determining whether an infection is uncomplicated or complicated is essential to guide the diagnostic and therapeutic plan.
- Recurrent infections are complicated infections and may be relapsing, refractory/persistent, reinfection, or superinfection.
- Antimicrobials are the cornerstone of treatment of bacterial UTI and, ideally, are selected based on culture and sensitivity.
- There is limited literature to support preventative therapies; identification and resolution of underlying causes are essential.

INTRODUCTION

Urinary tract infection (UTI) occurs when there is a compromise of host defense mechanisms and a virulent microbe adheres, multiplies, and persists in a portion of the urinary tract. Host defenses include normal micturition, anatomic structures, the mucosal barrier, properties of urine, and systemic immunocompetence. Most commonly UTIs are caused by bacteria, but fungi and viruses also may infect the urinary tract. UTIs may involve more than one anatomic location, and the infection should be categorized as upper urinary tract (kidneys and ureters) versus lower urinary tract (bladder, urethra, and vagina). Most bacterial UTI occur as a consequence of ascending migration of pathogens through the genital tract and urethra to the bladder, ureters, and one or both kidneys. Rectal, perineal, and genital bacteria serve as the principal reservoirs for infection.[1,2]

Disclosure Statement: The authors disclose no commercial or financial conflicts of interest.
[a] Department of Small Animal Clinical Sciences, College of Veterinary Medicine, University of Tennessee, 2407 River Drive, Knoxville, TN 37996, USA; [b] Cornell University Veterinary Specialists, 880 Canal Street, Stamford, CT 06902, USA
* Corresponding author.
E-mail address: solin@utk.edu

Bacterial Isolates

A single bacterial pathogen is isolated from approximately 75% infections; 20% of UTIs are caused by 2 coinfecting species, and approximately 5% are caused by 3 species.[3–5]

The bacteria that most commonly cause UTIs are similar in dogs and cats (**Fig. 1**).[3,6–8] *Escherichia coli* is most common, followed by gram-positive cocci, and then various others, including *Proteus, Klebsiella, Pasteurella, Pseudomonas, Corynebacterium*, and several other rarely reported genera.[3,6] *Mycoplasma* spp are isolated from urine of dogs with clinical signs of lower urinary tract in less than 5% of samples; whether *Mycoplasma* spp are associated with urinary tract disease in cats is controversial.[3,9–11]

Cats may be infected with a unique strain of *Staphylococcus, Staphylococcus felis*, and commercial phenotypic identification systems may not differentiate between *S felis* and other coagulase-negative *Staphylococcus* spp.[7,8] One study found that *S felis* was the third most common isolate based on 16S rDNA sequencing (n = 25/106, 19.8% of bacterial isolates cultured), suggesting *S felis* is the most common Staphylococcal species causing UTI in cats.[7]

Pyelonephritis

Pyelonephritis, or infection of the renal pelvis and parenchyma, is most commonly due to ascending infections from the lower urinary tract in dogs and cats (**Fig. 2**). In addition to the components of immunity that protect urinary tract in general, the kidneys are protected from bacterial infection by vesicoureteral flap valves, relatively long ureters that usually allow only one-way flow of urine via peristalsis, and generally hypoxic environment of the renal medulla.

Prostatitis

Inherent prostatic defense mechanisms against infection include local immune factors, such as immunoglobulin A and antibacterial proteins, retrograde flow of prostatic

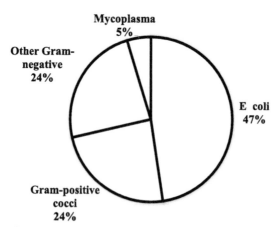

Fig. 1. Prevalence of common urinary pathogens: 33%–50% *E coli*, 25%–33% gram-positive cocci (*Staphylococcus* sp, *Streptococcus* sp, *Enterococcus* sp), 25%–33% other gram-negative (*Proteus* sp, *Klebsiella* sp, *Pasteurella* sp, *Pseudomonas* sp, *Corynebacterium* sp), less than 5% *Mycoplasma* sp. (*Data from* Ling GV, Norris CR, Franti CE, et al. Interrelations of organism prevalence, specimen collection method, and host age, sex, and breed among 8,354 canine urinary tract infections (1969–1995). J Vet Intern Med 2001;15:341–7; and Barsanti J. Genitourinary infections. In: Greene CE, editor. Infectious diseases of the dog and cat. 4th edition. St Louis (MO): Elsevier Saunders; 2012. p. 1013–31.)

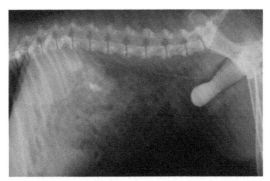

Fig. 2. Lateral abdominal excretory urography showing a pelvically displaced urinary bladder and renal pelvic dilation (pyelonephritis) due to ascending *E coli* urinary tract in a 4-year-old spayed female mixed breed dog.

fluid and urine, and urethral peristalsis, and the urethral high pressure zone.[12,13] Dogs with bacterial prostatitis often have alteration of normal defenses, such as underlying benign prostatic hyperplasia, prostatic cysts, or neoplasia.[14] Most commonly prostatitis develops from ascending bacterial infection and may result in prostatic abscessation in addition to prostatic parenchymal infection (**Fig. 3**). Hematogenous spread and prostatitis secondary to cystitis are also possible. Bacterial pathogens are similar to those causing bacterial cystitis with *E coli* being the most common (see **Fig. 1**). *Brucella canis* should also be considered, especially for intact male dogs, as a cause for both acute and chronic prostatitis.[14]

Catheter-associated urinary tract infection

Normal host defense mechanisms are effective in preventing bacterial UTIs; however, they are not impenetrable. Normal host defenses may be overwhelmed if large quantities of a virulent uropathogen are introduced into the urinary tract during diagnostic and therapeutic procedures. Catheter-associated bacterial UTI is a common complication of indwelling urinary catheters, especially if an open-ended system is used. In a

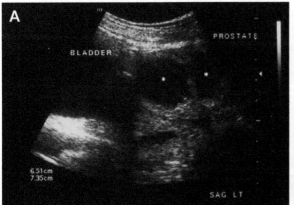
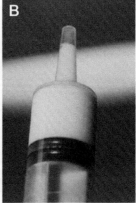

Fig. 3. (*A*) Sagittal ultrasonographic image of the prostate and urinary bladder showing 2 cystic lesions that were abscesses (*) and (*B*) purulent prostatic wash fluid due to *E coli* in a 6-year-old intact male Rhodesian ridgeback.

clinical study, infection developed in 30% to 52% of dogs and cats with indwelling urinary catheters; risk of infection increased with duration of catheterization.[15,16] The risk of infection is further compounded if the patient has pre-existing urinary tract disease. Use of indwelling urinary catheters during diuresis or corticosteroid administration is particularly dangerous.

Fungal Urinary Tract Infection

Fungal UTI is uncommon. As with bacterial UTI, fungal UTI occurs because of temporary or permanent breaches in local or systemic immunity of the lower urinary tract. Funguria may be due to primary infections of the lower urinary tract or secondary to shedding of fungal elements into the urine in animals with systemic infections. Primary fungal UTI is most commonly due to *Candida* spp, a commensal inhabitant of the genital mucosa, upper respiratory tract, and gastrointestinal tract.[17,18] *Candida albicans* is the most commonly identified species, followed by *Candida glabrata* and *Candida tropicalis*; other ubiquitous fungi may also occasionally cause primary fungal UTI, including *Aspergillus* spp, *Blastomycosis* spp (**Fig. 4**), and *Cryptococcus* spp.[19]

Viral Urinary Tract Infection

Viral-induced disease in humans is increasingly recognized, especially of the upper urinary tract. However, it can be difficult to determine cause-and-effect relationships because viral-induced disease may occur in the absence of detectable replicating virus. Several viruses have been implicated in canine and feline disease (**Box 1**).[20]

PATIENT EVALUATION OVERVIEW
Clinical Signs

Lower urinary tract infection: bacterial, fungal, viral
Lower UTI may be symptomatic or asymptomatic, and clinical signs are indistinguishable from other causes of lower urinary tract disease. Nonspecific clinical signs of lower urinary tract disease include, but are not limited to, pollakiuria, dysuria, stranguria, hematuria, and inappropriate urination.[21]

Prostatitis Acute prostatitis is usually associated with systemic illness, including fever, anorexia, vomiting, and lethargy. Dogs with acute disease may also have caudal abdominal pain, stiff gait, and preputial discharge and be unwilling to breed.[12–14] In contrast, dogs with chronic prostatitis are usually not systemically ill or febrile.[13]

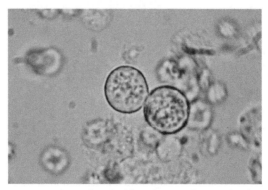

Fig. 4. *Blastomyces* spp organisms observed by microscopic examination of urine sediment from a 2-year-old castrated male Doberman pinscher.

Commonly, recurrent UTI or preputial bloody discharge is the only clinical sign of chronic prostatitis.[14] Other presentations include stiff gait, discomfort with rising, infertility, or orchiepididymitis, or dogs may be asymptomatic.[13]

Upper urinary tract infection

Pyelonephritis Pyelonephritis may have an acute or chronic presentation. Acute pyelonephritis is usually associated with signs of severe systemic illness (eg, uremia, fever, painful kidneys, possible nephromegaly, and/or sepsis). In contrast, chronic pyelonephritis usually has a more insidious presentation: slowly progressive azotemia that may not be associated with uremia, progressive kidney damage, and ultimately, renal failure if untreated. Bacterial pyelonephritis may be associated with hematuria only.

Diagnosis

Bacterial urinary tract infection

In addition to clinical signs, results of a complete urinalysis may provide evidence of a bacterial UTI. Hematuria, pyuria, and bacteriuria are often present unless there is suppression of immune response because of underlying disease or drugs (**Fig. 5**).

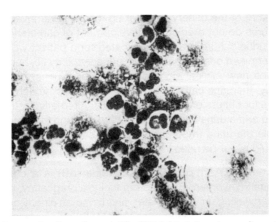

Fig. 5. Microscopic examination of a modified Wright stain urine sediment from a dog with *E coli* bacterial cystitis showing white blood cells and bacteria (×400).

Microscopic examination of unstained urine sediment is less sensitive and specific than examining urine sediment stained with a modified Wright stain.[22]

A positive urine culture is the "gold standard" for diagnosing bacterial UTI. A quantitative urine culture includes isolation and identification of the organism and determination of the number of bacteria (colony-forming units per unit volume). Quantitation of bacteria enables interpretation as to the significance of bacteria present in a urine sample. Caution should be exercised when interpreting quantitative urine cultures obtained by midstream voiding or manual expression of urine.[21]

Determining whether an infection is uncomplicated or complicated is essential to guide the diagnostic and therapeutic plan. A simple uncomplicated UTI occurs sporadically in an otherwise healthy animal with a normal structural and functional urinary tract.[23] In contrast, infections are complicated if there is (1) involvement of the upper urinary tract and/or prostate, (2) an underlying comorbidity that alters the structure or function of the urinary tract, such as an endocrinopathy or chronic kidney disease (CKD), or (3) recurrent infection.[23,24] Recurrent infections are further categorized as relapsing, refractory/persistent, reinfection, or superinfection (**Table 1**).[23,24] Most cats with bacterial UTI have complicated infections.[21] Additional laboratory testing and imaging studies are often required for complicated infections (**Box 2**).[21]

Pyelonephritis Pyelonephritis is an example of a complicated UTI. Diagnosis of pyelonephritis is usually presumptive based on positive urine culture, concurrent consistent renal diagnostic imaging abnormalities (eg, pyelectasia), and possible improvement in degree of azotemia following antimicrobial therapy. Although a positive culture is helpful for the diagnosis, a negative urine culture does not rule out pyelonephritis.

Prostatitis All dogs with suspected prostatic disease should have a complete physical examination, including rectal examination, and a minimum database with complete blood count, chemistry panel, urine analysis, and urine culture. Abdominal radiographs and ultrasound are useful to determine the size, shape, location, and architecture of the prostate as well as if any cysts or abscesses are present (see **Fig. 3**A).[14] Prostatic fluid should be evaluated for cytology and bacterial culture and sensitivity (see **Fig. 3**B). Options for prostatic fluid sampling are discussed elsewhere, but include semen evaluation of the third fraction, prostatic wash, fine-needle aspiration, and prostatic biopsy.[14]

Catheter-associated urinary tract infection There is no evidence to support routine urine culture or culture of the urinary catheter tip following removal in asymptomatic patients; such cultures do not predict the development of catheter-associated infection.[23] In contrast, urine culture is always indicated for a patient with clinical signs of UTI, fever of undetermined origin, or abnormal urine cytology (ie, hematuria, pyuria). If the patient develops new clinical signs or fever after a urinary catheter has been placed, then, ideally, the urine catheter is removed and a cystocentesis is performed to provide a sample for culture once the bladder fills. Alternatively, the original urinary catheter is replaced and a urine sample is collected through the second catheter. It is less ideal to sample the urine through the original catheter, and a sample from the collection bag should never be used.[23]

Asymptomatic bacteriuria Asymptomatic bacteriuria (AB) is a common and often benign finding in healthy women. Risk factors include pregnancy, diabetes mellitus, spinal cord injury, indwelling urinary catheter, and being an elderly nursing home resident.[25] Women with AB have more frequent symptomatic episodes, but antimicrobial treatment does not decrease the number of episodes. A benefit to treatment has not

Table 1
Uncomplicated and complicated urinary tract infections

	Definition	Underlying Cause
Uncomplicated UTI	• Healthy individual, normal urinary tract anatomy and function	• Sporadic infection
Complicated UTI		
Comorbidity	• Disease that alters the structure or function of the urinary tract • Relevant comorbidity predisposes to persistent infection, recurrent infection, or treatment failure	• Endocrinopathies ○ Diabetes mellitus ○ Hyperadrenocorticism ○ Hyperthyroidism • CKD • Urinary or reproductive tract anatomic abnormality • Immunocompromised • Neurogenic bladder • Pregnancy
Recurrent infection		
Relapsing	• Recurrence within weeks to months of a successfully treated infection • Sterile bladder during treatment • Same organism	Failure to eradicate pathogen • Deep-seated niche ○ Pyelonephritis ○ Prostatitis ○ Bladder submucosa ○ Stone ○ Neoplasia
Refractory/persistent	• Persistently positive culture with original pathogen despite in vitro antimicrobial susceptibility • No elimination of bacteriuria during or after treatment	Rare • Failure of host defenses • Structural abnormality • Patient/client incompliance • Abnormal metabolism/excretion of antimicrobial
Reinfection	• Recurrence with different organism • Variable time course after previous infection	• Poor systemic immune function ○ Endocrinopathy ○ Immunosuppressed • Loss urine antimicrobial properties ○ Glucosuria ○ Dilute urine • Anatomic abnormality • Physiologic predisposition ○ Neurogenic bladder ○ Urinary incontinence
Superinfection	• Infection with different pathogen during treatment of the original infection	• Cystotomy tube • Indwelling urinary catheter • Neoplasia

Adapted from Weese JS, Blondeau JM, Boothe D, et al. Antimicrobial use guidelines for treatment of urinary tract disease in dogs and cats: antimicrobial guidelines working group of the international society for companion animal infectious diseases. Vet Med Int 2011;2011:1–9; and Barsanti J. Multidrug-resistant urinary tract infection. In: Bonagura JD, Twedt DC, editors. Current veterinary therapy XIV. St Louis (MO): WB Saunders; 2009. p. 921–5.

Box 2
Diagnostic testing for complicated urinary tract infections

Extended diagnostic testing may be required for complicated infections.

- Urine analysis
- Urine culture (ideally, cystocentesis sample)
- Complete blood count
- Chemistry profile with electrolytes
- Digital rectal examination
- Feline leukemia virus/feline immunodeficiency virus (cats)
- Thyroid testing
  - Cats: total T4
- Adrenal testing
  - Low-dose dexamethasone suppression test
  - Adrenocorticotropic hormone stimulation test
- Abdominal radiographs
- Abdominal ultrasound
- Contrast radiology
  - Excretory urography
  - Contrast cystourethrography
  - Double-contrast cystography
  - Contrast vaginourethrography
- Prostatic wash
- Cystoscopy with bladder wall culture

Adapted from Bartges JW. Diagnosis of urinary tract infections. Vet Clin North Am Small Anim Pract 2004;34:927–29; and Weese JS, Blondeau JM, Boothe D, et al. Antimicrobial use guidelines for treatment of urinary tract disease in dogs and cats: antimicrobial guidelines working group of the international society for companion animal infectious diseases. Vet Med Int 2011;2011:2,4.

---

been found with clinical trials in humans, whereas potential complications include adverse drug reactions and the development of antimicrobial resistance.[25]

The prevalence of AB in healthy dogs and cats is low (2%–9%).[26–29] Animals with underlying comorbidities, such as hyperthyroidism, diabetes mellitus, or CKD, or recurrent infection have increased prevalence of AB, up to 30%[29–33] and 50%,[34] respectively. There are no prospective studies comparing clinical outcome in veterinary patients with or without antimicrobial treatment of AB. In one recent prospective study of dogs with AB, 50% had transient colonization and 50% had persistent bacteriuria over a 3-month time period; no dog developed clinical signs at any time point.[27] Similar to general recommendation in humans, treatment is not recommended for AB unless there is a high risk for ascending or systemic infection (eg, immunocompromised patients, CKD).[23]

Fungal urinary tract infection

Diagnosis of fungal UTI most commonly occurs by identification of fungal elements during routine or concentrated urine sediment examination. Fungal culture and sensitivity are ideal before treatment, especially in cases other than *C albicans*, which tend to be more resistant.[19]

Viral urinary tract infection
Routine diagnostic tests, including urine analysis and light microscopy, cannot identify viruses or viral-induced disease. Virus isolation is the gold standard for diagnosis, but this technique is expensive and time-consuming and requires live replicating virus. Diagnostic polymerase chain reaction assays are rapid and sensitive, but methods to optimize nucleic acid preparation are essential because the nucleic acids are easily degraded in urine.[20]

PHARMACOLOGIC TREATMENT OPTIONS
Antimicrobials

Antimicrobial drugs are the cornerstone of treatment of UTI. In most cases the antimicrobial agent chosen should be based on susceptibility testing of the uropathogen. Overuse and misuse of antimicrobial drugs may result in the emergence of resistant organisms, a situation that has implications for successful treatment of infections in the patient as well as overall veterinary and human health.

Patients with uncomplicated UTI and those with clinical signs severe enough to merit therapy before results of urine culture and sensitivity testing should receive a broad-spectrum antimicrobial that has excellent urine penetration. Suggested "first-line" antimicrobials for uncomplicated UTIs include amoxicillin, cephalexin, or trimethoprim-sulfamethoxazole (**Table 2**). The use of potentiated β-lactams (ie, amoxicillin-clavulanic acid), fluoroquinolones, or extended-release cephalexin (ie, cefovecin) is inappropriate for most uncomplicated UTIs and should be reserved for complicated or resistant infections (**Table 3**).

Combination therapies
If multiple bacteria are isolated, then the relative importance of each must be assessed based on quantification and suspected pathogenicity. Ideally, an antimicrobial effective against all pathogens is selected. If this is not possible, then combination therapy with multiple antimicrobials may be considered.[23] Assuming there is no evidence of pyelonephritis or increased risk of ascending infection, then targeting antimicrobial therapy against the pathogen with most clinical relevance is reasonable. For example,

Table 2
Summary of first-line antimicrobial options for urinary tract infections in the dog and cat

Infection	First-Line Drug Options
Uncomplicated UTI	Amoxicillin, trimethoprim-sulfonamide
Complicated	Guided by culture and susceptibility testing, but consider amoxicillin or trimethoprim-sulfonamide initially
Subclinical bacteriuria	Antimicrobial therapy not recommended unless high risk for ascending infection. If so, treat as per complicated UTI
Pyelonephritis	Start with a fluoroquinolone, with reassessment based on culture and susceptibility testing
Prostatitis	Trimethoprim-sulfonamide, enrofloxacin, chloramphenicol

Adapted from Weese JS, Blondeau JM, Boothe D, et al. Antimicrobial use guidelines for treatment of urinary tract disease in dogs and cats: antimicrobial guidelines working group of the International Society for Companion Animal Infectious Diseases. Vet Med Int 2011;2011:5,6.

Table 3
Antimicrobial treatment options for urinary tract infection in dogs and cats

Drug	Dose	Comments
Amoxicillin	11–15 mg/kg q8h, PO	Good first-line option for UTIs. Excreted in urine predominantly in active form if normal renal function is present. Ineffective against β-lactamase-producing bacteria.
Amikacin	Dogs: 15–30 mg/kg q24h, IV/IM/SC; Cats: 10–14 mg/kg q24h, IV/IM/SC	Not recommended for routine use but may be useful for treatment of multidrug-resistant organisms. Potentially nephrotoxic. Avoid in animals with renal insufficiency.
Amoxicillin/clavulanate	12.5–25 mg/kg q8h, PO (dose based on combination of amoxicillin + clavulanate)	Not established whether there is any advantage over amoxicillin alone.
Ampicillin		Not recommended because of poor oral bioavailability. Amoxicillin is preferred.
Cephalexin, Cefadroxil	12–25 mg/kg q12h, PO	Enterococci are resistant. Resistance may be common in *Enterobacteriaceae* in some regions
Cefovecin	8 mg/kg single SC injection. Can be repeated once after 7–14 d	Should only be used in situations where oral treatment is problematic. Enterococci are resistant. Pharmacokinetic data are available to support the use in dogs and cats, with a duration of 14 d (dogs) and 21 d (cats). The long duration of excretion in the urine makes it difficult to interpret posttreatment culture results.
Cefpodoxime proxetil	5 to 10 mg/kg q24h, PO	Enterococci are resistant.
Ceftiofur	2 mg/kg q12–24h, SC	Approved for treatment of UTIs in dogs in some regions. Enterococci are resistant.
Chloramphenicol	Dogs: 40–50 mg/kg q8h, PO; Cats: 12.5–20 mg/kg q12h, PO	Reserved for multidrug-resistant infections with few other options. Myelosuppression can occur, particularly with long-term therapy. Avoid contact by humans because of rare idiosyncratic aplastic anemia.
Ciprofloxacin	30 mg/kg q24h, PO	Sometimes used because of lower cost than enrofloxacin. Lower and more variable oral bioavailability than enrofloxacin, marbofloxacin, and orbifloxacin. Difficult to justify over approved fluoroquinolones. Dosing recommendations are empirical.
Doxycycline	3–5 mg/kg q12h, PO	Highly metabolized and excreted through intestinal tract, so urine levels may be low. Not recommended for routine uses.

Drug	Dose	Comments
Enrofloxacin	Dogs: 10–20 mg/kg q24h, PO Cats: 5 mg/kg q24h, PO	Excreted in urine predominantly in active form. Reserve for documented resistant UTIs but good first-line choice for pyelonephritis (dogs 20 mg/kg PO q24h). Limited efficacy against enterococci. Associated with risk of retinopathy in cats. Do not exceed 5 mg/kg/d of enrofloxacin in cats.
Imipenem-cilastatin	5 mg/kg q6–8h, IV/IM	Reserve for treatment of multidrug-resistant infections, particularly those caused by Enterobacteriaceae or P aeruginosa. Recommend consultation with a urinary or infectious disease veterinary specialist or veterinary pharmacologist before use.
Marbofloxacin	2.7–5.5 mg/kg q24h, PO	Excreted in urine predominantly in active form. Reserve for documented resistant UTIs but good first-line choice for pyelonephritis. Limited efficacy against enterococci.
Meropenem	8.5 mg/kg q12h, SC or q8h, IV	Reserve for treatment of multidrug-resistant infections, particularly those caused by Enterobacteriaceae or P aeruginosa. Recommend consultation with a urinary or infectious disease veterinary specialist or veterinary pharmacologist before use.
Nitrofurantoin	4.4–5 mg/kg q8h, PO	Good second-line option for simple uncomplicated UTI, particularly when multidrug-resistant pathogens are involved.
Orbifloxacin	Tablets: 2.5–7.5 mg/kg q24h, PO; oral suspension: 7.5 mg/kg q24h, PO (cats) or 2.5–7.5 mg/kg q24h, PO (dogs)	Excreted in urine predominantly in active form.
Pradofloxacin	Dogs: 3 mg/kg q24h, PO[a] Cats: 5 mg/kg q24h, PO[a]	May cause bone marrow suppression resulting in severe thrombocytopenia and neutropenia in dogs.
Trimethoprim-sulfadiazine	15 mg/kg q12h, PO Note: dosing is based on total trimethoprim + sulfadiazine concentration	Good first-line option. Concerns regarding idiosyncratic and immune-mediated adverse effects in some patients, especially with prolonged therapy. If prolonged (>7 d) therapy is anticipated, baseline Schirmer tear testing is recommended (dogs), with periodic re-evaluation and owner monitoring for ocular discharge. Avoid in dogs that may be sensitive to potential adverse effects such as keratoconjunctivitis sicca (KCS), hepatopathy, hypersensitivity, and skin eruptions.

[a] Dose extrapolated from previous studies.[37]

Adapted from Weese JS, Blondeau JM, Boothe D, et al. Antimicrobial use guidelines for treatment of urinary tract disease in dogs and cats: antimicrobial guidelines working group of the International Society for Companion Animal Infectious Diseases. Vet Med Int 2011;5,6.

anecdotally, resolution of *Enterococcus* sp infection is often possible after treatment of concurrent infection.[23]

Fluoroquinolone update

The use of fluoroquinolones for empiric treatment of bacterial UTI is discouraged because of the inherent resistance of many gram-positive organisms to this class of antimicrobials, and the developing resistance of many gram-negative organisms, including *E coli*, to this class of drugs.[35] Studies have found variable cross-resistance among different generations of fluoroquinolones, except pradofloxacin (Veraflox), and once fluoroquinolone resistance has developed, a later generation of drug may not be beneficial.[36] In vitro, pradofloxacin, a third-generation fluoroquinolone, outperformed other fluoroquinolones in terms of potency and efficacy; enrofloxacin was the least potent second only to ciprofloxacin. Molecular alterations of pradofloxacin allow increased bactericidal activity and decreased propensity for antimicrobial resistance.[35–37] These features make pradofloxacin an attractive choice for a susceptible fluoroquinolone-naïve isolate or pathogens with reduced fluoroquinolone susceptibility.[36,38] Currently, pradofloxacin is only licensed for feline skin infections in the United States, whereas the European license includes a wide range of indications for both dogs and cats. One prospective clinical trial (n = 78) found pradofloxacin was effective and well-tolerated for feline bacterial UTI.[38] In experimental studies, cats treated with 6 to 10 times the recommended dose did not experience retinal toxicity.[39]

Short-duration antimicrobials

In human medicine, short-duration antimicrobial therapy, commonly, trimethoprim-sulfamethoxazole or fluoroquinolone, has become the standard treatment of acute uncomplicated bacterial cystitis in women.[40] The recommendations are antimicrobial-specific because not all antimicrobials have comparable efficacy when given as only a 3-day treatment. Benefits of shorter therapy include better compliance, lower cost, and decreased adverse effects.[40] The goal of treatment is to decrease the bacterial load enough to control clinical signs with the immune system eliminating remaining organisms.

Two recent prospective, randomized studies evaluated short-duration treatment in dogs with uncomplicated bacterial UTI. The first study compared 3-day high-dose enrofloxacin (n = 35, 20 mg/kg orally every 24 hours) to standard doses of amoxicillin-clavulanic acid (n = 33, 13.75–20 mg/kg orally every 12 hours).[41] Clinical and microbiological cure was evaluated 7 days after antimicrobial discontinuation and short-term, high-dose treatment was not inferior to standard treatment. The second study was double-blinded and compared 3-day trimethoprim-sulfamethoxazole (n = 20, 15 mg/kg orally every 12 hours) plus 7-day placebo to 10 days of cephalexin (n = 18, 20 mg/kg orally every 12 hours).[42] There was no significant difference in the short-term (4-day after treatment) and long-term (30-day after treatment) clinical and microbiological cure rates between treatment groups. Clinical cure at 30 days was 50% to 65% and microbiological cure was 20% to 44%.[42] Additional studies are needed to determine the appropriate treatment duration for uncomplicated bacterial UTI.

Pyelonephritis

Antimicrobial therapy should be initiated while waiting for the culture and sensitivity results. Empirical antimicrobials should have efficacy against gram-negative bacteria, the most common pathogens; fluoroquinolones are a good first choice (see **Table 2**). Acute pyelonephritis requires hospitalization for parenteral antimicrobial therapy and intravenous fluids. Parenteral therapy should be continued until patients will eat and drink normally and azotemia is no longer improving with intensive therapy; infections should then be treated as complicated UTIs, with a minimum of 6 to 8 weeks of antibiotics and regular monitoring for recurrence of infections during and following therapy. Chronic pyelonephritis should be treated as complicated UTIs as well, but patients do not usually require hospitalization at initial diagnosis.

Prostatitis
The blood-prostate barrier is compromised with acute prostatitis and an appropriate antimicrobial should be selected based on culture and sensitivity. Treat as a complicated UTI for a minimum of 4 weeks.[12–14] Antimicrobials must be selected more carefully in cases of chronic prostatitis because the blood-prostate barrier is generally intact (see **Table 2**). Nonionized, basic, lipid-soluble antimicrobials have the best penetration into the prostatic tissue.[12–14] Drugs such as trimethoprim-sulfamethoxazole, chloramphenicol, and enrofloxacin (but not ciprofloxacin) are excellent choices. Examples of drugs with low-lipid solubility and poor diffusion across the blood-prostate barrier include penicillin and cephalothin.[12–14] Antimicrobials are given for a minimum of 6 to 8 weeks. Culture of prostatic fluid should be performed before and after discontinuation of antimicrobials.[12–14]

Castration is recommended as an adjunctive treatment to medical management to help reduce the prostatic size, speed recovery, and decrease recurrence.[12–14] Finasteride, 5α-reductase inhibitor, may be considered in valuable breeding animals or for owners that refuse surgery.[43]

Catheter-associated urinary tract infection
Although it seems logical to administer antimicrobial agents while an indwelling urinary catheter is inserted in an effort to decrease iatrogenic infection, the practice is strongly discouraged. Concomitant oral or parenteral administration of antimicrobial agents during indwelling urethral catheterization does not prevent development of bacterial UTI and promotes infection caused by multidrug-resistant bacteria.[15]

Antifungals
Fluconazole is recommended as initial treatment in most patients because of the high margin of safety, sensitivity of most strains of Candida spp, and excretion of active drug into urine in high concentrations (**Table 4**).[19] Candida spp other than C albicans are more likely to be resistant to fluconazole, and antifungal sensitivity testing is recommended to determine if a higher dose of fluconazole is appropriate or if another drug should be used. Although amphotericin B is renally excreted and achieves high concentration in urine, it is not often used because it is parenterally administered and nephrotoxic. Other commonly used antifungal drugs, including itraconazole and ketoconazole, are not renally excreted in active form.[19]

Secondary fungal UTI occurs because of shedding of organisms into urine in patients with systemic infections. Organisms most commonly associated with urine shedding are Aspergillus spp in dogs (particularly German shepherd dogs) and Cryptococcus spp in cats.[44–47] These patients should be treated with antifungal agents standardly recommended for systemic infections.

Antivirals
Antiviral drugs have not been evaluated for animals with viral-induced urinary tract disease, and management of these patients is limited to supportive care.[20]

Table 4
Treatment of fungal cystitis

For all cases	Identify and correct underlying predisposing factors	• Breaches in local or systemic immunity
If *C albicans*	Fluconazole 5–10 mg/kg PO q 12h for 4–6 wk	• Urine sediment and culture at 2- to 3-wk intervals to confirm resolution • Urine sediment and culture 1 and 2 mo after therapy discontinuation
If non-*C albicans*	Therapy based on culture and sensitivity	• Monitor as above • Consider drug penetration into urine when selecting therapy
If initial treatment fails	Repeat culture and sensitivity	Consider: • Intravesicular infusion 1% clotrimazole or amphotericin B • IV or SQ amphotericin B • Combination fluconazaole at maximum dose plus terbinafine • Benign neglect, regular monitoring for disease progression

Adapted from Pressler BM. Urinary tract infections—fungal. In: Polzin D, Bartges JW, editors. Nephrology and urology of small animals. Ames (IA): Blackwell Publishing; 2011. p. 719–21.

NONPHARMACOLOGIC TREATMENT OPTIONS
Bacterial Interference

Bacterial interference refers to the use of low-virulence, nonpathogenic bacteria to compete with and decrease the risk of colonization and infection with more pathogenic organisms.[48,49] Commonly used bacteria include *E coli* (strains 83972 and HU2117) and *Lactobacillus* sp. Proposed mechanisms of action include competition for nutrients and attachment sites, bacteriocidin (antibiotic-protein) production, biofilm prevention, and host immunomodulation.[48]

This treatment strategy is in its infancy even in human medicine, but preliminary studies are promising, especially in patients with spinal cord injury and neurogenic bladder.[48–50] An experimental protocol for colonizing the canine urinary tract with *E coli* 83972 has been described.[51] Another potential future application is the prevention of catheter-associated UTI.[49]

Probiotics

Alterations of vaginal microflora, in particular lactic acid–producing bacteria (LAB), may play a role in the establishment of UTI.[52] For example, women with recurrent UTI often have depletion of vaginal *Lactobacillus* sp, whereas increased vaginal colonization with *Lactobacillus* sp is associated with reduced numbers of recurrent UTI.[52] In humans, *Lactobacillus* sp are the most common LAB, whereas *Enterococcus canintestini* is the most common species in dogs.[53,54] LAB create an acidic environment that inhibits uropathogen colonization, modulates host immune function, and may downregulate virulence factor expression of pathogenic bacteria.[48]

Probiotics are a form of bacterial interference and recommended as a treatment and prophylaxis strategy in women. Probiotics restore *Lactobacillus* sp vaginal flora and displace potential uropathogens from the vagina.[48] Two studies in dogs have evaluated vaginal microflora before and after probiotic administration and found no significant differences.[53,54] However, more prospective studies are needed to evaluate the role of probiotics for lower urinary tract disease in veterinary species. Probiotics on the market vary by bacterial species, potency (number of colony-forming units), and viability. In addition, the gastrointestinal microbe has immunomodulatory effects throughout the body, and the impact of gastrointestinal probiotics on local urinary tract immune function has not been evaluated.

EVALUATION OF OUTCOME AND LONG-TERM RECOMMENDATIONS
Treatment Duration and Monitoring

Uncomplicated bacterial urinary tract infection
There is no consensus regarding the appropriate duration of treatment (**Table 5**).[23] Uncomplicated UTIs are usually successfully treated with a standard 7- to 14-day course of an appropriate antimicrobial agent.[23] There is some evidence that shorter treatment (ie, 3 days) is not inferior to standard durations of therapy, but more research is needed in this area.[23,41,42] If the proper antimicrobial is chosen and administered at the appropriate dosage and frequency, clinical signs and results of a complete urine analysis should resolve within 48 hours. If possible, a urine culture should be performed 5 to 7 days after cessation of antimicrobial therapy. Uncomplicated infections are rare in cats because of their inherent resistance to bacterial UTIs, and there is typically a predisposing cause.

Complicated bacterial urinary tract infection
Optimal duration of therapy is unknown. Antimicrobials are usually administered for a minimum of 3 to 6 weeks.[24] Urine should be evaluated with culture in the first week of treatment for response to therapy, before discontinuing therapy, 5 to 7 days and 1 month after therapy discontinuation.

Catheter-associated urinary tract infection
It is not necessary to treat bacteriuria associated with an indwelling catheter if there is no clinical or cytologic evidence of infection (**Fig. 6**). For patients that develop a catheter-associated UTI, treatment is more likely to be successful if the catheter can be removed. The infection may be treated as uncomplicated if there is not a history of recurrent infection and no relevant comorbidity. Otherwise, the infection should

Table 5 Treatment duration and monitoring		
	Treatment Duration	**Monitoring Urine Culture**
Uncomplicated bacterial UTI	7–14 d 3 d?	5–7 d after discontinue antimicrobials
Complicated bacterial UTI	Minimum 3–6 wk	• 1 wk into therapy • Before therapy discontinuation • 5–7 d after discontinue antimicrobial • 1 mo, 2 mo after treatment
AB	Treatment not recommended unless high risk for ascending or systemic infection	
Fungal UTI	Minimum 6–8 wk	As above for complicated bacterial UTI

Data from Refs.[19,23,24]

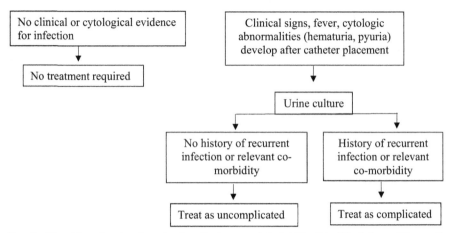

Fig. 6. Algorithm for treatment of catheter-associated UTI. (*Modified from* Weese JS, Blondeau JM, Boothe D, et al. Antimicrobial use guidelines for treatment of urinary tract disease in dogs and cats: antimicrobial guidelines working group of the international society for companion animal infectious diseases. Vet Med Int 2011;2011:1–9.)

be treated as complicated with 4 to 6 weeks of an appropriate antimicrobial based on the culture and sensitivity.[23]

Fungal urinary tract infection
Primary fungal UTIs should always be treated as complicated infections, with a minimum of 6 to 8 weeks of antifungal therapy and regular monitoring during and after cessation of therapy.[19]

Prevention

Catheter-associated urinary tract infection
There are several strategies to decrease the risk of catheter-associated UTI (**Box 3**).

Box 3
Strategies to prevent catheter-associated urinary tract infection

- Avoid indiscriminate use of urinary catheters. Carefully assess the need for placing and retaining catheter
- Always use hand hygiene
- Use a closed collection system for indwelling catheters
- Sterile catheter placement
- Minimize duration of catheterization
- Avoid indiscriminate antimicrobial use
- Try to avoid an indwelling urinary catheter in immunocompromised patients
- Be cautious with indwelling catheter use in patients undergoing diuresis

Adapted from Siddiq DM, Darouiche RO. New strategies to prevent catheter-associated urinary tract infections. Nat Rev Urol 2012;9:305–14; with permission.

Prophylactic antimicrobial therapy for recurrent infection There are no good studies evaluating pulse (intermittent) or chronic low-dose prophylactic antimicrobial therapy in animals with frequent reinfections, but anecdotally, some animals may benefit (**Box 3**). Careful patient selection is required and the impact of promoting antimicrobial resistance should be considered. Before prophylactic treatment is undertaken, urine culture and susceptibility testing should be done to ensure that the bacterial UTI has been eradicated. For long-term prophylaxis, a drug that is excreted in high concentration in urine and unlikely to cause adverse effects is selected. Often a fluoroquinolone, cephalosporin, or a β-lactam antimicrobial is chosen. The antimicrobial agent is administered at approximately one-third of the therapeutic daily dose immediately after the patient has voided, at a time when the drug and its metabolites will be retained in the urinary tract for 6 to 8 hours (typically at night). The drug is given for a minimum of 6 months. Urine samples, preferably collected by cystocentesis (not by catheterization because this may induce bacterial UTI), are collected every 4 to 8 weeks for urinalysis and quantitative urine culture. If the sample is free of infection, then prophylactic treatment is continued. If bacterial UTI is identified, active (breakthrough) infection is treated as a complicated bacterial UTI before returning to a prophylactic strategy. If a breakthrough bacterial UTI does not occur after 6 months of prophylactic antimicrobial therapy, then treatment may be discontinued and the patient should be monitored for reinfection.

Ancillary therapies

D-Mannose D-Mannose is used to prevent recurrent UTI, but there are no studies of clinical efficacy in veterinary patients. The D-mannose sugar competitively binds to mannose-fimbriae on certain E coli strains, thereby inhibiting adhesion to the uroepithelium.[55] There are little data available for other bacteria that may express mannose fimbriae. An extrapolated anecdotal dose for dogs is one-quarter teaspoon per 20 pounds 3 times daily.

Methenamine Methenamine salt is a urinary antiseptic that is converted to bacteriostatic formaldehyde in an acidic environment (urine pH <5.5). There is controversy in human medicine as to whether methenamine prevents UTI, although there is some evidence that it may be effective for short-term prophylaxis.[56] It is unknown if the 2 salts described in the literature, hippurate and mandelate, are equally effective; the mandelate salt is difficult to find.[56] There is limited veterinary literature on the use of methenamine in small animals, although there is a theoretic benefit.[23,34] Studies of safety, efficacy, and appropriate dosing are lacking. Commonly recommended doses are 10 to 20 mg/kg orally every 12 hours (dog) and 250 mg per cat orally every 12 hours.[57] Gastrointestinal upset and dysuria are the most commonly reported adverse events; methenamine is poorly tolerated by feline patients. Methenamine should not be used in cases of renal failure.[57] Concurrent use of a urinary acidifier, such as DL-methionine, is usually required for maximal effect.

Cranberry Proanthocyanidin, the "active ingredient" in cranberry, alters the genotypic or phenotypic expression of fimbriae, which subsequently inhibits E coli adherence to human bladder and vaginal epithelial cells.[58] Studies in humans reveal inconsistent efficacy for prevention of UTI. However, in meta-analysis (n = 1049), humans supplemented with cranberry products had less UTI over a 12-month period compared with placebo.[59]

There are few veterinary studies in healthy dogs and no feline studies.[60,61] In addition, quality and potency are variable among over-the-counter products; ideally each formulation would be tested in the species of interest. The Consensus of the Antimicrobial Guidelines Working Group of the International Society for Companion Animal Infectious Diseases is that there is insufficient evidence to support use of cranberry extract to prevent recurrent UTIs in dogs and cats.[23]

Local therapy Local infusions with antimicrobials, antiseptics, and dimethyl sulfoxide can be irritating and are not retained within the urinary bladder.[23] Anecdotally, instillation of dilute chlorhexidine (1:100, 0.02%) and/or ethylenediaminetetraacetic acid (EDTA)-tromethamine (EDTA-Tris)[62] via cystotomy tube may decrease the incidence of bacterial UTI (Bartges JW, personal communication, Knoxville, TN, 2014). In a small human study, bladder irrigation with dilute 0.02% chlorhexidine significantly decreased postoperative bacteriuria, although it did not eliminate pre-existing infection and did not appear to damage the bladder mucosa.[63] It has been postulated that EDTA-Tris has synergistic effects with systemic antimicrobials[64] as well as local chlorhexidine irrigation.[63] Proposed mechanisms included divalent ion binding causing alteration of bacterial DNA synthesis, cell wall permeability, and ribosomal stability. In additional, in vitro studies suggest that the presence of EDTA-Tris reduces the minimum inhibitory concentration for various antimicrobial drugs.[64] In a small study (n =17 dogs, n = 4 with chronic cystitis) daily local infusion via sterile urinary catheter (25 mL EDTA at 37°C) for 7 days was well tolerated and dogs had negative urine cultures up to 180 days after treatment.[64] Additional studies are needed to determine the short- and long-term effects of EDTA-Tris therapy.

TREATMENT RESISTANCE/COMPLICATIONS
Treatment Resistance

Bacterial resistance
The emergence of multidrug-resistant bacteria is concerning and has important implications for both the patient and public health. There are trends toward increasing resistance in both fecal and environmental reservoirs.[65] In addition to acquiring resistance genes via plasmids, there are other bacterial strategies for persistence within the urinary tract. For example, uropathogenic *E coli* can invade and persist within the superficial bladder wall epithelial cells.[65] These bacteria may remain dormant for a period of time followed by recrudescence.

Biofilms Some bacteria have the capacity for biofilm formation, which facilitates colonization.[66–68] A biofilm is composed of organisms adhered together by a self-produced polysaccharide matrix.[66] It has been suggested that the bacteria within the biofilm become sessile; they are protected from the immune system, are antimicrobial, and inherently are resistant to shear forces of removal.[66] In humans, bacteria with the capacity to produce biofilms have been associated with AB.[65,66] Biofilms are also implemented in the development of catheter-associated UTI.[69]

Strategies to prevent catheter-associated biofilms include using (1) materials that are less amendable to biofilm formation and (2) coatings or surface modifications that decrease biofilm formation. For example, silicone catheters are preferred over latex because scanning electron microscope imaging reveals that latex surfaces are more irregular and promote microbial adherence.[49] An example of an agent used for catheter coating is the antiseptic chlorhexidine. In a veterinary prospective study (n = 26 dogs) evaluating biofilm formation on indwelling urinary catheters, sustained-release varnish of chlorihexidine-coated urinary catheters statistically decreased biofilm formation.[69] There are an array of other catheter coatings and modifications to decrease bacterial adherence and biofilm formation that have primarily been studied in a research setting, including silver coating, nanoparticles, iontophoresis, antimicrobials, urease and other enzyme inhibitors, liposomes, and bacteriophages. Other novel strategies include quorum sensing inhibitors and vibroacoustic stimulation (**Box 4**). A detailed discussion of comparison is beyond the scope of this article and the reader is referred elsewhere.[49]

Some oral antimicrobials, in particular combination therapy with clarithromycin, have shown promise in vitro for antibiofilm activity. For example, *Pseudomonas aeruginosa* biofilm was eliminated by a synergistic combination of clarithromycin and ciprofloxacin.[70] Likewise, combination therapy of clarithromycin with fosfomycin was more effective than either treatment alone to reduce *Staphylococcus pseudintermedius* biofilm.[71] In vivo studies are needed to further evaluate the efficacy of these therapies.

Fungal resistance

Infections that fail to respond completely to fluconazole should be recultured and antifungal sensitivity testing performed (see **Table 4**). Some susceptible isolates may

Box 4 Strategies to prevent biofilm formation		
Strategy	**Definition**	**Mechanism of Action**
Silver coating		Bactericidal activity of silver ion by inhibiting enzymatic pathways and disrupting the cell wall
Nanoparticles	Nanometer-sized particles that attach to and penetrate bacterial cells	Disrupt cell membranes via lipid peroxidation and interacting with DNA
Iontophoresis	Application of an electrical field with low intensity direct current	Bioelectric effect—enhance antimicrobial efficacy against bacteria within biofilms
Urease and other enzyme inhibitors	Eg, acetohydroxamic acid, fluorofamide, N-acetyl-D-glucosamine-1-phosphate acetyltransferase inhibitors	In vitro, reduce encrustation and alter biofilm integrity
Liposomes	Act as carriers for hydrophobic and hydrophilic drugs	Increase drug half-life, decrease adverse effects, protect drug from environment
Bacteriophages	A virus that selectively infects bacteria	Bacteriophage rapidly divides within bacteria and lyses. Bacteria can develop resistance
Quorum sensing inhibitors	Quorum sensing describes a system of molecular signaling (ie, autoinducers) that controls population density and gene expression. Necessary for bacteria to develop the biofilm phenotype	Eg, *Delisea pulchra* algae produces a molecule that inhibits autoinducer signaling
Vibroacoustic stimulation	Low acoustic waves form a vibrating coat along the catheter surface	Inhibit bacterial adhesion and quorum-sensing electrical gradients

Adapted from Siddiq DM, Darouiche RO. New strategies to prevent catheter-associated urinary tract infections. Nat Rev Urol 2012;9:305–14; with permission.

respond to intravesicular administration of 1% clotrimazole or amphotericin B.[19,72,73] Urinary alkalinization has also been historically proposed as adjunctive therapy in patients with fungal UTI, because increased urine pH may inhibit fungal growth. However, this is not currently favored for treatment of fungal UTI in humans and is of questionable efficacy in veterinary patients.[19]

Complications

Magnesium ammonium phosphate (struvite) urolithiasis

Staphylococcus spp and *Proteus* spp, and more rarely *Corynebacterium* spp, *Klebsiella* spp, and *Ureaplasma* spp, may produce urease (**Box 5**). This enzyme hydrolyzes urea to ammonia, which buffers urine hydrogen ions, forming ammonium ions, increasing urine pH, and increasing dissolved ionic phosphate. In the presence of magnesium, magnesium ammonium phosphate (struvite) may precipitate around a nidus to form uroliths (**Fig. 7**). Bacteria are incorporated into the urolith matrix, and thus, should be considered complicated UTIs because of poor antimicrobial penetration. Greater than 90% of struvite uroliths in dogs are induced by urease-producing bacteria, whereas struvite uroliths in cats are commonly sterile (ie, not associated with bacterial UTI). Struvite uroliths can be dissolved through a combination of dietary therapy and appropriate antimicrobial therapy; following dissolution or removal, preventing urolith recurrence requires preventing reinfection. For dogs that are uncomfortably symptomatic from urocystolithiasis and/or fail medical management, minimally invasive procedures, such as laser lithotripsy, laparoscopic-assisted cystotomy, or cystotomy, may be considered.

Polypoid cystitis

Chronic bacterial infections may induce microscopic or macroscopic bladder mucosal proliferation and intramural accumulation of inflammatory cells. Polypoid cystitis occurs when epithelial proliferation is severe, resulting in masslike lesions or diffuse thickening of the bladder wall (**Fig. 8**).[74,75] Gross differentiation of polypoid cystitis from bladder wall neoplasms is not reliable; however, polypoid cystitis is more likely to develop in the bladder apex (vs transitional cell carcinomas, which are more commonly found in the bladder trigone), is more commonly botryoid in appearance rather than fimbriated, and is not as grossly vascular as transitional cell carcinomas. *Proteus* spp may be more commonly associated with development of these lesions.[74,75] Polypoid cystitis lesions are niduses of deep-seated bacterial infection and should be treated as complicated UTIs. In some cases long-term antimicrobial

---

Box 5
Complications of urinary tract infection

Potential complications of UTI

- Resistant infection
- Polypoid cystitis
- Emphysematous cystitis
- Magnesium ammonium phosphate (struvite) urolithiasis
- Pyelonephritis
- Prostatitis
- Prostatic abscess

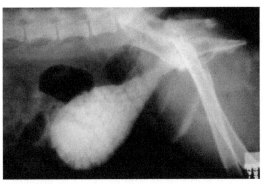

Fig. 7. Lateral survey abdominal radiograph of infection-induced struvite urocysto-urethroliths in a 3-year-old spayed female Irish setter.

therapy may result in successful resolution of lesions. However, partial cystectomy results in more rapid resolution of clinical signs, is likely associated with improved rates for long-term resolution of infection, and allows shorter antimicrobial treatment courses.[75]

Emphysematous cystitis

Emphysematous cystitis refers to accumulation of air within the bladder wall and lumen secondary to infection with glucose-fermenting bacteria. Most cases are due to *E coli* infection, but *Proteus* spp, *Clostridum* spp, and *Aerobacter aerogenes* have also been reported.[76,77] Emphysematous cystitis most commonly develops in dogs and cats with diabetes mellitus because of the high concentration of fermentable substrate.[77] Treatment of emphysematous cystitis should be as described for complicated UTI; if glucosuria is present, then appropriate treatment should be initiated for the underlying cause.

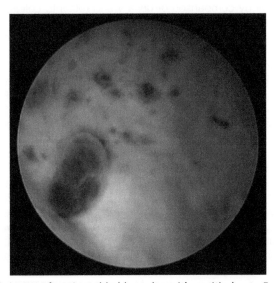

Fig. 8. Cystoscopic image of a urinary bladder polyp with cystitis due to *E coli* in a 6-year-old spayed female Irish setter.

Pyelonephritis

Although no systematic reviews of pyelonephritis in dogs or cats have been performed, animals with systemically compromised immunity (ie, hyperadrenocorticism, diabetes mellitus), dogs or cats with CKD, and patients with any cause of vesicoureteral reflux are likely predisposed to development of pyelonephritis. Chronic pyelonephritis is likely underdiagnosed as a cause of renal failure in dogs and cats and should be especially considered in patients with previously stable CKD that have unexpected worsening of azotemia (ie, "acute-on-chronic" renal failure).

Prostatic abscessation

Prostatic abscessation is a sequela to prostatitis and is characterized by purulent fluid accumulations within the prostatic tissue. Clinical signs are variable and dependent on the size and extent of the abscess as well as systemic involvement. Prostatic abscesses are generally easily identified with ultrasonography and the goal of therapy is to provide drainage either through ultrasound-guided percutaneous drainage or surgery. Surgical options include partial prostatectomy and prostate omentalization.[14]

SUMMARY

- Determining whether an infection is uncomplicated or complicated is essential to guide the diagnostic and therapeutic plan.
- Recurrent infections are complicated infections and may be relapsing, refractory/persistent, reinfection, or superinfection.
- Antimicrobials are the cornerstone of treatment of bacterial UTI and, ideally, selected based on culture and sensitivity.
- There is limited literature to support preventative therapies; identification and resolution of underlying causes are essential.

REFERENCES

1. Johnson JR, Kaster N, Kuskowski MA, et al. Identification of urovirulence traits in Escherichia coli by comparison of urinary and rectal E. coli isolates from dogs with urinary tract infection. J Clin Microbiol 2003;41:337–45.
2. Osborne C, Caywood D, Johnston G, et al. Perineal urethrostomy versus dietary management in prevention of recurrent lower urinary tract disease. J Small Anim Pract 1991;32:296–305.
3. Ling GV, Norris CR, Franti CE, et al. Interrelations of organism prevalence, specimen collection method, and host age, sex, and breed among 8,354 canine urinary tract infections (1969–1995). J Vet Intern Med 2001;15:341–7.
4. Bartges D, Blanco L. Bacterial urinary tract infections in cats. Compend Std Care 2001;3:1–5.
5. Davidson A, Ling G, Stevens F, et al. Urinary tract infection in cats: a retrospective study 1977–1989. Calif Vet 1992;46:32–4.
6. Barsanti J. Genitourinary infections. In: Greene CE, editor. Infectious diseases of the dog and cat. 4th edition. St Louis (MO): Elsevier Saunders; 2012. p. 1013–31.
7. Litster A, Moss SM, Honnery M, et al. Prevalence of bacterial species in cats with clinical signs of lower urinary tract disease: recognition of Staphylococcus felis as a possible feline urinary tract pathogen. Vet Microbiol 2007;121:182–8.
8. Litster A, Thompson M, Moss S, et al. Feline bacterial urinary tract infections: an update on an evolving clinical problem. Vet J 2011;187:18–22.
9. Jang S, Ling G, Yamamoto R, et al. Mycoplasma as a cause of canine urinary tract infection. J Am Vet Med Assoc 1984;185:45–7.

10. Ülgen M, Cetin C, ŞEntürk S, et al. Urinary tract infections due to Mycoplasma canis in dogs. J Vet Med A Physiol Pathol Clin Med 2006;53:379–82.
11. Abou N, van Dongen A, Houwers D. PCR-based detection reveals no causative role for Mycoplasma and Ureaplasma in feline lower urinary tract disease. Vet Microbiol 2006;116:246–7.
12. Kustritz MR. Prostatic disease. In: Polzin D, Bartges JW, editors. Nephrology and urology of small animals. 1st edition. Ames (IA): Blackwell Publishing; 2011. p. 787–96.
13. Feldman EC, Nelson RW. Prostatitis. In: Kersey R, LeMelledo D, editors. Canine and feline endocrinology and reproduction. St Louis (MO): Elsevier Publishing; 2004. p. 977–86.
14. Smith J. Canine prostatic disease: a review of anatomy, pathology, diagnosis, and treatment. Theriogenology 2008;70:375–83.
15. Barsanti J, Blue J, Edmunds J. Urinary tract infection due to indwelling bladder catheters in dogs and cats. J Am Vet Med Assoc 1985;187:384–8.
16. Hugonnard M, Chalvet-Monfray K, Dernis J, et al. Occurrence of bacteriuria in 18 catheterised cats with obstructive lower urinary tract disease: a pilot study. J Feline Med Surg 2013;10:843–8.
17. Jin Y, Lin D. Fungal urinary tract infections in the dog and cat: a retrospective study (2001–2004). J Am Anim Hosp Assoc 2005;41:373–81.
18. Pressler BM, Vaden SL, Lane IF, et al. Candida spp. urinary tract infections in 13 dogs and seven cats: predisposing factors, treatment, and outcome. J Am Anim Hosp Assoc 2003;39:263–70.
19. Pressler BM. Urinary tract infections—fungal. In: Polzin D, Bartges JW, editors. Nephrology and urology of small animals. Ames (IA): Blackwell Publishing; 2011. p. 717–24.
20. Kruger JM, Osborne CA, Wise AG, et al. Viruses and urinary tract disease. In: Polzin D, Bartges JW, editors. Nephrology and urology of small animals. Chichester (United Kingdom): Blackwell Publishing Ltd; 2011. p. 725–33.
21. Bartges JW. Diagnosis of urinary tract infections. Vet Clin North Am Small Anim Pract 2004;34:923–33.
22. Swenson CL, Boisvert AM, Kruger JM, et al. Evaluation of modified Wright-staining of urine sediment as a method for accurate detection of bacteriuria in dogs. J Am Vet Med Assoc 2004;224:1282–9.
23. Weese JS, Blondeau JM, Boothe D, et al. Antimicrobial use guidelines for treatment of urinary tract disease in dogs and cats: antimicrobial guidelines working group of the international society for companion animal infectious diseases. Vet Med Int 2011;2011:263768. Available at: http://www.hindawi.com/journals/vmi/2011/263768/.
24. Barsanti J. Multidrug-resistant urinary tract infection. In: Bonagura JD, Twedt DC, editors. Current veterinary therapy XIV. St Louis (MO): WB Saunders; 2009. p. 921–5.
25. Nicolle LE. Asymptomatic bacteriuria: review and discussion of the IDSA guidelines. Int J Antimicrob Agents 2006;28:42–8.
26. McGhie J, Stayt J, Hosgood G. Prevalence of bacteriuria in dogs without clinical signs of urinary tract infection presenting for elective surgical procedures. Aust Vet J 2014;92:33–7.
27. Wan SY, Hartmann FA, Jooss MK, et al. Prevalence and clinical outcome of sub-clinical bacteriuria in female dogs. J Am Vet Med Assoc 2014;245:106–12.
28. Eggertsdóttir AV, Sævik BK, Halvorsen I, et al. Occurrence of occult bacteriuria in healthy cats. J Feline Med Surg 2011;13:800–3.
29. Litster A, Moss S, Platell J, et al. Occult bacterial lower urinary tract infections in cats—urinalysis and culture findings. Vet Microbiol 2009;136:130–4.

30. Mayer-Roenne B, Goldstein RE, Erb HN. Urinary tract infections in cats with hyperthyroidism, diabetes mellitus and chronic kidney disease. J Feline Med Surg 2007;9:124–32.
31. White JD, Stevenson M, Malik R, et al. Urinary tract infections in cats with chronic kidney disease. J Feline Med Surg 2013;15(6):459–65.
32. McGuire NC, Schulman R, Ridgway MD, et al. Detection of occult urinary tract infections in dogs with diabetes mellitus. J Am Anim Hosp Assoc 2002; 38:541–4.
33. Koutinas A, Heliadis N, Saridomichelakis M, et al. Asymptomatic bacteriuria in puppies with canine parvovirus infection: a cohort study. Vet Microbiol 1998;63: 109–16.
34. Seguin MA, Vaden SL, Altier C, et al. Persistent urinary tract infections and reinfections in 100 dogs (1989–1999). J Vet Intern Med 2003;17:622–31.
35. Boothe D, Smaha T, Carpenter DM, et al. Antimicrobial resistance and pharmacodynamics of canine and feline pathogenic E. coli in the United States. J Am Anim Hosp Assoc 2012;48:379–89.
36. Liu X, Boothe DM, Jin Y, et al. In vitro potency and efficacy favor later generation fluoroquinolones for treatment of canine and feline Escherichia coli uropathogens in the United States. World J Microbiol Biotechnol 2013;29:347–54.
37. Lees P. Pharmacokinetics, pharmacodynamics and therapeutics of pradofloxacin in the dog and cat. J Vet Pharmacol Ther 2013;36:209–21.
38. Litster A, Moss S, Honnery M, et al. Clinical efficacy and palatability of pradofloxacin 2.5% oral suspension for the treatment of bacterial lower urinary tract infections in cats. J Vet Intern Med 2007;21:990–5.
39. Messias A, Gekeler F, Wegener A, et al. Retinal safety of a new fluoroquinolone, pradofloxacin, in cats: assessment with electroretinography. Doc Ophthalmol 2008;116:177–91.
40. Nicolle LE. Short-term therapy for urinary tract infection: success and failure. Int J Antimicrob Agents 2008;31:40–5.
41. Westropp J, Sykes J, Irom S, et al. Evaluation of the efficacy and safety of high dose short duration enrofloxacin treatment regimen for uncomplicated urinary tract infections in dogs. J Vet Intern Med 2012;26:506–12.
42. Clare S, Hartmann F, Jooss M, et al. Short-and long-term cure rates of short-duration trimethoprim-sulfamethoxazole treatment in female dogs with uncomplicated bacterial cystitis. J Vet Intern Med 2014;28:818–26.
43. Niżański W, Levy X, Ochota M, et al. Pharmacological treatment for common prostatic conditions in dogs–benign prostatic hyperplasia and prostatitis: an update. Reprod Domest Anim 2014;49:8–15.
44. Gerds-Grogan S, Dayrell-Hart B. Feline cryptococcosis: a retrospective evaluation. J Am Anim Hosp Assoc 1997;33:118–22.
45. Kabay M, Robinson W, Huxtable C, et al. The pathology of disseminated Aspergillus terreus infection in dogs. Vet Pathol 1985;22:540–7.
46. Kahler J, Leach M, Jang S, et al. Disseminated aspergillosis attributable to Aspergillus deflectus in a springer spaniel. J Am Vet Med Assoc 1990;197: 871–4.
47. Jang S, Dorr T, Biberstein E, et al. Aspergillus deflectus infection in four dogs. Med Mycol 1986;24:95–104.
48. Darouiche RO, Hull RA. Bacterial interference for prevention of urinary tract infection. Clin Infect Dis 2012;55(10):1400–7.
49. Siddiq DM, Darouiche RO. New strategies to prevent catheter-associated urinary tract infections. Nat Rev Urol 2012;9:305–14.

50. Darouiche RO, Green BG, Donovan WH, et al. Multicenter randomized controlled trial of bacterial interference for prevention of urinary tract infection in patients with neurogenic bladder. Urology 2011;78:341–6.
51. Thompson MF, Schembri MA, Mills PC, et al. A modified three-dose protocol for colonization of the canine urinary tract with the asymptomatic bacteriuria Escherichia coli strain 83972. Vet Microbiol 2012;158:446–50.
52. Petricevic L, Unger FM, Viernstein H, et al. Randomized, double-blind, placebo-controlled study of oral lactobacilli to improve the vaginal flora of postmenopausal women. Eur J Obstet Gynecol Reprod Biol 2008;141:54–7.
53. Hutchins R, Vaden S, Jacob M, et al. Vaginal microbiota of spayed dogs with or without recurrent urinary tract infections. J Vet Intern Med 2014;28:300–4.
54. Hutchins R, Bailey C, Jacob M, et al. The effect of an oral probiotic containing lactobacillus, bifidobacterium, and bacillus species on the vaginal microbiota of spayed female dogs. J Vet Intern Med 2013;27:1368–71.
55. Kranjčec B, Papeš D, Altarac S. D-mannose powder for prophylaxis of recurrent urinary tract infections in women: a randomized clinical trial. World J Urol 2014; 32:79–84.
56. Lee B, Simpson JM, Craig JC, et al. Methenamine hippurate for preventing urinary tract infections. Cochrane Database Syst Rev 2007;(4):CD003265.
57. Plumb DC. Plumb's veterinary drug handbook. Ames (IA): Blackwell Publishing; 2005.
58. Gupta K, Chou M, Howell A, et al. Cranberry products inhibit adherence of p-fimbriated Escherichia coli to primary cultured bladder and vaginal epithelial cells. J Urol 2007;177:2357–60.
59. Wang CH, Fang CC, Chen NC, et al. Cranberry-containing products for prevention of urinary tract infections in susceptible populations: a systematic review and meta-analysis of randomized controlled trials. Arch Intern Med 2012;172: 988–96.
60. Howell AB, Griffin DW, Whalen MO. Inhibition of p-fimbriated Escherichia coli adhesion in an innovational ex-vivo model in dogs receiving a bioactive cranberry tablet (Crananidin TM). In: Programs and abstracts of the Am College Vet Intern Med. Anaheim (CA): 2010. p. 660.
61. Smee N, Grauer GF, Schermerhorn T. Investigations into the effect of cranberry extract on bacterial adhesion to canine uroepithelial cells. In: Programs and abstracts of the Am College Vet Intern Med. Denver (CO): 2011. p. 722–3.
62. King J, Stickler D. The effect of repeated instillations of antiseptics on catheter-associated urinary tract infections: a study in a physical model of the catheterized bladder. Urol Res 1992;20:403–7.
63. Ball A, Carr T, Gillespie W, et al. Bladder irrigation with chlorhexidine for the prevention of urinary infection after transurethral operations: a prospective controlled study. J Urol 1987;138:491–4.
64. Farca A, Piromalli G, Maffei F, et al. Potentiating effect of EDTA-Tris on the activity of antibiotics against resistant bacteria associated with otitis, dermatitis and cystitis. J Small Anim Pract 1997;38:243–5.
65. Thompson MF, Litster AL, Platell JL, et al. Canine bacterial urinary tract infections: new developments in old pathogens. Vet J 2011;190:22–7.
66. DiCicco M, Neethirajan S, Singh A, et al. Efficacy of clarithromycin on biofilm formation of methicillin-resistant Staphylococcus pseudintermedius. BMC Vet Res 2012;8:225.
67. Nam EH, Chae JS. Characterization and zoonotic potential of uropathogenic Escherichia coli isolated from dogs. J Microbiol Biotechnol 2013;23:422–9.

68. Hancock V, Ferrieres L, Klemm P. Biofilm formation by asymptomatic and virulent urinary tract infectious Escherichia coli strains. FEMS Microbiol Lett 2007;267: 30–7.

69. Segev G, Bankirer T, Steinberg D, et al. Evaluation of urinary catheters coated with sustained-release varnish of chlorhexidine in mitigating biofilm formation on urinary catheters in dogs. J Vet Intern Med 2013;27:39–46.

70. Elkhatib W, Noreddin A. Efficacy of ciprofloxacin-clarithromycin combination against drug-resistant pseudomonas aeruginosa mature biofilm using in vitro experimental model. Microb Drug Resist 2014;20(6):575–82.

71. DiCicco M, Neethirajan S, Weese JS, et al. In vitro synergism of fosfomycin and clarithromycin antimicrobials against methicillin-resistant Staphylococcus pseudintermedius. BMC Microbiol 2014;14:129.

72. Forward ZA, Legendre AM, Khalsa HD. Use of intermittent bladder infusion with clotrimazole for treatment of candiduria in a dog. J Am Vet Med Assoc 2002;220: 1496–8.

73. Toll J, Ashe CM, Trepanier LA. Intravesicular administration of clotrimazole for treatment of candiduria in a cat with diabetes mellitus. J Am Vet Med Assoc 2003;223:1156–8.

74. Johnston S, Osborne C, Stevens J. Canine polypoid cystitis. J Am Vet Med Assoc 1975;166:1155–60.

75. Martinez I, Mattoon JS, Eaton KA, et al. Polypoid cystitis in 17 dogs (1978–2001). J Vet Intern Med 2003;17:499–509.

76. Petite A, Busoni V, Heinen MP, et al. Radiographic and ultrasonographic findings of emphysematous cystitis in four nondiabetic female dogs. Vet Radiol Ultrasound 2006;47:90–3.

77. Root C, Scott R. Emphysematous cystitis and other radiographic manifestations of diabetes mellitus in dogs and cats. J Am Vet Med Assoc 1971;158:721.

Urolithiasis

Joseph W. Bartges, DVM, PhD*, Amanda J. Callens, BS, LVT

KEYWORDS

- Lower urinary tract • Urolithiasis • Urinary calculi • Struvite • Calcium oxalate
- Purine • Cystine

KEY POINTS

- Urolithiasis occurs commonly in dogs and cats, and most uroliths occur in the lower urinary tract.
- More than 80% to 90% of lower urinary tract uroliths are struvite or calcium oxalate.
- Some uroliths, such as struvite, cysteine, and urate, are amenable to medical dissolution, whereas others, such as calcium oxalate, are not.

INTRODUCTION

Formation of uroliths is not a disease but rather a complication of several disorders. Some disorders can be identified and corrected (such as infection-induced struvite urolith formation), some can be identified but not corrected (such as hyperuricosuria, which occurs in Dalmatians that excrete high levels of uric acid, which forms ammonium urate uroliths), whereas for others the underlying etiopathogenesis is not known (such as calcium oxalate urolith formation in miniature schnauzers). A common denominator of these disorders is that they can from time to time create oversaturation of urine with 1 or more crystal precursors, resulting in formation of crystals. To develop rational and effective approaches to treatment, abnormalities that promote urolith formation must be identified, with the goal of eliminating or modifying them. It is important, therefore, to understand several basic concepts associated with urolithiasis and the factors that promote urolith formation that may be modified with medical treatment, including the state of urinary saturation, modifiers of crystal formation, presence of multiple crystal types, and presence of bacterial infection, urinary obstruction, or foreign compounds.[1] Urolith formation, dissolution, and prevention involve complex physical processes. Major factors include (1) supersaturation resulting in crystal formation, (2) effects of inhibitors of crystallization and inhibitors of crystal aggregation and growth, (3) crystalloid complexors, (4) effects of promoters of crystal aggregation and growth, and (5) effects of noncrystalline matrix.[1]

The authors have nothing to disclose.
Cornell University Veterinary Specialists, 880 Canal Street, Stamford, CT 06902, USA
* Corresponding author.
E-mail address: jbartges@cuvs.org

DIAGNOSIS OF UROLITHS

Imaging is the most definitive diagnostic tool for detection of uroliths. Abdominal radiography is generally the first diagnostic imaging modality used to detect radiopaque uroliths (**Fig. 1**). Ultrasonography (**Fig. 2**) or double contrast cystography (**Fig. 3**) can be used to detect uroliths, including those that are radiolucent.[2] These abdominal imaging techniques are used to verify the presence of uroliths and location, number, size, shape, and density.

In patients with suspected urinary tract disorders, urinalysis is an important part of diagnostic evaluation. Crystalluria can be an important finding (**Fig. 4**). Crystals do not confirm the presence of uroliths, but they do suggest crystalline oversaturation, and some patients may have active urocystoliths present but not have crystalluria.[3] Temperature change caused by elapsed time between urine collection and urinalysis can cause crystals to form in urine, resulting in a false-positive crystalluria.[4] Therefore, in patients with suspected urolithiasis, freshly collected urine should be evaluated.[5]

Urine specific gravity and urine pH can help assess the chemical environment of urine. The chemical environment of the urine determines urolith formation and can suggest which type of urolith is present. A high urine specific gravity suggests an increase in concentration of urolithic precursors.[6] Calcium oxalate, purines, and cystine uroliths form typically in urine with a pH less than 7.0, whereas struvite calculi form typically in urine with a pH greater than 7.0.[5]

Urine culture and sensitivity testing are indicated because urinary tract infections may occur secondarily in patients with urolithiasis or may induce urolith formation in

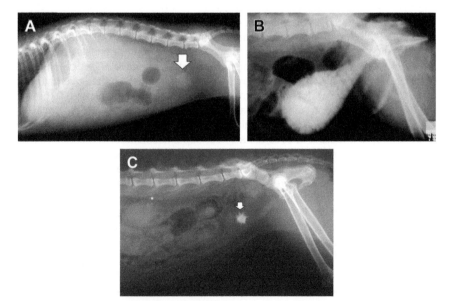

Fig. 1. Radiographic appearance of struvite and calcium oxalate uroliths by abdominal radiography. (*A*) Lateral abdominal radiograph of a 4-year-old castrated male domestic shorthaired cat showing a single round radiopaque sterile struvite urocystolith (*arrow*). (*B*) Lateral abdominal radiograph of a 3-year-old spayed female Irish setter with numerous variably sized and shaped infection-induced struvite urocystoliths. (*C*) Lateral abdominal radiograph of an 8-year-old castrated male domestic shorthaired cat showing 1 calcium oxalate dehydrate urocystolith (*arrow*). Renal mineralization is also present (*asterisk*).

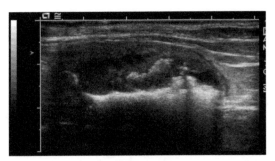

Fig. 2. Images from a 14 year-old, castrated male domestic shorthaired cat with urolithiasis. Urocystoliths appear as shadowing hyperechoic objects on ultrasonographic image of the urinary bladder.

the case of infection-induced struvite uroliths.[7–9] Factors contributing to this situation include mucosal damage induced by the stones, incomplete urine voiding, or microorganism entrapment in the stone.

When uroliths are found, it is important to obtain a blood biochemical profile. Blood biochemical results can sometimes suggest presence of underlying diseases such as hypercalcemia that can predispose patients to urolith formation.[10–13] Because uroliths occasionally cause obstruction, electrolyte, mineral, creatinine, and blood urea nitrogen concentrations should be monitored. Urate calculi may be caused by underlying liver disease, particularly congenital vascular anomalies; therefore, hepatic function should be determined in patients with suspected or confirmed urate uroliths.[14,15]

DESCRIPTION OF UROLITHS

Determining the composition of uroliths is essential to prevent recurrence. Although many types of uroliths have a characteristic appearance, guessing composition by appearance is unreliable and subject to error.[16] All removed or voided uroliths should be analyzed to determine mineral composition, which aids in developing a successful treatment and prevention plan. Analysis results report the chemical makeup of the different components of the urolith. In cases of recurrence, uroliths should be resubmitted, because mineral composition can change from 1 episode to another.[16]

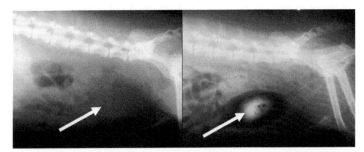

Fig. 3. Survey abdominal radiograph (*left*) and double contrast cystogram (*right*) of a 2 year-old castrated male Pomeranian with radiolucent urate urocystoliths secondary to a portosystemic shunt. The arrows point to the urinary bladder (*left*) and filling defects (urocystoliths, *right*).

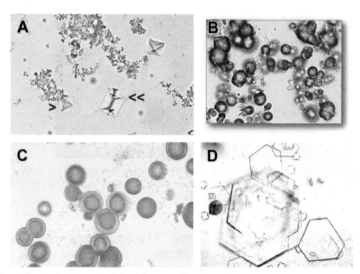

Fig. 4. Crystalluria. (*A*) Struvite (*double arrowhead*) and calcium oxalate (*single arrowhead*) crystals in a urine sample collected from a 6-year-old castrated male domestic shorthaired cat. (*B*) Ammonium urate crystals in a urine sample collected from a 1.5-year-old castrated male English bulldog. (*C*) Xanthine crystals in a urine sample collected from a 3-year-old spayed female beagle administered allopurinol. (*D*) Cystine crystals in a urine sample collected from a 2-year-old male English bulldog.

A urolith is composed primarily of 1 or more minerals in combination with small quantities of organic matrix. The composition of uroliths may be mixed, with uneven mixtures of minerals throughout the stone or minerals deposited in layers. The different layers of stone are the nidus, stone, shell, and surface crystals. The nidus is the area of obvious initiation of stone growth. The stone refers to the major portion of the urolith. The shell is the material that surrounds the body of the stone and the surface crystals are an incomplete coating of the outer surface of the stone.[7] A urolith may be defined by a single mineral type, as mixed if the composition consists of more than 1 mineral type, or as a compound stone if there are mineral layers.

MANAGEMENT OF UROCYSTOLITHS

Uroliths may result in clinical signs of lower urinary tract disease, including urethral obstruction. Often, urethral obstruction is associated with azotemia, hyperkalemia, metabolic acidosis, and dehydration.[17] Treatment of urethral obstruction involves relieving the obstruction and correcting the metabolic imbalances as quickly as possible. If urethral obstructions are recurrent, perineal urethrostomy in male cats and scrotal urethrostomy in male dogs may be considered; however, these procedures are associated with increased risk of lower urinary tract disease and bacterial urinary tract infections.[18]

Surgical Treatment

Detection of urocystoliths does not necessarily warrant surgical intervention; however, obstruction of urine outflow, an increase in size or number of calculi, persistent clinical signs, and a lack of response to therapy are indications for calculi removal.[7] Surgery is required in patients with nondissolvable calculi and clinical signs. Traditional open surgical options are available for treatment of urolithiasis, including cystotomy, ure-throtomy, and urethrostomy.

Minimally Invasive Techniques

There are several minimally invasive treatment options for retrieval of bladder and urethral stones. These options include voiding urohydropropulsion, transurethral cystoscopic stone removal with or without use of laser lithotripsy, and minilaparotomy-assisted cystoscopic stone removal, also called percutaneous cystolithotomy (PCCL).

In catheter-assisted retrieval or voiding urohydropropulsion of calculi, the patient is sedated or anesthetized, the bladder is filled with sterile crystalloid solution, and a catheter is passed into the urinary bladder transurethrally.[19] In cats, a 3.5-French or 5-French catheter is used and in dogs a 5-French, 8-French, or 10-French catheter is used, depending on patient size. During catheter retrieval, the contents of the bladder are aspirated while the bladder is agitated by palpating and manipulating it or rotating the patient's body. This procedure is difficult in most male cats and in small male dogs because of the limiting size of the urethra and the size of the catheter. With voiding urohydropropulsion, the patient is held vertically while the distended bladder is manually expressed (**Fig. 5**).[19] Sizes of uroliths that may be retrieved with this technique are approximately 1 mm in male cats, up to 5 mm in female cats, 1 to 3 mm in male dogs, and up to 10 mm in female dogs. These methods are used to eliminate small calculi and to collect them for analysis to plan further treatment. However, these techniques are not successful if a patient presents with urethral obstruction, because this situation indicates that there is at least 1 urolith that is too large to pass through the urethra.

PCCL is a procedure by which the bladder is temporarily fastened to the incised linea, allowing cystoscopic stone removal through a stab incision or a laparoscopic port placed in the urinary bladder (**Fig. 6**).[20,21] This method is an effective, safe, and efficient means for managing urocystoliths. Cystoscopy produces magnified images of the fluid-distended urinary bladder, allowing identification of abnormalities such as strictures, masses, and calculi.[22,23] This is the minimally invasive procedure of choice for male dogs and cats, because the diameter of the male urethra limits insertion of a cystoscope with operating channel. Cystoscopic techniques are more

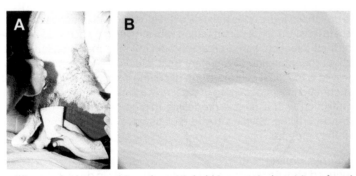

Fig. 5. In voiding urohydropropulsion, the cat is held in a vertical position after the urinary bladder is distended by infusion of fluid through a transurethral catheter. (A) The transurethral catheter is removed and the urinary bladder is gently agitated by grasping it through the abdominal wall. (B) The urinary bladder is gently compressed, inducing micturition and voiding of the urocystoliths.

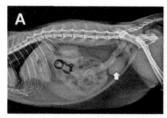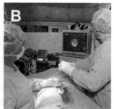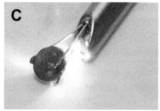

Fig. 6. Minilaparotomy-assisted cystotomy. (*A*) Lateral abdominal radiograph of an 8-year-old castrated male domestic shorthaired cat with a single urocystolith (*arrow*). (*B*) The urinary bladder is grasped through a small incision and tacked to the body wall. A stab incision is made through the bladder wall, and a rigid cystoscope is inserted. Urocystoliths are retrieved using retrieval devices. Cystoscopy provides magnification and better visualization. The urocystolith grasped with 4-prong nitinol graspers is projected on the endoscopic monitor. (*C*) Urocystolith retrieved via the procedure.

efficient than surgical procedures, decreasing the risk of trauma and abdominal contamination.[22,23]

In transurethral cystoscopy, a cystoscope is inserted into the urethra and passed into the urinary bladder. This procedure is preferred for use in females but has been described in male dogs because it is less invasive than other diagnostic and treatment methods. If calculi are small enough, they can be removed using stone retrieval devices such as stone baskets and graspers. For larger calculi, lithotripsy may be used if available.[23] Lithotripsy uses a laser fiber, which is passed through the operating channel on the cystoscope. The fiber emits light at an infrared wavelength to fragment calculi,[24–29] and the resulting fragments are removed transurethrally. This procedure is possible in female dogs and cats and male dogs, but not male cats, because of the limiting size of the male cat urethra and inability to insert a large enough scope with an operating channel.

Medical Management

Struvite
Struvite is another name for crystals or uroliths composed of magnesium ammonium phosphate hexahydrate ($Mg^{2+}NH_4^+PO_4^{3-} \cdot 6H_2O$). For uroliths to form, urine must be oversaturated with respect to the minerals that precipitate to form that type of urolith. For struvite uroliths to form, urine must be oversaturated with magnesium, ammonium, and phosphate ions. Urinary oversaturation with struvite may occur as a consequence of a urinary tract infection with a urease-producing microbe (infection-induced struvite) or without the presence of a urinary tract infection (sterile struvite).[30] Infection-induced struvite is the most common form occurring in dogs,[31] whereas sterile struvite is the most common form occurring in cats. Any animal that develops a bacterial urinary tract infection with a urease-producing microorganism can develop infection-induced struvite uroliths. Sterile struvite uroliths have been documented to occur in dogs,[32] but they are rare.

Infection-induced struvite
Infection-induced struvite uroliths occur more commonly in dogs and in cats less than 1 year and greater than 10 years of age.[8,9,33] There is no published information on gender predilection for infection-induced struvite uroliths in cats; however, they occur more commonly in female dogs, because of their increased risk of urinary tract infection. Infection-induced struvite uroliths form because of an infection with a

urease-producing microbe in a fashion similar to human beings.[34] In this situation, dietary composition is not important, because the production of the enzyme, urease, by the microbial organism is the driving force behind struvite urolith formation. *Staphylococcus* spp, *Enterococcus* spp, and *Proteus* spp are the most common organisms associated with urease production and infection-induced struvite urolith formation.

Infection-induced struvite uroliths can be dissolved by feeding a struvite dissolution diet and administering an appropriate antimicrobial agent based on bacteriologic culture and sensitivity, although there is a case report[35] of dissolution with administration of an antimicrobial agent only. Average dissolution time for infection-induced struvite uroliths was 79 days (range, 64–92 days) in 3 cats reported in a study.[30] An alternative dissolution protocol was shown to be effective in 8 of 11 dogs with presumed infection-induced struvite.[36] In this protocol, the diet was not changed; instead a urinary acidifier, D,L-methionine, was administered at a dosage of 75 to 100 mg/kg by mouth every 12 hours in combination with an appropriate antibiotic for the organism responsible for struvite formation (typically *Staphylococcus*).[36] Median time to dissolution was 2 months, with a range of 1 to 4 months.

It is important that the patient receives an appropriate antimicrobial agent during the entire time of medical dissolution because bacteria become trapped in the matrix of the urolith, and as the urolith dissolves, bacteria are released into urine. If therapeutic levels of an appropriate antimicrobial agent are not present in urine, then an infection will recur, and dissolution will cease.

Prevention of infection-induced struvite does not require feeding a special diet, because the infection causes these struvite uroliths to form. It involves preventing a bacterial urinary tract infection from recurring and treating bacterial infections as they arise. Dietary modification does not prevent infection-induced struvite uroliths from recurring, because diet does not prevent recurrence of a bacterial urinary tract infection.

Sterile struvite

Sterile struvite uroliths form typically in cats between 1 and 10 years of age.[33] Risk for struvite urolith formation decreases after approximately 6 to 8 years of age in cats.[37] Struvite uroliths occur with equal frequency in male and female cats. Sterile struvite uroliths form because of dietary composition as well as innate risks for urolith formation. Experimentally, magnesium phosphate and struvite uroliths formed in healthy cats consuming calculogenic diets containing 0.15% to 1.0% magnesium (dry matter basis).[34,38,39] However, these data are difficult to interpret, because the amount of magnesium consumption by cats in these studies may be different from that by cats that spontaneously form sterile struvite uroliths consuming commercial diets, because of differences in caloric density, palatability, and digestibility.[40] The influence of magnesium on struvite formation depends on urine pH[41] and influence of ions, minerals, and other components in urine.[42] Alkaluria is associated with increased risk for struvite formation.[43,44] In a clinical study including 20 cats with naturally occurring struvite urocystoliths and no detectable bacterial urinary tract infection,[30] the mean urinary pH at the time of diagnosis was 6.9 ± 0.4. An additional factor is water intake and urine volume. Consumption of increased quantities of water may result in decreasing concentrations of calculogenic substances in urine, thus decreasing risk of urolith formation.[45] Consumption of small quantities of food frequently rather than 1 or 2 large meals per day is associated with production of more acidic urine and a lesser degree of struvite crystalluria by cats.[46,47]

Sterile struvite uroliths can be dissolved by feeding a diet that is restricted in magnesium, phosphorous, and protein and that induces aciduria relative to maintenance adult cat foods.[30,48] In a clinical study including 22 cats with sterile struvite urocysto-liths,[30] urocystoliths dissolved in 20 cats in a mean of 36.2 ± 26.6 days (range, 14–141 days). The cats were fed a high-moisture (canned), calorically dense diet containing 0.058% magnesium (dry matter basis) and increased sodium chloride (0.79% dry matter basis). Similar results have been found in another study.[49] In a more recent study of 32 cats with presumed struvite urocystoliths comparing 2 low magnesium acidifying diets, one a struvite dissolution diet and the other a struvite prevention diet, the mean (± standard deviation [SD]) times for a 50% reduction in urolith size (0.69 ± 0.1 weeks) and complete urolith dissolution (13.0 ± 2.6 days) were significantly shorter for cats fed the struvite dissolution diet, compared with those (1.75 ± 0.27 weeks and 27.0 ± 2.6 days, respectively) for cats fed the struvite prevention diet. At study termination, mean ± SD urine pH (6.083 ± 0.105) for cats fed the struvite dissolution diet was lower than that (6.431 ± 0.109) for cats fed the struvite prevention diet.[50] Therefore, sterile struvite urocystoliths often dissolve in 2 to 4 weeks.

Prevention of sterile struvite uroliths involves inducing a urine pH less than approximately 6.8,[41,51] increasing urine volume, and decreasing excretion of magnesium, ammonium, and phosphorous. There are many diets available that are formulated to be struvite preventive.[33]

Calcium oxalate

Calcium oxalate accounts for 40% to 50% of all uroliths. Risk factors for calcium oxalate formation include increased urinary or oxalate excretion and aciduria. Certain breeds of dogs and cats are predisposed to formation of calcium oxalate uroliths, including long-haired cats (Burmese, Persian, and Himalayan breeds) and small breeds dogs (miniature schnauzer, Lhasa apso, shih tzu, and Yorkshire terrier breeds).[52–54] Calcium oxalate urolith formation occurs when urine is oversaturated with calcium and oxalate.[1] In addition to these alterations in activities of ions, large-molecular-weight proteins occurring in urine, such as nephrocalcin, uropontin, and Tamm-Horsfall mucoprotein, influence calcium oxalate formation.[55] We have a limited understanding of the role of these macromolecular and ionic inhibitors of calcium oxalate formation in cats. Certain metabolic factors are known to increase risk of calcium oxalate urolith formation in several species, including cats and dogs. Medical and nutritional strategies for stone prevention have focused on amelioration of these factors.

Calcium homeostasis is achieved through actions of parathyroid hormone (PTH) and 1,25-dihydroxycholecalciferol (1,25-vitamin D) on bones, intestines, and kidneys. When serum ionized calcium concentration decreases, PTH and 1,25-vitamin D activities increase, resulting in mobilization of calcium from bone, increased absorption of calcium from intestine, and increased reabsorption of calcium by renal tubules. Conversely, high serum ionized calcium concentration suppresses release of PTH and production of 1,25-vitamin D, resulting in decreased bone mobilization, decreased intestinal absorption of calcium, and increased urinary excretion of calcium. Therefore, hypercalciuria can result from hypercalcemia, excessive intestinal absorption of calcium (gastrointestinal [GI] hyperabsorption), impaired renal reabsorption of calcium (renal leak), or excessive skeletal mobilization of calcium (resorptive).

Hypercalcemia is associated with increased risk of calcium oxalate urolith formation. In cats with calcium oxalate uroliths, hypercalcemia was observed in 35% of the cases,[56] whereas in dogs with calcium oxalate uroliths, it occurs in approximately 4%, usually associated with primary hyperparathyroidism.[57] Conversely, uroliths developed in 35% of cats with idiopathic hypercalcemia.[12] Hypercalcemia results in increased calcium fractional excretion and hypercalciuria when severe.

Hypercalciuria is a significant risk factor, but not necessarily the cause of calcium oxalate urolith formation in human beings, dogs, and cats.[58] In miniature schnauzers, GI hyperabsorption seems to occur most commonly, although renal leak hypercalciuria has also been observed.[59] Hypercalciuria has not been well defined in normocalcemic cats with calcium oxalate uroliths but is believed to occur. Although excessive dietary intake of calcium may result in hypercalciuria, studies in human beings refute this. Apparently, dietary calcium may bind to dietary oxalic acid, resulting in calcium oxalate formation in the lumen of the GI tract, thereby preventing absorption of calcium and oxalate. Hypercalciuria may also occur with administration of loop diuretics, glucocorticoids, urinary acidifiers, and vitamin D or C.

Metabolic acidosis promotes hypercalciuria by promoting bone turnover (release of calcium with buffers from bone), increasing serum ionized calcium concentration, resulting in increased urinary calcium excretion and decreased renal tubular reabsorption of calcium. Consumption of diets supplemented with the urinary acidifier ammonium chloride by cats has been associated with increased urinary calcium excretion.[60] In addition, consumption by human beings of diets containing high amounts of animal protein results in metabolic acidosis and increased urinary calcium excretion. Metabolic acidosis promotes hypercalciuria by promoting bone turnover (release of calcium with buffers from bone), increasing serum ionized calcium concentration, resulting in increased urinary calcium excretion and decreased renal tubular reabsorption of calcium. In addition, acidic urine alters function and concentration of crystal inhibitors. Low urine pH decreases urinary citrate concentration by increasing renal proximal tubular citrate reabsorption. Acidic urine is known to impair function of macromolecular protein inhibitors. In dogs, hypercalciuria resulting from ammonium chloride administration was decreased by bicarbonate administration.[61] In cats, magnesium supplementation as magnesium chloride was associated with increased urinary calcium excretion and aciduria, whereas magnesium supplementation as magnesium oxide was associated with alkaluria and a lesser degree of urinary calcium excretion.[41] Urine pH has a direct effect on solubility of calcium oxalate. In a study of healthy cats fed similar diets that differed in only their acidifying or alkalinizing properties, urinary saturation with calcium oxalate was lower when the urine pH was greater than 7.2 and greater when urine pH was less than 6.5.[51]

Inhibitors, such as citrate, magnesium, and pyrophosphate, form soluble salts with calcium or oxalic acid and reduce availability of calcium or oxalic acid for precipitation. Other inhibitors, such as Tamm-Horsfall glycoprotein and nephrocalcin, interfere with the ability of calcium and oxalic acid to combine minimizing crystal formation, aggregation, and growth.

Oxalic acid is a metabolic end product of ascorbic acid (vitamin C) and several amino acids, such as glycine and serine, derived from dietary sources. Oxalic acid forms soluble salts with sodium and potassium ions, but a relatively insoluble salt with calcium ions. Therefore, any increased urinary concentration of oxalic acid may promote calcium oxalate formation. Dietary increases of oxalate and vitamin B_6 deficiency are known factors increasing urinary oxalate. Hyperoxaluria has been observed experimentally in kittens consuming vitamin B_6-deficient diets[11] but has not been associated with formation of naturally occurring calcium oxalate uroliths in adults. Genetic anomalies may also increase urine oxalic acid concentration. Hyperoxaluria has also been recognized in a group of related cats with reduced quantities of hepatic D-glycerate dehydrogenase, an enzyme involved in metabolism of oxalic acid precursors (primary hyperoxaluria type II).[62] Hyperoxaluria has also been associated with defective peroxisomal alanine/glyoxylate aminotransferase activity (primary hyperoxaluria type I) and intestinal disease in human beings (enteric hyperoxaluria). These conditions have not been evaluated in cats or dogs. *Oxalobacter formigenes* is an enteric bacterial organism that metabolizes oxalic acid in the GI tract. It has recently been shown that dogs that have less enteric colonization with *Oxalobacter formigenes* have a higher risk of calcium oxalate urolith formation than dogs that are colonized.[63] Compared with the situation in human beings, urinary oxalate seems to have a lesser role in calcium oxalate formation in dogs and cats and urinary calcium seems to have a greater role.[64,65]

Decreased urine volume results in increased calcium and oxalic acid saturation and an increased risk for urolith formation. Cats can achieve urine specific gravities in excess of 1.065, indicating a marked ability to produce concentrated urine. Many cats affected with calcium oxalate uroliths have a urine specific gravity greater than 1.040 unless there is some impairment of renal function or concentrating ability.[58] Detection of calcium oxalate crystals indicates that urine is supersaturated with calcium oxalate and, if persistent, represents an increased risk for calcium oxalate urolith formation. However, calcium oxalate crystalluria is present in less than 50% of feline and canine cases at time of diagnosis of urolithiasis.[58]

Medical protocols that promote dissolution of calcium oxalate uroliths are not available; therefore, uroliths must be removed physically, either surgically or by voiding urohydropropulsion.[66]

Calcium oxalate uroliths are recurrent; therefore, preventive measures are warranted. There is an approximate 10% recurrence at 6 months and 35% recurrence at 12 months in dogs,[7] and many cats have recurrence within 2 years of removal if preventive measures are not undertaken.[67] Because the cause of calcium oxalate urolith formation is not completely known, no treatment has been shown to be completely effective. If possible, metabolic factors known to increase calcium oxalate risk should be corrected or minimized. Goals of dietary prevention include (1) reducing urine calcium and oxalate concentration, (2) promoting high concentrations and activity of urolith inhibitors, (3) reducing urine acidity, and (4) promoting dilute urine.

Increasing urine volume is a mainstay of preventive therapy for calcium oxalate urolithiasis. By increasing water intake, urinary concentrations of calculogenic minerals are reduced. In addition, larger urine volumes typically increase urine transit time and voiding frequency, thereby reducing retention time for crystal formation and growth. Feeding a canned food is the most practical means of increasing water intake and decreasing calcium oxalate urine saturation. The goal is to dilute urine to a specific gravity of 1.040 or less in cats and 1.030 or less in dogs.[7,68] Flavoring water, enhancing water access, and adding water to dry foods may be used in patients that refuse to eat canned foods. Sodium chloride may be used to increase water intake, and several calcium oxalate preventive diets contain greater than 1% sodium chloride (dry matter basis).[69,70] However, increased dietary sodium may increase urinary calcium excretion and can contribute to ongoing renal damage in cats with marginal renal function,[68] although this has not been a consistent finding.[71,72]

Epidemiologic studies consistently identify acidifying diets among the most prominent risk factors for calcium oxalate urolithiasis.[52,53,73] Solubility of calcium oxalate in urine is minimally influenced by pH; however, there is a linear relationship between increasing calcium oxalate solubility and urine pH in healthy cats, with alkaluria inducing a lower relative supersaturation for calcium oxalate when compared with aciduria.[51] Persistent aciduria may be associated with low-grade metabolic acidosis, which promotes bone mobilization and increases urinary calcium excretion; however, this effect has not been reported in studies of cats for up to 1 year.[51] In a case series of 5 cats with hypercalcemia and calcium oxalate uroliths,[53] discontinuation of acidifying diets or urinary acidifiers was associated with normalization of serum calcium concentration. In dogs, the influence of urine pH on risk of calcium oxalate formation is less clear.[74] Furthermore, aciduria promotes hypocitraturia and functional impairment of endogenous urolith inhibitors. Thus, feeding an acidifying diet or administering urinary acidifiers to cats at risk for calcium oxalate is contraindicated. A target urine pH of 6.6 to 7.5 is suggested in dogs and cats at risk for recurrence of calcium oxalate uroliths.[68]

Potassium citrate is often included in diets designed for calcium oxalate prevention. In urine, citric acid combines with calcium to form soluble complexes, thereby reducing ionic calcium concentration. Citric acid also directly inhibits nucleation of calcium and oxalate crystals. When oxidized within the tricarboxylic acid cycle, supplemental citrate results in urine alkalinization caused by production of bicarbonate. The metabolic alkalinization increases endogenous renal citrate excretion and reduces calcium absorption and urinary excretion.[68] Commercial products that add citrate but continue to acidify the urine (pH <6.5) negate the benefit of citrate therapy.

Although reduction of urine calcium and oxalic acid concentrations by restriction of dietary calcium and oxalic acid seems logical, it is not without risk. Reducing consumption of only one of these constituents may increase availability and intestinal absorption of the other, resulting in increased urinary excretion. Conversely, increasing dietary calcium levels in normal cats contributes directly to increased urine calcium concentration. Because epidemiologic data in cats suggest that marked dietary calcium restriction increases urolith risk, moderate levels of dietary calcium are advised in nonhypercalcemic cats.[68]

Dietary phosphorus should not be restricted in dogs or cats with calcium oxalate urolithiasis. Low dietary phosphorus is a risk factor for calcium oxalate urolith formation in cats.[75] Reduction in dietary phosphorus may be associated with activation of vitamin D, which in turn promotes intestinal calcium absorption and hypercalciuria. In addition, phosphate status determines pyrophosphate urinary concentrations, an inhibitor of calcium oxalate urolith formation in human beings and rodents. If calcium oxalate urolithiasis is associated with hypophosphatemia and normal calcium concentration, oral phosphorus supplementation may be considered. However, caution should be used because excessive dietary phosphorus may predispose to formation of calcium phosphate uroliths. Whether this occurs in dogs or cats is unknown.

Urinary magnesium forms complexes with oxalic acid, reducing the amount of oxalic acid available to form calcium oxalate. Studies in cats associate low dietary magnesium with calcium oxalate risk.[37,53,73,75-77] In human beings, supplemental magnesium has been used to minimize recurrence of calcium oxalate uroliths; however, supplemental magnesium may increase the risk of struvite formation in cats. Risks and benefits of magnesium supplementation to dogs and cats with calcium oxalate urolithiasis have not been evaluated and it is not advised. It seems logical that magnesium should not be highly restricted in diets that are consumed by dogs or cats with calcium oxalate urolithiasis.

Consumption of high amounts of animal protein by human beings is associated with an increased risk of calcium oxalate formation. Dietary protein of animal origin may increase urinary calcium and oxalic acid excretion, decrease urinary citrate excretion, and promote bone mobilization to buffer the acid intake from metabolism of animal proteins. However, a case control study[75] showed that higher protein concentration in cat foods appeared protective against calcium oxalate uroliths. Although several coassociations (eg, higher protein in canned foods) might explain this finding, cats are obligatory carnivores and dietary protein restriction in the management of calcium oxalate urolithiasis is not advised.

Excess intake of vitamin C, a metabolic oxalate precursor, should be avoided.[68] Although normal dietary vitamin C levels are not considered a risk in human beings, very small increases in urinary oxalate are a concern in urolith formers. Because dogs and cats do not have a dietary vitamin C requirement, supplementation should be avoided in foods fed to dogs or cats at risk for calcium oxalate uroliths. Cranberry concentrate tablets are also contraindicated. They provide mild acidification and are high in oxalate, as well as vitamin C.[78]

The diet should be adequately fortified with vitamin B_6, because vitamin B_6 deficiency promotes endogenous production and subsequent urinary excretion of oxalic acid.[79] There is no evidence that providing increased vitamin B_6 beyond meeting the nutritional requirement provides a benefit in cats. Because most commercial diets designed for dogs and cats are well fortified with vitamin B_6, it is unlikely additional supplementation is beneficial except in homemade diets. Regardless, vitamin B_6 is reasonably safe and sometimes provided to patients with persistent calcium oxalate crystalluria or frequent recurrences.

Increased dietary fiber intake is associated with decreasing risk of calcium oxalate recurrence in some human beings but not in cats unless they are hypercalcemic. Certain types of fiber (soy or rice bran) decrease calcium absorption from the GI tract, which may decrease urinary calcium excretion. Also, higher-fiber diets tend to be less acidifying. In 5 cats with idiopathic hypercalcemia and calcium oxalate uroliths, feeding a high-fiber diet with supplemental potassium citrate resulted in normalization of serum calcium concentrations[11]; however, efficacy of increased fiber intake is unproved. There are no studies in dogs evaluating dietary fiber and calcium oxalate urolithiasis.

In dogs, feeding a protein-restricted and sodium-restricted alkalinizing diet has been shown to decrease recurrence of calcium oxalate uroliths.[77] If a neutral to slightly alkaline urine pH is not accomplished by diet, potassium citrate may be administered (initial dose: 75 mg/kg by mouth every 12 hours; adjust to induce a urine pH of 7.0–7.5). Because protein-restricted and sodium-restricted alkalinizing diet is also high in fat, some dogs cannot tolerate the diet. In these dogs, feeding a low-fat, higher-fiber diet with supplemental potassium citrate seems to be effective.

In cats, several diets are available that are formulated to reduce calcium and oxalic acid concentrations in urine, promote high concentration and activity of inhibitors of calcium oxalate crystal growth and aggregation in urine, and maintain dilute urine. Consumption of these diets by healthy cats results in production of urine that is undersaturated with calcium oxalate.[37,45] In 1 study of cats with naturally occurring calcium oxalate uroliths,[67] consumption of 1 oxalate preventive diet resulted in a decrease of urine saturation from the oversaturated state to a metastable state; cats did not reform uroliths. In cats with hypercalcemia and calcium oxalate uroliths, prevention seems to be more successful when feeding a higher-fiber diet, and administering potassium citrate (initial dose: 75 mg/kg by mouth every 12 hours; adjust to induce a urine pH of 7.0–7.5).[11] Other treatments that have been proposed include vitamin B_6 (2 mg/kg by mouth every 24 hours) and hydrochlorothiazide (2–4 mg/kg by mouth every 12 hours).

Calcium oxalate uroliths are recurrent. Serial monitoring of a dog or cat with a history of calcium oxalate urolithiasis should be part of the preventive protocol. Periodically, a complete urinalysis should be performed to monitor urine specific gravity, pH, and presence of calcium oxalate crystalluria. Ideally, urine should be dilute, urine pH in the neutral to alkaline range, and calcium oxalate crystalluria should not be present. Survey abdominal radiography should be performed approximately every 6 months to evaluate for recurrence. If calcium oxalate urocystoliths are detected while small, they may be retrieved nonsurgically and adjustment to the preventive protocol can be made.

Purines

Urates Most information concerning urate uroliths is derived from dogs, with little information available for cats. Uric acid is one of several biodegradation products of purine nucleotide metabolism.[80] Purines are made up of 3 groups of compounds: oxypurines (hypoxanthine, xanthine, uric acid, allantoin), aminopurines (adenine, guanine), and methylpurines (caffeine, theophylline, theobromine). In most dogs and cats, allantoin is the major metabolic end product; it is the most soluble of the purine metabolic products excreted in urine. Uroliths that are composed of uric acid (anhydrous uric acid, uric acid dihydrate, sodium urate, ammonium urate) or xanthine form because urine is oversaturated with these substances. Ammonium urate (also known as ammonium acid urate and ammonium biurate) is the monobasic ammonium salt of uric acid. It is the most common form of naturally occurring purine uroliths observed in dogs and cats. Other naturally occurring purine uroliths include sodium urate (also known as sodium acid urate or monosodium urate), sodium calcium urate, potassium urate, and uric acid dihydrate.

Urate is the third most common mineral found in uroliths in dogs and cats, accounting for 5% to 8% of uroliths, and the second most common urolith, occurring in dogs and cats less than 1 year of age (infection-induced struvite is the most common urolith in these patients). Urate uroliths form when urine is oversaturated with urate and usually ammonium. These uroliths form because of liver disease (usually a portosystemic vascular shunt)[14,15] or because of an inborn error of metabolism resulting in hyperuricosuria (eg, Dalmatians and English bulldogs).[81,82] They are more common in dogs and cats less than 7 years of age.[81–83]

Dalmatian dogs are predisposed to urate uroliths because of the unique metabolism of purines.[81,84] The ability of Dalmatians to oxidize uric acid to allantoin is intermediate between human beings and most non-Dalmatian dogs.[85] Human beings have a serum uric acid concentration of approximately 3 to 7 mg/dL, and excrete approximately 500 to 700 mg of uric acid in their urine per day.[86] Most non-Dalmatian dogs have a serum uric acid concentration of less than 0.5 mg/dL and excrete approximately 10 to 60 mg of uric acid in their urine per day. Dalmatians have a serum uric acid concentration that is 2 to 4 times that of non-Dalmatians and excrete more than 400 to 600 mg of uric acid in their urine per day.[80]

Studies of the fate of uric acid in Dalmatians have shown unique hepatic and renal pathways of metabolism.[84,87] Of these 2 metabolic sites, reciprocal allogenic renal and hepatic transplantations between Dalmatians and non-Dalmatians indicate that the hepatic mechanism is quantitatively the most significant. The liver of Dalmatians does not completely oxidize available uric acid, even although it contains a sufficient concentration of uricase.[88] It has been shown that Dalmatians, English bulldogs, and black Russian terriers have a mutation in the SLC2A9 gene that encodes for a transporter of uric acid, and homozygous mutation results in lack of hepatic conversion of uric acid to allantoin.[89,90] The definitive mechanism of urate urolith formation in Dalmatian dogs remains unknown. Increased uric acid excretion is a risk factor rather than a primary cause. Urate uroliths are reported more commonly in males than females; the average age of urolith diagnosis is 4.5 years.[80,81] Although all Dalmatians excreting high uric acid excrete relatively increased quantities of uric acid in their urine, apparently, only a small percentage form urate stones.[91]

Dissolution is not possible in dogs and cats with uncorrected liver disease (eg, nonsurgical portovascular anomalies or microvascular dysplasia). Surgical removal, voiding urohydropropulsion, or cystoscopy ± laser lithotripsy remains the treatment of choice for symptomatic urate stones that cannot be dissolved. It is logical to hypothesize that elimination of hyperuric aciduria and reduction of urine ammonium concentration after surgical correction of anomalous shunts would result in spontaneous dissolution of uroliths composed primarily of ammonium urate. Appropriate clinical studies are needed to prove or disprove this hypothesis. We have occasionally been successful in medically dissolving urate uroliths in dogs with portal vascular anomalies but have not attempted dissolution in cats with ammonium urate uroliths and portal vascular anomalies. Additional clinical studies are needed to evaluate the relative value of calculolytic diets, allopurinol, or alkalinization of urine in dissolving ammonium urate uroliths in cats with portal vascular anomalies. The pharmacokinetics and efficacy of allopurinol may be altered in cats with portal vascular anomalies, because biotransformation of this drug, which has a very short half-life, to oxypurinol, which has a longer half-life, requires adequate hepatic function. Xanthine uroliths have been observed to form in dogs with portovascular anomalies given allopurinol; therefore, allopurinol had an effect on xanthine oxidase conversion of xanthine to uric acid.

In dogs and cats without underlying liver disease, dissolution may be attempted. Dissolution of urate uroliths in dogs is accomplished by feeding a purine-restricted, alkalinizing, diuresing diet and administering the xanthine oxidase inhibitor, allopurinol (15 mg/kg by mouth every 12 hours)[80,92–96]; allopurinol has not been evaluated in cats and should not be used. Although renal failure diets are protein restricted and thus lower in purines, there are 2 commercially available diets formulated to be low in purines: Prescription Diet u/d (Hill's Pet Products) and UC Low Purine (Royal Canin). Canned diets may be better than dry diets. In 1 study,[80] medical dissolution was effective in approximately 40% of Dalmatians, partial dissolution occurred in approximately 30%, and no dissolution of growth of uroliths caused by xanthine formation occurred in approximately 30%. Although no studies have been performed evaluating the efficacy or safety of medical dissolution of urate uroliths in cats with idiopathic urate urolithiasis, we have successfully dissolved urate uroliths in cats using a renal failure diet (Prescription Diet k/d, Hill's Pet Products) and allopurinol (7.5 mg/kg by mouth every 12 hours). Until further studies are performed to confirm the safety and efficacy of medical dissolution, surgical removal remains the treatment of choice for urate uroliths in cats.

Prevention of urate uroliths in dogs without liver disease involves continued feeding of the low purine diet. If necessary, allopurinol may be administered at a lower dose (7–10 mg/kg by mouth every 12–24 hours). Periodic abdominal ultrasonography or double contrast cystography may be necessary. Determination of 24-hour urinary uric acid excretion may also be useful, although data are limited and collection of 24-hour urine samples can be difficult. The goal is to achieve 24-hour urinary acid excretion of approximately 250 to 350 mg/dog/24 h. Use of urine uric acid/urine creatinine ratios may be useful for diagnosis of risk of urate urolith formation[90] but are inaccurate for predicting success of dissolution or prevention.[80] Prevention of urate urolith recurrence in cats has been greater than 90% when using a protein-restricted alkalinizing diet.

Xanthine Xanthine urolithiasis may occur with allopurinol administration to dogs, especially when dietary purines are not restricted. Management involves adjusting dosage of allopurinol and changing diet. Spontaneously occurring xanthine uroliths have been reported rarely in cats (0.14% of uroliths analyzed at the Minnesota Urolith Center). They are composed typically of pure xanthine, and they have been reported to occur in cats less than 5 years of age, with approximately even distribution between males and females. Often, xanthine uroliths occur in multiple numbers but are smaller than 5 mm; they are radiolucent. Of 64 cats that formed xanthine uroliths in 1 report, none of the cats had been treated with the xanthine oxidase inhibitor allopurinol. Sixty-one xanthine uroliths were obtained from the lower urinary tract, whereas xanthine uroliths from 3 cats came from the upper urinary tract. Xanthine uroliths occurred in 30 neutered and 8 nonneutered males and 25 neutered females (the gender of 1 cat was not specified). Mean age of cats at time of diagnosis of xanthine uroliths was 2.8 ± 2.3 years (range, 4 months to 10 years). Eight of the 64 cats were less than 1 year old. Urinary uric acid excretion was similar between 8 xanthine urolith-forming cats and healthy cats (2.09 ± 0.8 mg/kg/d vs 1.46 ± 0.56 mg/kg/d); however, urinary xanthine excretion (2.46 ± 1.17 mg/kg/d) and urinary hypoxanthine excretion (0.65 ± 0.17 mg/kg/d) were higher (neither is detectable in urine from healthy cats). Xanthine uroliths have also been found in a few Cavalier King Charles spaniels.[97–99] No medical dissolution protocol for naturally occurring xanthine uroliths exists. Prevention involves feeding a purine-restricted, alkalinizing, diuresing diet. Without preventive measures, xanthine uroliths often recur within 3 to 12 months after removal.

No medical dissolution protocol for feline xanthine uroliths exists. Prevention involves feeding a protein-restricted alkalinizing diet. Without preventive measures, xanthine uroliths often recur within 3 to 12 months after removal. In an unpublished observational study (JW Bartges, personal communication, 2014), 10 cats with confirmation of xanthine uroliths by quantitative analysis had been consuming the protein-restricted alkalinizing diet and followed for at least 2 years; only one had had recurrence.

Cystine

Cystinuria occurs when there is a proximal renal tubular defect in reabsorption and often occurs with other amino acids (notably, ornithine, lysine, and arginine).[100–105] Affected animals also show altered intestinal transport of cystine.[106–108] Several genetic mutations have been identified in dogs and cats that are associated with cystinuria.[109–112] Cystinuria is associated only with urolith formation and is not associated with protein malnutrition or amino acid deficiency, although it can be associated with hypercarnitinuria or hypertaurinuria and associated dilated cardiomyopathy.[113] However, cystinuria by itself does not result in urolithiasis, and many cystinuric dogs and human beings do not form uroliths.[114]

Canine cystine uroliths can be dissolved medically. Feed a diet that is low protein, alkalinizing, and induces a diuresis. Although renal failure diets are protein restricted and thus lower in amino acids, there are 2 commercially available diets formulated to be low in sulfur-containing amino acids: Prescription Diet u/d (Hill's Pet Products) and UC Low Purine (Royal Canin). Canned diets may be better than dry diets. Administer 2-mercaptopropionylglycine (2-MPG, Tiopronin, Thiola).[100,101,115] This drug is similar to D-penicillamine in that it binds to the individual cysteine molecules, preventing formation of the disulfide bond of cystine; however, it is associated with fewer side effects and complications than D-penicillamine. Dosage is 15 mg/kg by mouth every 12 hours for dissolution. There are studies showing that administration of 2-MPG without modifying diet may result in dissolution of cystine uroliths. Cats do not tolerate 2-MPG well and it is associated with GI signs, liver disease, and anemia; therefore, it should not be used in cats; dissolution of cystine uroliths has not been successful.

Prevention of cystine uroliths involves inducing undersaturation of urine with cystine. Continued feeding of the low sulfur-containing amino acid diets to dogs and feeding a renal failure diet to cats has been successful in prevention of cystine urolith recurrence. Cystine solubility in urine is dependent on pH and the solubility increases exponentially when the urine pH is greater than 7.2; therefore, maintain an alkaline urine pH. If additional alkalinization is required, potassium citrate may be administered (initial dosage: 75 mg/kg by mouth every 12 hours; adjust to urine pH >7.2). 2-MPG may be used for prevention; however, many dogs do not require it and, as mentioned, it should not be used in cats.

Mixed and compound uroliths
Between 5% and 15% of uroliths may be mixed or compound stones. This observation refers to a situation in which more than 1 mineral is present within the stone, either mixed within all layers or different parts of the stone are composed of different minerals (nidus vs major volume of the stone vs the outer layer or shell). As mentioned earlier, ammonium urate and calcium carbonate (or calcium apatite) may be mixed with struvite as part of infection-induced struvite stone formation. In this situation, the struvite caused by the infection is the primary focus for prevention. Some stones may be composed of both struvite and calcium oxalate. In this situation, usually calcium oxalate is the nidus (inner part of the stone), and struvite is layered around it. This compound stone forms because the patient first formed a calcium oxalate stone and then developed a urinary tract infection and layered infection-induced struvite around the calcium oxalate nidus. In this situation, preventive therapy is directed toward the inner calcium oxalate component, because calcium oxalate formed first and this led to infection-induced struvite formation. Management of infection is also important; however, dietary prevention is focused on the calcium oxalate component. Ammonium urate uroliths may contain xanthine in patients that receive allopurinol for dissolution or prevention. This situation may be because of (1) too high a dose of allopurinol, (2) lack of restriction of dietary protein/purine, or (3) individual patient metabolism of allopurinol despite appropriate allopurinol dosage and dietary management. Prevention is directed to (1) decreasing or discontinuing allopurinol, (2) changing the diet to a more protein-/purine-restricted diet, or (3) both.

REFERENCES

1. Bartges JW, Osborne CA, Lulich JP, et al. Methods for evaluating treatment of uroliths. Vet Clin North Am Small Anim Pract 1999;29:45–57.
2. Feeney DA, Anderson KL. Radiographic imaging in urinary tract disease. In: Bartges J, Polzin DJ, editors. Nephrology and urology of small animals. Ames (IA): Wiley-Blackwell; 2011. p. 97–127.
3. Osborne CA, Lulich JP, Kruger JM, et al. Analysis of 451,891 canine uroliths, feline uroliths, and feline urethral plugs from 1981 to 2007: perspectives from the Minnesota Urolith Center. Vet Clin North Am Small Anim Pract 2009;39:183–97.
4. Sturgess CP, Hesford A, Owen H, et al. An investigation into the effects of storage on the diagnosis of crystalluria in cats. J Feline Med Surg 2001;3:81–5.
5. Langston C, Gisselman K, Palma D, et al. Diagnosis of urolithiasis. Compend Contin Educ Vet 2008;30:447–50, 452–4; [quiz: 455].
6. Bartges JW. Urinary saturation testing. In: Bartges J, Polzin DJ, editors. Nephrology and urology of small animals. Ames (IA): Wiley-Blackwell; 2011. p. 75–85.
7. Lulich JP, Osborne CA, Albasan H. Canine and feline urolithiasis: diagnosis, treatment, and prevention. In: Bartges J, Polzin DJ, editors. Nephrology and urology of small animals. West Sussex (United Kingdom): Wiley-Blackwell; 2011. p. 687–706.

8. Seaman R, Bartges JW. Canine struvite urolithiasis. Compen Contin Educ Pract Vet 2001;23:407–29.
9. Palma D, Langston C, Gisselman K, et al. Canine struvite urolithiasis. Compend Contin Educ Vet 2013;35:E1 [quiz: E1].
10. Gisselman K, Langston CE, Douglas P, et al. Calcium oxalate urolithiasis. Compend Contin Educ Vet 2009;31:496–502.
11. McClain HM, Barsanti JA, Bartges JW. Hypercalcemia and calcium oxalate urolithiasis in cats: a report of five cases. J Am Anim Hosp Assoc 1999;35:297–301.
12. Midkiff AM, Chew DJ, Randolph JF, et al. Idiopathic hypercalcemia in cats. J Vet Intern Med 2000;14:619–26.
13. Savary KC, Price GS, Vaden SL. Hypercalcemia in cats: a retrospective study of 71 cases (1991–1997). J Vet Intern Med 2000;14:184–9.
14. EH GC, Phillips H, Underwood L, et al. Risk factors for urolithiasis in dogs with congenital extrahepatic portosystemic shunts: 95 cases (1999–2013). J Am Vet Med Assoc 2015;246:530–6.
15. Bartges JW, Cornelius LM, Osborne CA. Ammonium urate uroliths in dogs with portosystemic shunts. In: Bonagura JD, editor. Current veterinary therapy XIII. Philadelphia: WB Saunders; 1999. p. 872–4.
16. Koehler LA, Osborne CA, Buettner MT, et al. Canine uroliths: frequently asked questions and their answers. Vet Clin North Am Small Anim Pract 2009;39: 161–81.
17. Bartges JW, Finco DR, Polzin DJ, et al. Pathophysiology of urethral obstruction. Vet Clin North Am Small Anim Pract 1996;26:255–64.
18. McLoughlin MA. Complications of lower urinary tract surgery in small animals. Vet Clin North Am Small Anim Pract 2011;41:889–913, v.
19. Lulich JP, Osborne CA. Voiding urohydropropulsion. In: Bartges J, Polzin DJ, editors. Nephrology and urology of small animals. Ames (IA): Wiley-Blackwell; 2011. p. 375–8.
20. Bartges J, Sura P, Callens A. Minilaparotomy-assisted cystoscopy for urocystoliths. In: Bonagura J, Twedt DC, editors. Kirk's current veterinary therapy. St Louis (MO): Elsevier; 2014. p. 905–9.
21. Runge JJ, Berent AC, Mayhew PD, et al. Transvesicular percutaneous cystolithotomy for the retrieval of cystic and urethral calculi in dogs and cats: 27 cases (2006–2008). J Am Vet Med Assoc 2011;239:344–9.
22. Rawlings C. Diagnostic rigid endoscopy: otoscopy, rhinoscopy, and cystoscopy. Vet Clin North Am Small Anim Pract 2009;39:849–68.
23. Rawlings C. Surgical views: endoscopic removal of urinary calculi. Compend Contin Educ Vet 2009;31:476–84.
24. Lulich JP, Osborne CA, Albasan H, et al. Efficacy and safety of laser lithotripsy in fragmentation of urocystoliths and urethroliths for removal in dogs. J Am Vet Med Assoc 2009;234:1279–85.
25. Lulich JP, Adams LG, Grant D, et al. Changing paradigms in the treatment of uroliths by lithotripsy. Vet Clin North Am Small Anim Pract 2009;39:143–60.
26. Bevan JM, Lulich JP, Albasan H, et al. Comparison of laser lithotripsy and cystotomy for the management of dogs with urolithiasis. J Am Vet Med Assoc 2009;234:1286–94.
27. Grant DC, Werre SR, Gevedon ML. Holmium: YAG laser lithotripsy for urolithiasis in dogs. J Vet Intern Med 2008;22:534–9.
28. Adams LG, Berent AC, Moore GE, et al. Use of laser lithotripsy for fragmentation of uroliths in dogs: 73 cases (2005–2006. J Am Vet Med Assoc 2008;232: 1680–7.

29. Davidson EB, Ritchey JW, Higbee RD, et al. Laser lithotripsy for treatment of canine uroliths. Vet Surg 2004;33:56–61.

30. Osborne CA, Lulich JP, Kruger JM, et al. Medical dissolution of feline struvite urocystoliths. J Am Vet Med Assoc 1990;196:1053–63.

31. Okafor CC, Pearl DL, Lefebvre SL, et al. Risk factors associated with struvite urolithiasis in dogs evaluated at general care veterinary hospitals in the United States. J Am Vet Med Assoc 2013;243:1737–45.

32. Bartges JW, Osborne CA, Pozin DJ. Recurrent sterile struvite urocystolithiasis in three related cocker spaniels. J Am Anim Hosp Assoc 1992;28:459–69.

33. Palma D, Langston C, Gisselman K, et al. Feline struvite urolithiasis. Compend Contin Educ Vet 2009;31:542–52.

34. Osborne CA, Polzin DJ, Abdullahi SU, et al. Struvite urolithiasis in animals and man: formation, detection, and dissolution. Adv Vet Sci Comp Med 1985;29: 1–101.

35. Rinkardt NE, Houston DM. Dissolution of infection-induced struvite bladder stones by using a noncalculolytic diet and antibiotic therapy. Can Vet J 2004; 45:838–40.

36. Bartges J, Moyers T. Evaluation of d,l-methionine and antimicrobial agents for dissolution of spontaneously-occurring infection-induced struvite urocystoliths in dogs. ACVIM Forum. Anaheim (CA); 2010.

37. Smith BH, Moodie SJ, Wensley S, et al. Differences in urinary pH and relative supersaturation values between senior and young adult cats. J Vet Intern Med 1997;11:127.

38. Buffington T. Struvite urolithiasis in cats. J Am Vet Med Assoc 1989;194:7–8.

39. Finco DR, Barsanti JA, Crowell WA. Characterization of magnesium-induced urinary disease in the cat and comparison with feline urologic syndrome. Am J Vet Res 1985;46:391–400.

40. Osborne CA, Kruger JM, Lulich JP, et al. Feline lower urinary tract diseases. In: Ettinger SJ, Feldman EC, editors. Textbook of veterinary internal medicine. 5th edition. Philadelphia: WB Saunders; 1999. p. 1710–46.

41. Buffington CA, Rogers QR, Morris JG. Effect of diet on struvite activity product in feline urine. Am J Vet Res 1990;51:2025–30.

42. Buffington CA, Blaisdell JL, Sako T. Effects of Tamm-Horsfall glycoprotein and albumin on struvite crystal growth in urine of cats. Am J Vet Res 1994;55:965–71.

43. Tarttelin MF. Feline struvite urolithiasis: factors affecting urine pH may be more important than magnesium levels in food. Vet Rec 1987;121:227–30.

44. Bartges JW, Tarver SL, Schneider C. Comparison of struvite activity product ratios and relative supersaturations in urine collected from healthy cats consuming four struvite management diets. Ralston Purina Nutrition Symposium. St. Louis (MO); 1998.

45. Smith BH, Stevenson AE, Markwell PJ. Urinary relative supersaturations of calcium oxalate and struvite in cats are influenced by diet. J Nutr 1998;128: 2763S–4S.

46. Finke MD, Litzenberger BA. Effect of food intake on urine pH in cats. J Small Anim Pract 1992;33:261–5.

47. Tarttelin MF. Feline struvite urolithiasis: fasting reduced the effectiveness of a urinary acidifier (ammonium chloride) and increased the intake of a low magnesium diet. Vet Rec 1987;121:245–8.

48. Roudebush P, Forrester SD, Padgelek T. What is the evidence? Therapeutic foods to treat struvite uroliths in cats instead of surgery. J Am Vet Med Assoc 2010;236:965–6.

49. Houston DM, Rinkardt NE, Hilton J. Evaluation of the efficacy of a commercial diet in the dissolution of feline struvite bladder uroliths. Vet Ther 2004;5: 187–201.
50. Lulich JP, Kruger JM, Macleay JM, et al. Efficacy of two commercially available, low-magnesium, urine-acidifying dry foods for the dissolution of struvite uroliths in cats. J Am Vet Med Assoc 2013;243:1147–53.
51. Bartges JW, Kirk CA, Cox SK, et al. Influence of acidifying or alkalinizing diets on bone mineral density and urine relative supersaturation with calcium oxalate and struvite in healthy cats. Am J Vet Res 2013;74:1347–52.
52. Kirk CA, Ling GV, Franti CE, et al. Evaluation of factors associated with development of calcium oxalate urolithiasis in cats. J Am Vet Med Assoc 1995;207: 1429–34.
53. Thumchai R, Lulich J, Osborne CA, et al. Epizootiologic evaluation of urolithiasis in cats: 3,498 cases (1982–1992). J Am Vet Med Assoc 1996;208:547–51.
54. Lekcharoensuk C, Lulich JP, Osborne CA, et al. Patient and environmental factors associated with calcium oxalate urolithiasis in dogs. J Am Vet Med Assoc 2000;217:515–9.
55. Balaji KC, Menon M. Mechanism of stone formation. Urol Clin North Am 1997;24: 1–11.
56. Bartges JW. Calcium oxalate urolithiasis. In: August JR, editor. Consultations in feline internal medicine. 4th edition. Philadelphia: WB Saunders; 2001. p. 352–64.
57. Lulich JP, Osborne CA, Koehler LA. Canine calcium oxalate urolithiasis: changing paradigms in detection, management and prevention. In: Hand MS, Thatcher CD, Remillard RL, et al, editors. Small animal clinical nutrition. 5th edition. Topeka (KS): Mark Morris Institute; 2010. p. 855–70.
58. Bartges JW, Kirk C, Lane IF. Update: management of calcium oxalate uroliths in dogs and cats. Vet Clin North Am Small Anim Pract 2004;34:969–87, vii.
59. Lulich JP, Osborne CA, Nagode LA, et al. Evaluation of urine and serum metabolites in miniature schnauzers with calcium oxalate urolithiasis. Am J Vet Res 1991;52:1583–90.
60. Ching SV, Fettman MJ, Hamar DW, et al. The effect of chronic dietary acidification using ammonium chloride on acid-base and mineral metabolism in the adult cat. J Nutr 1989;119:902–15.
61. Sutton RA, Wong NL, Dirks J. Effects of metabolic acidosis and alkalosis on sodium and calcium transport in the dog kidney. Kidney Int 1979;15:520–33.
62. McKerrell RE, Blakemore WF, Heath MF, et al. Primary hyperoxaluria (L-glyceric aciduria) in the cat: a newly recognised inherited disease. Vet Rec 1989;125: 31–4.
63. Gnanandarajah JS, Abrahante JE, Lulich JP, et al. Presence of *Oxalobacter formigenes* in the intestinal tract is associated with the absence of calcium oxalate urolith formation in dogs. Urol Res 2012;40:467–73.
64. Dijcker JC, Kummeling A, Hagen-Plantinga EA, et al. Urinary oxalate and calcium excretion by dogs and cats diagnosed with calcium oxalate urolithiasis. Vet Rec 2012;171:646.
65. Dijcker JC, Plantinga EA, van Baal J, et al. Influence of nutrition on feline calcium oxalate urolithiasis with emphasis on endogenous oxalate synthesis. Nutr Res Rev 2011;24:96–110.
66. Lulich JP, Osborne CA, Sanderson SL, et al. Voiding urohydropropulsion: lessons from 5 years of experience. Vet Clin North Am Small Anim Pract 1999;29:283–92.

67. Lulich JP, Osborne CA, Lekcharoensuk C, et al. Effects of diet on urine composition of cats with calcium oxalate urolithiasis. J Am Anim Hosp Assoc 2004;40: 185–91.
68. Kirk CA, Ling GV, Osborne CA, et al. Clinical guidelines for managing calcium oxalate uroliths in cats: medical therapy, hydration, and dietary therapy. In: Managing urolithiasis in cats: recent updates and practice guidelines. Topeka (KS): Hill's Pet Nutrition Inc; 2003. p. 10–9.
69. Lulich JP, Osborne CA, Sanderson SL. Effects of dietary supplementation with sodium chloride on urinary relative supersaturation with calcium oxalate in healthy dogs. Am J Vet Res 2005;66:319–24.
70. Stevenson AE, Hynds WK, Markwell PJ. Effect of dietary moisture and sodium content on urine composition and calcium oxalate relative supersaturation in healthy miniature schnauzers and Labrador retrievers. Res Vet Sci 2003;74: 145–51.
71. Xu H, Laflamme DP, Long GL. Effects of dietary sodium chloride on health parameters in mature cats. J Feline Med Surg 2009;11:435–41.
72. Chetboul V, Reynolds BS, Trehiou-Sechi E, et al. Cardiovascular effects of dietary salt intake in aged healthy cats: a 2-year prospective randomized, blinded, and controlled study. PLoS One 2014;9:e97862.
73. Lekcharoensuk C, Lulich JP, Osborne CA, et al. Association between patient-related factors and risk of calcium oxalate and magnesium ammonium phosphate urolithiasis in cats. J Am Vet Med Assoc 2000;217:520–5.
74. Stevenson AE, Wrigglesworth DJ, Smith BH, et al. Effects of dietary potassium citrate supplementation on urine pH and urinary relative supersaturation of calcium oxalate and struvite in healthy dogs. Am J Vet Res 2000;61:430–5.
75. Lekcharoensuk C, Osborne CA, Lulich JP, et al. Association between dietary factors and calcium oxalate and magnesium ammonium phosphate urolithiasis in cats. J Am Vet Med Assoc 2001;219:1228–37.
76. Robertson WG. Urinary calculi. In: Nordin BE, Need AG, Morris HA, editors. Metabolic bone and stone disease. Edinburgh (Scotland): Churchill Livingstone; 1993. p. 249–311.
77. Lulich JP, Osborne CA, Bartges JW, et al. Canine lower urinary tract disorders. In: Ettinger SJ, Feldman EC, editors. Textbook of veterinary internal medicine. 5th edition. Philadelphia: WB Saunders; 1999. p. 1747–83.
78. Terris MK, Issa MM, Tacker JR. Dietary supplementation with cranberry concentrate tablets may increase the risk of nephrolithiasis. Urology 2001;57:26–9.
79. Bai SC, Sampson DA, Morris JG, et al. Vitamin B_6 requirement of growing kittens. J Nutr 1989;119:1020–7.
80. Bartges JW, Osborne CA, Lulich JP, et al. Canine urate urolithiasis. Etiopathogenesis, diagnosis, and management. Vet Clin North Am Small Anim Pract 1999;29:161–91.
81. Bartges JW, Osborne CA, Lulich JP, et al. Prevalence of cystine and urate uroliths in bulldogs and urate uroliths in Dalmatians. J Am Vet Med Assoc 1994;204:1914–8.
82. Case LC, Ling GV, Ruby AL, et al. Urolithiasis in Dalmations: 275 cases (1981–1990). J Am Vet Med Assoc 1993;203:96–100.
83. Albasan H, Osborne CA, Lulich JP, et al. Risk factors for urate uroliths in cats. J Am Vet Med Assoc 2012;240:842–7.
84. Giesecke D, Kraft W, Tiemeyer W. Why Dalmatians excrete uric acid. Causes and consequences of a classical metabolic disorder. Tierarztl Prax 1985;13: 331–41.

85. Matsumoto M, Zhang CH, Kosugi C, et al. Gas chromatography-mass spectrometric studies of canine urinary metabolism. J Vet Med Sci 1995;57:205–11.
86. Williams AW, Wilson DM. Uric acid metabolism in humans. Semin Nephrol 1990; 10:9–14.
87. Giesecke D, Tiemeyer W. Defect of uric acid uptake in Dalmatian dog liver. Experientia 1984;40:1415–6.
88. Cohn R, Cibbell DG, Laub DR, et al. Renal allotransplantation and allantoin excretion of Dalmatian. Arch Surg 1965;91:911–2.
89. Bannasch D, Safra N, Young A, et al. Mutations in the SLC2A9 gene cause hyperuricosuria and hyperuricemia in the dog. PLoS Genet 2008;4:e1000246.
90. Karmi N, Safra N, Young A, et al. Validation of a urine test and characterization of the putative genetic mutation for hyperuricosuria in bulldogs and black Russian terriers. Am J Vet Res 2010;71:909–14.
91. Sorenson JL, Ling GV. Metabolic and genetic aspects of urate urolithiasis in Dalmatians. J Am Vet Med Assoc 1993;203:857–62.
92. Bartges JW, Osborne CA, Felice LJ, et al. Influence of four diets containing approximately 11% protein (dry weight) on uric acid, sodium urate, and ammonium urate urine activity product ratios of healthy beagles. Am J Vet Res 1995;56:60–5.
93. Bartges JW, Osborne CA, Felice LJ, et al. Diet effect on activity product ratios of uric acid, sodium urate, and ammonium urate in urine formed by healthy beagles. Am J Vet Res 1995;56:329–33.
94. Bartges JW, Osborne CA, Felice LJ, et al. Influence of chronic allopurinol administration on urine activity product ratios of uric acid, sodium urate, ammonium urate, and xanthine. J Vet Intern Med 1994;8:168A.
95. Bartges JW, Osborne CA, Felice LJ, et al. Influence of allopurinol and two diets on 24-hour urinary excretions of uric acid, xanthine, and ammonia by healthy dogs. Am J Vet Res 1995;56:595–9.
96. Bartges JW, Osborne CA, Koehler LA, et al. An algorithmic approach to canine urate uroliths. 12th Annual Veterinary Medical Forum of the American College of Veterinary Internal Medicine. San Francisco (CA); 1994;476–477.
97. Jacinto AM, Mellanby RJ, Chandler M, et al. Urine concentrations of xanthine, hypoxanthine and uric acid in UK Cavalier King Charles spaniels. J Small Anim Pract 2013;54:395–8.
98. van Zuilen CD, Nickel RF, van Dijk TH, et al. Xanthinuria in a family of Cavalier King Charles spaniels. Vet Q 1997;19:172–4.
99. Gow AG, Fairbanks LD, Simpson JW, et al. Xanthine urolithiasis in a Cavalier King Charles spaniel. Vet Rec 2011;169:209.
100. Hoppe A, Denneberg T. Cystinuria in the dog: clinical studies during 14 years of medical treatment. J Vet Intern Med 2001;15:361–7.
101. Osborne CA, Sanderson SL, Lulich JP, et al. Canine cystine urolithiasis. Cause, detection, treatment, and prevention. Vet Clin North Am Small Anim Pract 1999; 29:193–211.
102. Hoppe A, Denneberg T, Jeppsson JO, et al. Urinary excretion of amino acids in normal and cystinuric dogs. Br Vet J 1993;149:253–68.
103. Osborne CA, Lulich JP, Bartges JW, et al. Metabolic uroliths in cats. In: Kirk RW, Bonagura JD, editors. Current veterinary therapy XI. Philadelphia: WB Saunders Co; 1992. p. 909–10.
104. DiBartola SP, Chew DJ, Horton ML. Cystinuria in a cat. J Am Vet Med Assoc 1991;198:102–4.
105. Bovee KC, Thier SO, Rea C, et al. Renal clearance of amino acids in canine cystinuria. Metabolism 1974;23:51–8.

106. Tsan MF, Jones TC, Wilson TH. Canine cystinuria: intestinal and renal amino acid transport. Am J Vet Res 1972;33:2463–8.
107. Holtzapple PG, Rea C, Bovee K, et al. Characteristics of cystine and lysine transport in renal jejunal tissue from cystinuric dogs. Metabolism 1971;20: 1016–22.
108. Treacher RJ. Intestinal absorption of lysine in cystinuric dogs. J Comp Pathol 1965;75:309–22.
109. Mizukami K, Raj K, Giger U. Feline cystinuria caused by a missense mutation in the SLC3A1 gene. J Vet Intern Med 2015;29:120–5.
110. Brons AK, Henthorn PS, Raj K, et al. SLC3A1 and SLC7A9 mutations in autosomal recessive or dominant canine cystinuria: a new classification system. J Vet Intern Med 2013;27(6):1400–8.
111. Harnevik L, Hoppe A, Soderkvist P. SLC7A9 cDNA cloning and mutational analysis of SLC3A1 and SLC7A9 in canine cystinuria. Mamm Genome 2006;17: 769–76.
112. Henthorn PS, Liu J, Gidalevich T, et al. Canine cystinuria: polymorphism in the canine SLC3A1 gene and identification of a nonsense mutation in cystinuric Newfoundland dogs. Hum Genet 2000;107:295–303.
113. Sanderson SL, Osborne CA, Lulich JP, et al. Evaluation of urinary carnitine and taurine excretion in 5 cystinuric dogs with carnitine and taurine deficiency. J Vet Intern Med 2001;15:94–100.
114. Brand E, Cahill GF, Kassell B. Canine cystinuria V. Family history of cystinuric Irish terriers and cystine determinations in urine. J Biol Chem 1940;133:430.
115. Hoppe A, Denneberg T, Kågedal B. Treatment of clinically normal and cystinuric dogs with 2-mercaptopropionylglycine. Am J Vet Res 1988;49:923–8.

Micturition Disorders

Julie K. Byron, DVM, MS

KEYWORDS

- Incontinence • Dysuria • Urethral obstruction • Overactive bladder • Urine retention

KEY POINTS

- Differentiation of conscious versus unconscious voiding is important to determine the cause of micturition disorders.
- It is important to determine whether the clinical signs are caused by a disorder of storage or a disorder of voiding.
- Observation of the patient while urinating is key to diagnosing disorders of voiding.
- Patients with disorders of voiding have difficulty fully emptying the bladder and can have overflow incontinence.
- Patients with disorders of storage can have urinary incontinence or increased frequency of urination caused by decreased storage capability.

 Video of functional outflow obstruction accompanies this article at www. vetsmall.theclinics.com/

INTRODUCTION
Physiology of Micturition

The primary purpose of the lower urinary tract is to store urine and to facilitate its elimination at an appropriate time. The bladder is in storage phase 99% of the time and in emptying phase only 1% of the time. Coordination of storage and emptying requires a complex interaction between the somatic and autonomic nervous systems, as well as normal function of the organs and tissues involved.

All 3 components of the peripheral nervous system are involved in the micturition cycle (**Table 1**). In addition, conscious voiding involves the lumbar and sacral spinal cord as well as the brainstem and cerebral cortex (**Fig. 1**).

During filling and storage, stretch receptors in the bladder wall send afferent signals along the pelvic nerve, which activate a reflex arc through the hypogastric nerve to the urethra (**Fig. 2**). Norepinephrine is released by postganglionic neurons to activate

Disclosure: The author discloses that Merck Animal Health Division, manufacturers of estriol (Incurin, Merck) has supported her research in the past.
Department of Veterinary Clinical Sciences, College of Veterinary Medicine, The Ohio State University, 601 Vernon Tharp Street, Columbus, OH 43210, USA
E-mail address: byron.7@osu.edu

Vet Clin Small Anim 45 (2015) 769–782
http://dx.doi.org/10.1016/j.cvsm.2015.02.006
0195-5616/15/$ – see front matter © 2015 Elsevier Inc. All rights reserved.

Table 1
Peripheral nervous system components of micturition

Type (Receptor)	Location	Nerve	Function When Stimulated	Function When Blocked	Function When Inappropriately Stimulated	Function When Inappropriately Blocked
Parasympathetic (M_3 muscarinic)	Bladder body (detrusor)	Pelvic nerve (S1–S3)	Contraction and bladder emptying	Detrusor relaxation and bladder filling	Overactive bladder	Bladder atony, urine retention
Sympathetic (beta$_3$-adrenergic)	Bladder body (detrusor)	Hypogastric nerve (L1–L4)	Detrusor relaxation and filling	Detrusor contraction and urination	Urine retention	Decreased bladder compliance and increased filling pressure
Sympathetic (alpha$_1$-adrenergic)	Bladder neck/urethra	Hypogastric nerve (L1–L4)	Contraction and continence	Urination	Urine retention	Open urethra, incontinence
Somatic (nicotinic)	Distal urethra/pelvic floor	Pudendal nerve (S1–S2)	Conscious/reflex contraction and continence	Urination	Urine retention	Open urethra, incontinence

Storage Phase

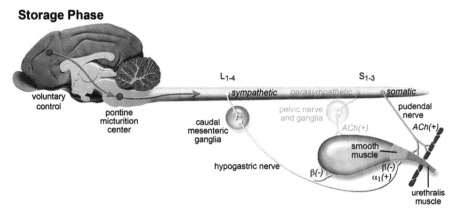

Fig. 1. Innervation and signal pathways during the storage phase of the micturition cycle. The symbol (+) denotes stimulation of muscular contraction, and (−) denotes inhibition of muscular contraction. ACh, acetylcholine-mediated receptors; α, alpha-adrenergic receptors; β, beta-adrenergic receptors; L_{1-4}, lumbar spinal cord segments 1 to 4; S_{1-3}, sacral spinal cord segments 1 to 3. (Drawing by Tim Vojt, MA. Used with permission from The Ohio State University.)

beta$_3$-adrenergic receptors in the bladder wall, allowing relaxation and continued filling. Norepinephrine also stimulates alpha$_1$-adrenergic receptors in the urethra and causes contraction of the urethral smooth muscle, thus preventing urine leakage. During initiation of micturition, stretch receptors send afferent signals along myelinated fibers of the pelvic nerve to the lumbar spinal cord and cranial to the pontine micturition center in the brain. Signals from the cerebral cortex and the hypothalamus are processed to determine whether the situation is appropriate for urination. If so, signals are sent down the pelvic nerve, which leads to acetylcholine release at the postganglionic parasympathetic neurons. Acetylcholine binds to M_3 receptors and stimulates bladder smooth muscle contraction. At the same time, inhibitory signals are sent to the sympathetic reflexes and the urethra relaxes, allowing normal emptying.

A local urethral reflex arc is the somatic-mediated contraction of the striated muscle surrounding the urethra in response to a sudden increase in abdominal pressure and movement of urine into the urethra, such as during a cough or sneeze.

Voiding Phase

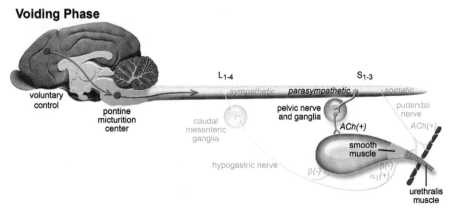

Fig. 2. Innervation and signal pathways during the voiding phase of the micturition cycle. (Drawing by Tim Vojt, MA. Used with permission from The Ohio State University.)

In addition to normal neurologic mechanisms, several other factors are important for the normal function of the micturition cycle in dogs and cats. The integrity of the smooth muscle of the urethra, normal urethral mucosa that creates a watertight seal, associated vasculature, and the support of connective tissues are also key.[1,2] In females, estrogen seems to have a significant impact on these tissues.[3,4] Its decline after neutering seems to play a role in the urethral sphincter mechanism incompetence (USMI) seen in neutered female dogs.[5,6] Alternatively, prostatic hyperplasia in intact male dogs can lead to functional urethral obstruction and urinary retention.

Disorders of Storage

Storage disorders primarily occur because of an inability to maintain adequate urethral tone if there are normal or increased bladder pressures. These disorders may result from an anatomic or developmental abnormality or acquired dysfunction in the spinal cord, urinary bladder, or urethra and surrounding tissues. Disorders of storage generally result in the unconscious loss of urine: urinary incontinence. These disorders include USMI, lower motor neuron bladder (LMB), and overactive bladder (OAB).

Urethral Sphincter Mechanism Incompetence

USMI is the most common storage disorder in dogs.[7] The urethral sphincter mechanism involves the smooth muscle of the urethra as well as the surrounding support tissues, submucosal vasculature, and urothelium. USMI is thought to result from the breakdown in this complex through reduced muscular responsiveness and tone, and structural changes in the periurethral tissues. In female dogs these changes seem to be associated with a reduction in estrogen and alterations in follicle-stimulating hormone and luteinizing hormone after neutering; hence the term hormone-responsive incontinence.[8,9] The pathophysiology of its development in male dogs is poorly understood; however, there may be a relationship with decreased testosterone levels, and increased follicle-stimulating hormone and luteinizing hormone levels, because it appears more frequently in neutered than in intact males.[10,11]

USMI is most common among neutered female dogs. It is less common in neutered males and rare in cats.[11] It seems to affect up to 20% of neutered females and up to 30% of large breed dogs weighing more than 20 kg. Several breeds have been found to have increased risk, including the Doberman pinscher, giant schnauzer, Old English sheepdog, rottweiler, Weimaraner, and boxer, but any breed may be affected.[12] Recent literature has shown an increased risk of development of USMI in dogs neutered before 3 months of age.[13,14] However, this finding remains controversial because other studies have found no relationship with age at neuter.[15] It is possible that this is related to the development and sensitivity of the sphincter mechanism tissues to estrogen and other hormones, but the mechanism is incompletely understood.

Predisposing factors such as a pelvic bladder, short urethra, or recessed vulva may also be associated with increased risk of developing USMI; however, the presence of one of these does not necessarily lead to incontinence. A reduction in pressure transmission from the abdomen to the proximal urethra has the potential to lead to urinary incontinence in animals with a short urethra or pelvic bladder by setting up a negative pressure gradient from the bladder to the urethra.

Clinical Presentation and Diagnosis of Urethral Sphincter Mechanism Incompetence

Signs of incontinence may begin at any time, but appear most often within a few years of neutering. Dogs with USMI usually have normal bladder capacity and are able to urinate normally with complete emptying of the bladder. Although most of these dogs are otherwise healthy, clinical signs can worsen dramatically if comorbidities develop, leading to polyuria or difficulty posturing to urinate. The increased volumes of urine in the bladder, and for longer periods of time, may lead to increased pressure on the already weakened sphincter mechanism and leakage. Lower urinary tract infection (UTI) can also lead to increased frequency of clinical signs. It is suspected that USMI, and urinary incontinence of any cause, is associated with increased risk of UTI; however, no studies have been conducted to fully evaluate this.

Owners often seek veterinary care when the frequency becomes bothersome, although, in the author's experience, the incontinence may have been present for months or years. It is essential to establish that the animal is passing urine unconsciously. Many owners complain of incontinence when the animal is showing submissive urination or is otherwise consciously urinating in inappropriate places. Dogs with USMI may leak urine when recumbent, sleeping, or after exertion. Although the passage of urine is involuntary, dogs may increase grooming of the perivulvar or preputial area. USMI is an acquired condition, so questioning of the owner regarding the onset of clinical signs is important. Animals that have been incontinent from birth or before neutering should be assessed for congenital malformations such as ectopic ureters before making a diagnosis of USMI.

Physical examination of these animals is often normal, with the exception of perivulvar or preputial urine staining. As mentioned earlier, the conformation of the vulva should be noted, although its contribution to USMI is unclear. The presence of perivulvar dermatitis, regardless of conformation, may increase the risk of UTI. Rectal examination and palpation of the urethra are usually normal. Urination is observed to be normal and complete, with little or no residual volume. The assessment of residual urine is essential in male dogs to differentiate USMI from detrusor urethral dyssynergia, which is a disorder of incomplete bladder emptying (discussed later).

The presence of urinary incontinence in an otherwise healthy neutered female dog that was previously continent is often adequate for presumptive diagnosis of USMI and a trial of empiric therapy. Because of its lower incidence, intact females, intact or neutered males, and cats with similar histories and clinical signs require additional evaluation before making a diagnosis of USMI.

The animal should be observed urinating, if possible. Normal posturing and a full stream without stranguria should be noted. Assessment of residual urine volume may be made by bladder catheterization or estimated using abdominal ultrasonography of the bladder. A urinalysis and urine culture should be performed. The presence of isosthenuria or hyposthenuria may contribute to severity of incontinence and may require additional evaluation for an underlying cause. Animals with polyuria may not respond to medical treatment as well as those making normal volumes of urine. As noted earlier, the risk of UTI in animals with USMI has not been evaluated, but its presence may lead to worsening signs. Therefore, screening for, and treating of, an infection may increase therapeutic success. A complete blood count and serum biochemistry panel may be indicated but are not always necessary for diagnosis of USMI, although they may be helpful when making therapeutic choices, and are important in evaluating animals with polyuria.

If anatomic abnormalities are suspected, imaging, such as contrast radiography, abdominal ultrasonography, or contrast computed tomography, is indicated. Cystoscopic evaluation of the lower urinary tract allows assessment of the entire urethra, ureter placement, and bladder mucosa. It also allows detailed investigation of vestibular and vaginal conformation. Advanced diagnostics, such as urodynamic studies, are designed to quantify the pressure produced along the urethra and the compliance and detrusor function of the urinary bladder. These diagnostics are available at many referral institutions and are most often indicated in patients with equivocal signs and poor response to therapy.

Medical Treatment of Urethral Sphincter Mechanism Incompetence

Medical therapy for USMI is generally considered the first line of management; only after failure or intolerance of medical therapy are surgical options considered. Medical treatment of USMI in neutered female dogs consists of increasing the number and sensitivity to estrogen of alpha receptors in the urethral sphincter, or stimulating those receptors with an alpha-agonist (**Table 2**).

The most commonly used estrogens are diethylstilbestrol (DES) and estriol (Incurin, Merck Animal Health, Madison, NJ). DES is not available commercially so it must be compounded. Adverse effects associated with estrogen use include mammary gland development, vulvar swelling, and attractiveness to males.[16] These effects are usually dose related and subside with dose reduction. A more serious adverse event associated with estrogen use is irreversible bone marrow suppression.[17] It is considered standard of care to monitor the complete blood count in animals receiving estrogen compounds; however, the doses most associated with bone marrow suppression are much higher than those recommended to treat USMI. The author recommends performing a complete blood count before starting treatment with an estrogen compound, and then rechecking it 1 month into treatment. Estriol seems to have a higher response rate among female dogs than DES (89% and 65% respectively).[16,18]

Phenylpropanolamine (PPA; Proin, PRN Pharmacal, Pensacola, FL) is the most widely used alpha-agonist for the treatment of USMI. It is commercially available in sizes designed for use in dogs. The dose and frequency needed for each animal tend to vary widely and may need to be increased over time to maintain continence. Adverse effects associated with PPA include restlessness, aggression, changes in sleeping patterns, and gastrointestinal signs. These effects are also usually alleviated by a reduction in dose or frequency.[19,20] Clinical response to PPA administration ranges from 75% to 90%.[20,21] Both an estrogen and PPA are often used in the same patient for severe or refractory incontinence. There is little evidence supporting a synergistic increase in efficacy; however, there are anecdotal reports of greater improvement than on a single-medication regimen.[22]

PPA is also frequently used in male dogs and cats with USMI. In addition, neutered male dogs may be treated with testosterone cypionate as monthly injections however its efficacy is not well documented. Although male dogs with USMI are most responsive to PPA, it is at a rate of only 43% showing good to excellent response, which is much lower than in female dogs.[11] Estrogen compounds should not be used in males because of the risk of prostatic metaplasia and feminization. They are rarely used in cats, and care should be taken to monitor the mammary glands for neoplasia in cats receiving estrogens.

Surgical Treatment of Urethral Sphincter Mechanism Incompetence

In patients that fail medical therapy, it may be necessary to consider surgical intervention. Surgery is generally only pursued if the animal does not respond to, or cannot tolerate, medical treatment. Several surgical procedures have been used to treat USMI, many based on the theory of increasing the transmission of abdominal pressure to the proximal urethra. These procedures include colposuspension, transobturator vaginal tape, and urethropexy. These procedures have had variable outcomes and are considered to have poor long-term efficacy, particularly in animals with normal bladder position.[23] The most promising surgical procedure for USMI is placement of an artificial urethral sphincter that may be adjusted via a subcutaneous port. Recent studies have shown it to lead to a significant increase in continence in male and female dogs that had failed medical therapy for USMI.[24–26]

Table 2
Drugs frequently used to treat USMI

Drug	Class	Dose	Side Effects	Caution
Phenylpropanolamine	Alpha-agonist	1.0–1.5 mg/kg PO q 8–12 h	Hypertension, aggression, restlessness, gastrointestinal upset, anxiety	Hypertension, hyperadrenocorticism, renal disease
DES	Estrogen	0.1–1.0 mg/dog PO q 24 h for 5–7 d then weekly or as needed	Myelosuppression (rare at these doses), attractiveness to males, mammary/vulvar swelling, behavior changes	Males (can develop prostatic metaplasia)
Conjugated estrogen	Estrogen	0.02 mg/kg PO q 24 h for 5–7 d then q 2–4 d as needed	Same as DES	Same as DES
Estriol	Estrogen	2 mg/dog PO q 24 h × 14 d, then reduce to 1 mg q 24 h	Same as DES	Same as DES
Testosterone cypionate	Androgen	2.2 mg/kg IM q 4–8 wk	Behavior change, aggression, perianal adenoma, prostatic hyperplasia	Cardiac disease, renal disease, hepatic disease, prostatic disease

Abbreviations: DES, diethylstilbestrol; IM, intramuscular; PO, orally; q, every.
Data from Papich MG. Saunders handbook of veterinary drugs, small and large animal. 3rd edition. Philadelphia: Elsevier; 2010.

In the past, injectable urethral bulking agents have been used, particularly bovine cross-linked collagen, to increase resting urethral pressure in dogs with USMI. In 2009 the manufacturers of the most commonly used product removed it from the market, so, at the time of writing, injectable bulking agent therapy for USMI is considered unavailable, except in some research studies.

Lower Motor Neuron Bladder

Incontinence as a disorder of storage can also occur secondary to spinal cord injury or disease. Lesions in the S1 to S2 region lead to weakness of the striated muscular sphincter. Disruption of the local reflex arc at these segments leads to an easily expressible bladder that may empty with minor increases in abdominal pressure. These animals are identified by decreased anal tone and a poor perineal reflex as well as their easily expressible bladder. Most of these animals are unable to voluntarily void and require intermittent catheterization or manual expression by the owner. Correction of the underlying cause may lead to some return to normal function. Because of the tendency to have incomplete emptying of the bladder with manual expression, these animals are at increased risk of developing UTI and appropriate monitoring must be in place. The muscarinic agonist bethanechol has been used in these patients to increase detrusor contraction; however, the evidence for its efficacy remains controversial.[27,28]

Detrusor Hyperreflexia/Overactive Bladder

Detrusor hyperreflexia/OAB is the most common form of urinary incontinence in people, but it has been poorly characterized in domestic species. The incidence of OAB and its importance as a cause of urinary incontinence in dogs and cats are unknown. In people it is characterized by sudden urgency to urinate and involuntary loss of urine associated with bursts of detrusor contractions at bladder volumes far less than capacity. In dogs it may manifest as an animal that loses bladder compliance and capacity and thus may need to urinate more often than before without an increase in urine production or inflammation of the lower urinary tract. OAB may be a cause of treatment failure in some dogs treated for USMI, and should be considered in these cases. Diagnosis of OAB in animals can be challenging and is only definitively made using urodynamic studies such as cystometrography. Response to therapy with antimuscarinic drugs is often used to presumptively diagnose OAB in veterinary species. The most commonly used include oxybutynin and imipramine, the latter of which also has alpha-agonist effects, potentially increasing urethral sphincter tone. Adverse effects of these medications include gastrointestinal abnormalities such as diarrhea and constipation, as well as parasympatholytic signs like tachycardia and hyposalivation.

Disorders of Emptying

The inability to completely empty the bladder during a normal void can result from either a functional or mechanical obstruction of the outflow tract and urethra, or an abnormality of the detrusor muscle that impairs its complete contraction. Overflow incontinence can result from the lack of complete emptying, often when the animal is at rest. An owner may not be able to differentiate this from an animal with a storage disorder (eg, USMI), and it is up to the clinician to determine the underlying process so that appropriate therapy can be instituted. Inability to completely empty the bladder is a risk factor for UTI, and these animals should be monitored for infection.

Detrusor Atony

Complete emptying of the urinary bladder depends on the normal contraction of the detrusor muscle. In the normal animal, the bladder relaxes during filling with only small increases in intravesical pressure. As the bladder continues to fill, the pressure increases to a threshold that triggers a detrusor contraction and emptying. Loss of adequate detrusor contraction can result from neurogenic or nonneurogenic abnormalities. Injury to the sacral spinal cord S1 to S3 or pelvic nerves can lead to bladder atony, and is often associated with weakened urethral tone. These animals often have decreased perineal reflexes and easily expressed bladders (LMB). Treatment of the underlying lesion, if possible, may lead to improved voiding function. However, until normal function returns, careful management of urination must be followed. Male dogs are manually expressed or aseptically catheterized 2 to 4 times a day either in the hospital or at home, and cats and female dogs are often manually expressed.

Direct damage to the detrusor muscle can occur from overdistension caused by mechanical or functional outflow obstruction of an acute or chronic nature. The muscle fibers of the detrusor transmit action potentials that initiate contraction via tight junctions. With overdistension, these tight junctions are interrupted, leading to an absent or ineffective contraction. The overdistension may be acute, as with obstructive feline idiopathic cystitis in a male cat, or chronic, as with a dog with a functional obstruction of the urethra. Relief of the obstruction and maintenance of a small bladder volume for up to 2 weeks may allow the junctions to reestablish and the return of coordinated detrusor function. This condition is usually managed by either indwelling or frequent sterile catheterization of the bladder. Bethanechol may be used in these patients to enhance stimulation of the detrusor contraction because the pelvic nerve is intact. Other medications that have been shown to enhance detrusor function are cisapride and metoclopramide; however, the individual response varies widely.[29,30] It is essential that relief of any urethral obstruction, functional or mechanical, be attained before starting medical therapy to enhance detrusor contraction.

Functional Obstruction: Detrusor Urethral Dyssynergy

Functional urethral obstruction, or detrusor urethral dyssynergy (DUD), arises from an abnormality in the reflex arc that allows the urethral sphincter to relax at the initiation of detrusor contraction and urination. The lesion is thought to be in the reticulospinal tract, Onuf nucleus, or the caudal mesenteric ganglion, and it is possible that the lesion involves the loss of inhibitory signals to the pudendal and hypogastric nerves.[31] It is unknown whether there is a more local lesion to the nerves, the neuromuscular junction, or the smooth or striated urethral sphincters.[32] Unlike the upper motor neuron bladder seen in animals with thoracolumbar intervertebral disc disease and other spinal cord lesions, these animals typically have an otherwise normal neurologic examination.

The disorder affects primarily middle-aged large and giant-breed male dogs, although female dogs and cats can be affected. One case series of 22 dogs reported a mean age of 4.9 years.[33] Clinical signs are similar to those of mechanical obstruction. The animal often postures to urinate and is able to produce a urine stream that quickly becomes attenuated or stops completely. The animal may continue to posture to urinate or make several attempts without fully emptying the bladder (Video 1). The presence of large amounts of residual urine typically leads to overflow incontinence and may be mistaken for USMI. This leakage can occur because the hypertonicity of the involved sphincter is often dynamic and is triggered by the act of voiding. In chronic cases, bladder overdistension and subsequent atony may develop. Unlike animals with mechanical obstruction, these dogs are typically easy to catheterize and usually do not show increases in urethral pressure on urodynamic evaluation unless actively voiding. Contrast urethrography may be normal or reveal areas of narrowing of the urethra (urethrospasm).

Presumptive diagnosis of DUD is often made by observing the dog urinate with a typical interrupted pattern, documentation of a large residual urine volume, easy passage of a urinary catheter, and ruling out of a mechanical obstruction. Normal residual urine volumes in 48 normal dogs were reported to be 0.1 to 3.4 mL/kg body weight with a mean of 0.2 mL/kg.[34] The author uses less than 0.5 mL/kg as a general guideline. Ultrasonography is recommended to assess the ureters and renal pelves for dilatation secondary to chronic obstruction and ureterorenal reflux of urine. Additional diagnostics, including contrast urethrography, urethroscopy, or urodynamic evaluation, may be necessary to verify the diagnosis in patients that fail to respond to medical therapy.

Treatment of the hypertonic urethral sphincter generally consists of alpha-adrenergic blockade with prazosin, an $alpha_1$-specific antagonist with demonstrated effects on both the internal and external urethral sphincters.[35] Tamsulosin, which is specific for the $alpha_{1A}$ subtype found in the internal urethral sphincter, has also been successful in these dogs. Some dogs require additional therapy if the striated muscle is more significantly affected. Benzodiazepines, such as diazepam, or other skeletal muscle relaxants, including acepromazine and methocarbamol, may be more effective if the external urethral sphincter is involved. Diazepam is typically administered 30 minutes before voiding to decrease external urethral sphincter pressure. Dantrolene and baclofen have been used in the past as skeletal muscle relaxants; however, the potential for adverse effects has decreased their use in veterinary patients.[35,36] In severe and refractory cases, intermittent sterile catheterization by the owner at home may be necessary. Medical therapy for associated bladder atony should only be started after adequate relief of the functional urethral obstruction has been reached (**Table 3**). Close monitoring of these patients for residual urine volume and UTI is needed to assess the efficacy of treatment and prevent complications.

Prognosis for recovery of normal voiding is good, but most dogs require lifelong therapy for DUD. Attempts to taper medications to the lowest effective dose may be hampered by relapse of clinical signs after months of normal voiding.[33] Prognosis seems to be worse in patients with bladder atony or UTI secondary to urine retention. Anecdotally, urethral stenting may improve clinical signs; however, this is considered a salvage procedure with several potential complications, and is indicated only in the most refractory of cases.

Functional Obstruction: Upper Motor Neuron Bladder

Neurogenic functional urethral obstruction is generally caused by spinal cord lesions cranial to the sacral segment, which leads to loss of inhibitory signals to the hypogastric and pudendal nerves, which prevents sphincter relaxation on voiding. This condition is the classic upper motor neuron bladder in which the patient is unable to urinate normally and is difficult to manually express. The most commonly affected patients are those with intervertebral disc disease and associated paresis. These animals typically have additional neurologic deficits, including paresis and nociceptive loss. Treatment of the underlying lesion typically leads to partial or complete return to normal voiding function after days to weeks. Until normal voiding resumes, the patients are managed as for DUD with alpha-adrenergic blockade and manual expression or catheterization. Monitoring for overdistension and UTI is critical in these patients, as is nursing care, particularly because the overflow incontinence that can accompany this process may lead to skin breakdown in these recumbent patients.

Table 3
Drugs frequently used to treat disorders of emptying

Drug	Mechanism	Dose	Side Effects/Caution
Prazosin	Alpha₁-antagonism, smooth muscle relaxant	1 mg/animal <15 kg q 8–12 h PO 2 mg/animal >15 kg q 8–12 h PO	Hypotension, weakness, syncope, GI upset/renal disease, cardiac disease
Tamsulosin[a]	Alpha₁ₐ-antagonism, smooth muscle relaxant	0.01–0.2 mg/kg PO q 24 h	Hypotension
Phenoxybenzamine	Nonspecific Alpha-antagonism, smooth muscle relaxant	Dog: 0.25 mg/kg q 8–12 h Cat: 1.25–7.5 mg/cat q 8–12 h PO	Hypotension, tachycardia, miosis/first dose hypotension
Acepromazine	Nonspecific Alpha-antagonism Skeletal muscle relaxant Anxiolytic	Dog: 0.5–2.2 mg/kg q 6–8 h PO Cat: 1.1–2.2 mg/kg q 6–8 h PO	Sedation, hypotension
Diazepam	Skeletal muscle relaxant Anxiolytic	Dog: 0.5–2 mg/kg q 8 h PO or 30 min before voiding	Sedation, ataxia/liver dysfunction Do not use in cats
Methocarbamol	Skeletal muscle relaxant	22–44 mg/kg q 8 h PO	CNS sedation, weakness, hypersalivation
Baclofen[a]	Skeletal muscle relaxant	Dog: 1–2 mg/kg q 8 h PO	Weakness, GI upset; do not use in cats
Dantrolene	Skeletal muscle relaxant	Dog: 1–5 mg/kg q 8 h PO Cat: 1–2 mg/kg q 8 h PO	Weakness/liver disease
Bethanechol	Parasympathomimetic	Dog: 2.5–15 mg/dog q 8 h PO Cat: 1.25–5 mg/cat q 8 h PO	Diarrhea/GI or urethral obstruction
Cisapride	Prokinetic	Dog: 0.1–0.5 mg/kg q 8–12 h PO Cat: 2.5–5 mg/cat q 8–12 h PO	Ataxia, GI upset/GI obstruction

Abbreviations: CNS, central nervous system; GI, gastrointestinal.
[a] *From* Lane IF, Westropp JL, Urinary incontinence and micturition disorders: pharmacologic management, Kirk's Current Veterinary Therapy. 14th edition. St Louis (MO): Elsevier; 2009. p. 955–9.
Data from Papich MG. Saunders handbook of veterinary drugs, small and large animal. 3rd edition. Philadelphia: Elsevier; 2010.

Dysautonomia

Dysautonomia is a rare condition involving the degeneration of the neurons of the autonomic nervous ganglia, leading to sympathetic and parasympathetic dysfunction. It has been most commonly reported in both dogs and cats in the United Kingdom and Scandinavia, but small clusters of cases in both species have been seen in the United State.[37] Its underlying cause is unknown, but neurotoxin exposure is strongly suspected. In addition to the classic findings of unresponsive mydriasis and prolapsed nictitans, the abnormalities seen with dysautonomia can range from ileus and constipation to decreased systolic function of the heart. These dogs and cats often have significant voiding dysfunction and urine retention caused by bladder atony and overflow incontinence secondary to urethral sphincter incompetence. There is no specific treatment of dysautonomia and spontaneous remission is uncommon. The prognosis is related to the severity of the clinical signs and the specific organ functions affected. Management of the urinary complications is usually possible, involving bladder expression and/or urethral catheterization, along with parasympathomimetic agents. It is the challenging management of the gastrointestinal components of the disease that often leads to euthanasia.

SUMMARY

The accurate determination of a micturition disorder as one of storage or voiding is essential to selecting appropriate medical and surgical therapy. Differentiation between conscious and unconscious voiding, as well as observation of the patient urinating, can greatly increase success in diagnosis and management of these disorders. Therapy often relies on pharmacologic manipulation of neurologic control of storage and voiding, with surgical options pursued if medical management is unsuccessful.

SUPPLEMENTARY DATA

Supplementary data related to this article can be found online at http://dx.doi.org/10.1016/j.cvsm.2015.02.006.

REFERENCES

1. Robinson D, Cardozo LD. The role of estrogens in female lower urinary tract dysfunction. Urology 2003;62(4 Suppl 1):45–51.
2. Schreiter F, Fuchs P, Stockamp K. Estrogenic sensitivity of alpha-receptors in the urethra musculature. Urol Int 1976;31(1–2):13–9.
3. Augsburger HR, Oswald M. Immunohistochemical analysis of collagen types I, III, IV and alpha-actin in the urethra of sexually intact and ovariectomized beagles. Int Urogynecol J Pelvic Floor Dysfunct 2007;18(9):1071–5.
4. Byron JK, Graves TK, Becker MD, et al. Evaluation of the ratio of collagen type III to collagen type I in periurethral tissues of sexually intact and neutered female dogs. Am J Vet Res 2010;71(6):697–700.
5. Veronesi MC, Rota A, Battocchio M, et al. Spaying-related urinary incontinence and oestrogen therapy in the bitch. Acta Vet Hung 2009;57(1):171–82.
6. Augsburger HR, Fuhrer C. Immunohistochemical analysis of estrogen receptors in the urethra of sexually intact, ovariectomized, and estrogen-substituted ovariectomized sheep. Int Urogynecol J 2014;25(5):657–62.

7. Noel S, Claeys S, Hamaide A. Acquired urinary incontinence in the bitch: update and perspectives from human medicine. Part 2: the urethral component, pathophysiology and medical treatment. Vet J 2010;186(1):18–24.

8. Arnold S, Hubler M, Reichler I. Urinary incontinence in spayed bitches: new insights into the pathophysiology and options for medical treatment. Reprod Domest Anim 2009;44(Suppl 2):190–2.

9. Reichler IM, Hubler M, Jochle W, et al. The effect of GnRH analogs on urinary incontinence after ablation of the ovaries in dogs. Theriogenology 2003;60(7):1207–16.

10. Power SC, Eggleton KE, Aaron AJ, et al. Urethral sphincter mechanism incompetence in the male dog: importance of bladder neck position, proximal urethral length and castration. J Small Anim Pract 1998;39(2):69–72.

11. Aaron A, Eggleton K, Power C, et al. Urethral sphincter mechanism incompetence in male dogs: a retrospective analysis of 54 cases. Vet Rec 1996;139(22):542–6.

12. Holt PE, Thrusfield MV. Association in bitches between breed, size, neutering and docking, and acquired urinary incontinence due to incompetence of the urethral sphincter mechanism. Vet Rec 1993;133(8):177–80.

13. Thrusfield MV, Holt PE, Muirhead RH. Acquired urinary incontinence in bitches: its incidence and relationship to neutering practices. J Small Anim Pract 1998;39(12):559–66.

14. Stocklin-Gautschi NM, Hassig M, Reichler IM, et al. The relationship of urinary incontinence to early spaying in bitches. J Reprod Fertil Suppl 2001;57:233–6.

15. Beauvais W, Cardwell JM, Brodbelt DC. The effect of neutering on the risk of urinary incontinence in bitches - a systematic review. J Small Anim Pract 2012;53(4):198–204.

16. Mandigers PJ, Nell T. Treatment of bitches with acquired urinary incontinence with oestriol. Vet Rec 2001;149(25):764–7.

17. Sontas HB, Dokuzeylu B, Turna O, et al. Estrogen-induced myelotoxicity in dogs: a review. Can Vet J 2009;50(10):1054–8.

18. Nendick PA, Clark WT. Medical therapy of urinary incontinence in ovariectomised bitches: a comparison of the effectiveness of diethylstilboestrol and pseudoephedrine. Aust Vet J 1987;64(4):117–8.

19. Hill K, Jordan D, Ray J, et al. Medical therapy for acquired urinary incontinence in dogs. Int J Pharm Compd 2012;16(5):369–75.

20. Byron JK, March PA, Chew DJ, et al. Effect of phenylpropanolamine and pseudoephedrine on the urethral pressure profile and continence scores of incontinent female dogs. J Vet Intern Med 2007;21(1):47–53.

21. Scott L, Leddy M, Bernay F, et al. Evaluation of phenylpropanolamine in the treatment of urethral sphincter mechanism incompetence in the bitch. J Small Anim Pract 2002;43(11):493–6.

22. Hamaide AJ, Grand JG, Farnir F, et al. Urodynamic and morphologic changes in the lower portion of the urogenital tract after administration of estriol alone and in combination with phenylpropanolamine in sexually intact and spayed female dogs. Am J Vet Res 2006;67(5):901–8.

23. Rawlings C, Barsanti JA, Mahaffey MB, et al. Evaluation of colposuspension for treatment of incontinence in spayed female dogs. J Am Vet Med Assoc 2001;219(6):770–5.

24. Delisser PJ, Friend EJ, Chanoit GP, et al. Static hydraulic urethral sphincter for treatment of urethral sphincter mechanism incompetence in 11 dogs. J Small Anim Pract 2012;53(6):338–43.

25. Reeves L, Adin C, McLoughlin M, et al. Outcome after placement of an artificial urethral sphincter in 27 dogs. Vet Surg 2013;42(1):12–8.

26. Currao RL, Berent AC, Weisse C, et al. Use of a percutaneously controlled urethral hydraulic occluder for treatment of refractory urinary incontinence in 18 female dogs. Vet Surg 2013;42(4):440–7.

27. Noel S, Massart L, Hamaide A. Urodynamic investigation by telemetry in Beagle dogs: validation and effects of oral administration of current urological drugs: a pilot study. BMC Vet Res 2013;9:197.

28. Buranakarl C, Kijtawornrat A, Angkanaporn K, et al. Effects of bethanechol on canine urinary bladder smooth muscle function. Res Vet Sci 2001;71(3):175–81.

29. Mitchell WC, Venable DD. Effects of metoclopramide on detrusor function. J Urol 1985;134(4):791–4.

30. Kullmann FA, Kurihara R, Ye L, et al. Effects of the 5-HT4 receptor agonist, cisapride, on neuronally evoked responses in human bladder, urethra, and ileum. Auton Neurosci 2013;176(1–2):70–7.

31. de Groat WC, Fraser MO, Yoshiyama M, et al. Neural control of the urethra. Scand J Urol Nephrol Suppl 2001;(207):35–43 [discussion: 106–25].

32. Gookin JL, Bunch SE. Detrusor-striated sphincter dyssynergia in a dog. J Vet Intern Med 1996;10(5):339–44.

33. Espineira MM, Viehoff FW, Nickel RF. Idiopathic detrusor urethral dyssynergia in dogs: a retrospective analysis of 22 cases. J Small Anim Pract 1998;39(6):264–70.

34. Atalan G, Barr FJ, Holt PE. Frequency of urination and ultrasonographic estimation of residual urine in normal and dysuric dogs. Res Vet Sci 1999;67(3):295–9.

35. Fischer JR, Lane IF, Cribb AE. Urethral pressure profile and hemodynamic effects of phenoxybenzamine and prazosin in non-sedated male beagle dogs. Can J Vet Res 2003;67(1):30–8.

36. Khorzad R, Lee JA, Whelan M, et al. Baclofen toxicosis in dogs and cats: 145 cases (2004–2010). J Am Vet Med Assoc 2012;241(8):1059–64.

37. Kidder AC, Johannes C, O'Brien DP, et al. Feline dysautonomia in the Midwestern United States: a retrospective study of nine cases. J Feline Med Surg 2008;10(2):130–6.

Feline Idiopathic Cystitis

S. Dru Forrester, DVM, MS[a],*, Todd L. Towell, DVM, MS[b]

KEYWORDS

- Lower urinary tract signs • Diagnosis • Evidence-based treatment • Stress
- Nutrition • Environmental enrichment

KEY POINTS

- Complex interactions between the bladder, neuroendocrine system, and the cat's environment seem to be involved in the pathogenesis of feline idiopathic cystitis (FIC).
- FIC is diagnosed by excluding other causes of LUT signs.
- For cats with FIC, the highest grade of evidence supports nutritional management with a multipurpose therapeutic urinary food, environmental enrichment, and feeding moist food.

INTRODUCTION—DEFINITION/TERMINOLOGY

It has been said that a well-defined problem is half solved. Perhaps feline idiopathic cystitis (FIC) remains the most common cause of feline lower urinary tract (LUT) signs, in part, because it is so difficult to define. Historically, the term feline urologic syndrome was used to describe cats with the typical clinical signs of LUT dysfunction as well as partial or complete urethral obstruction.[1] In the early 1990s, results of studies focused on identifying abnormalities of the LUT led to the suggestion that affected cats represented a naturally occurring model of interstitial cystitis (IC), a chronic LUT syndrome in people. By 1996, the term "feline interstitial cystitis" was proposed to describe cats with idiopathic LUT signs.[2] Although it remains a diagnosis of exclusion, studies over the last 2 decades suggest that FIC is a result of complex interactions between the urinary bladder, nervous system, adrenal glands, husbandry practices, and the environment in which the cat lives.[3] This syndrome is further complicated by the fact that signs can be acute or chronic and have been associated with various combinations of abnormalities in the lumen of the LUT, the LUT itself, and other organ systems that cause LUT dysfunction.[4] Comorbid conditions related to the gastrointestinal tract, respiratory system, skin, central nervous system, cardiovascular

Disclosures: S.D. Forrester is a full-time employee at Hill's Pet Nutrition, and T.L. Towell is a former employee of Hill's Pet Nutrition.
[a] Department of Global Professional & Veterinary Affairs, Hill's Pet Nutrition Inc, 400 Southwest 8th Avenue, Topeka, KS 66603, USA; [b] Global Veterinary Consulting, Erie, CO 80516, USA
* Corresponding author.
E-mail address: Dru_Forrester@hillspet.com

system, and the immune system are also recognized in cats with FIC.[5-9] Despite decades of research, it is still unclear if FIC is a single disease entity or a syndrome with multiple causes. The increasing evidence for multisystem involvement and evolving complexity of this diagnosis has recently led one investigator to suggest use of the term "Pandora syndrome."[4] A diagnosis of Pandora syndrome would apply to those cats that exhibit the following:

- Signs of LUT dysfunction and clinical signs in other organ systems
- Waxing and waning of clinical signs associated with stressful events
- Undergone resolution of severity of clinical signs following effective environmental enrichment

It is postulated that by broadening the name used to describe cats with chronic FIC, clinicians will be encouraged to conduct more comprehensive diagnostic and therapeutic evaluations. Ultimately, this may lead to better outcomes for affected cats and their owners.

EPIDEMIOLOGY/RISK FACTORS

A variety of identifiable causes of LUT dysfunction have been reported in cats, including urolithiasis, urethral plugs or strictures, trauma, bacterial cystitis, and neoplasia. When standard diagnostic evaluation fails to identify an underlying cause, cats are classified as having idiopathic feline LUT disease or FIC. Remarkably, in well over half of nonobstructed cats with signs of LUT dysfunction, the exact cause is unknown. In the last 25 years, 8 studies representing data from 23,837 affected cats from North America, Europe, and the Far East have identified underlying causes of LUT dysfunction.[10-17] FIC is the single most common diagnosis in these prospective (n = 627), retrospective (n = 302), and case-controlled (n = 23,019) studies (**Fig. 1**).

Although the aforementioned studies grouped together all unobstructed cats without an identified underlying cause, it is important to understand that cats ultimately diagnosed with FIC may have a variety of clinical presentations, including urethral obstruction (15%–20%) or nonobstructive disease with acute self-limiting episodes (80%–90%), frequently recurring episodes (2%–15%), or chronic persistent episodes (2%–15%).[18] Whether these presentations represent a spectrum of clinical manifestations associated with similar etiologic factors or entirely different disease mechanisms remains to be determined.

At least 5 studies have reported risk factors for development of LUT signs in general without differentiating the underlying causes.[14,16,17,19,20] Recognized breed predispositions are variable and appear to be somewhat dependent on the geography/breed popularity. One large study in the United States found that compared with domestic shorthair cats, Persian, Manx, and Himalayan cats had increased risk, and Siamese cats had decreased risk for LUT signs.[14] A similar pattern of risk was observed in Sweden for Persian (increased) and Siamese (decreased) cats.[21] Conversely, Siamese, along with Persian cats, were the most common purebred breeds affected in a New Zealand study, and the first epidemiologic study of LUT signs in Thailand reported that most cats (81.4%) were Siamese-mixed breed.[17,19] In most studies, middle-aged (4–7 years), neutered, and overweight cats are at increased risk for LUT signs.

In studies that have evaluated risk factors specifically for cats with FIC,[6,22,23] or as part of studies evaluating all causes of LUT dysfunction,[11,12,14,16] numerous risk factors have been identified (**Table 1**). Most of these studies report that male, middle-aged (~2–7 years), overweight cats are at increased risk. A variety of husbandry/environmental risk factors, most indicative of indoor housing and increased

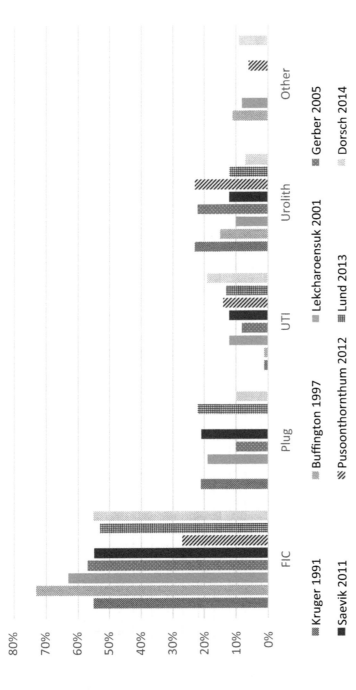

Fig. 1. Prevalence of different causes of LUT dysfunction in 8 studies from North America, Europe, and Thailand. Other, trauma, neoplasia, anatomic abnormality, urinary incontinence, chemical-induced or drug-induced inflammation, and neurogenic causes; Plug, urethral plug or obstruction; UTI, bacterial urinary tract infection. (*Data from* Refs.[10–17])

Table 1
Summary of risk factors for feline idiopathic cystitis

Risk Factor	Lekcharosensuk[14]	Cameron[22]	Gerber[12]	Buffington[6]	Saevik[16]	Defauw[23]	Dorsch[11]
Neutered	Yes	No	Yes	No	Yes	No	NA
~2–7 y	Yes	No	Yes	Yes	Yes	Yes	Yes
Breed	No	Yes	NA	No	Yes	No	No
Gender	Male	Male	Male	No	Male	Male	Male
Dry food[a]	NA	No	Yes	No	No	No	No
Overweight	NA	Yes	Yes	NA	NA	Yes	Yes
Environment[b]	NA	Yes	Yes	Yes	Yes	Yes	Yes
Comorbid disease	NA	NA	NA	Yes	NA	NA	NA
Stress[c]	NA	Yes	NA	Yes	NA	Yes	NA

Abbreviation: NA, not available.
[a] >50% of diet dry food.
[b] Factors include indoor only, litter box use, time owned, multicat household, low activity, no hunting behavior, lower water intake.
[c] Stress defined as conflict with other cats, nervous, fearful, house move.

stress, are also consistent findings. Interestingly, one investigator has demonstrated that there are deficiencies in the way most owners manage indoor cats. As a result, in the absence of specific environmental enrichment, it is likely that modern household environments are inherently stressful to most cats.[24] It is becoming increasingly evident that the interaction between cat-related factors and environmental factors is important for expression of LUT dysfunction, especially FIC.[6] Although the effect of environment/husbandry and stress in cats with LUT signs alone is not enough to cause FIC, when susceptible cats are housed in deficient environments, FIC is more likely to occur.[23]

PATHOPHYSIOLOGY

The underlying cause of FIC is unknown, and given the spectrum of presentations and manifestations, it is probable that FIC is a syndrome with multiple causes rather than a single entity. Although it is not yet possible to differentiate cause from effect or incidental finding, there is a growing body of evidence that suggests both local bladder abnormalities and neuroendocrine changes are important in the pathophysiology of FIC.

Bladder Abnormalities

Studies suggesting that human IC patients have an abnormal degree of urothelial permeability have led to similar investigations in cats with FIC.[25–28] In a healthy bladder, the mucus layer contains glycosaminoglycans (GAGs) and glycoproteins, which form a barrier preventing leakage of urine through the urothelium. One proposed pathogenic mechanism in human patients with IC involves disruption of the mucus layer, which allows the migration of urinary solutes across the epithelium. Of particular concern is potassium, which is thought to depolarize nerves and muscles and cause tissue injury.[27] Studies in cats with FIC have documented decreased concentrations of urinary GAGs.[29–31] Similar to human IC patients, the epithelial barrier of bladders from FIC cats has been shown to be compromised, allowing increased penetration of irritating protons and potassium ions from urine to the submucosa, which may stimulate sensory neurons.[32,33] Decreased urine volume and frequency of urination may further complicate FIC by allowing increased contact time of highly concentrated urine with uroepithelial tissue. Numerous cat-related and environmental factors may contribute to altered voiding frequency and increased urine concentration, including decreased water consumption (taste, availability, temperature), confinement, impaired mobility (obesity, arthritis, or illness), dirty or poorly available litter boxes, and intercat aggression. A growing number of additional local bladder abnormalities have been identified in cats with FIC (**Table 2**).[34–42] Although it is not yet understood if these changes are a cause or effect or both, these studies provide additional insight into potential pathologic processes and therapeutic targets.

Neuroendocrine Abnormalities

Recent studies suggest that stress is integrally involved in the pathogenesis of FIC. As first described by Dr Hans Selye, stress is the nonspecific response of the body to any nocuous agent or "stressor."[43] Stressors may be physical, chemical, or psychological in nature. In both humans and animals, physical and emotional stresses are involved in the pathophysiology of a variety of chronic relapsing conditions, such as irritable bowel syndrome (IBS), inflammatory bowel disease (IBD), and IC/painful bladder syndrome.[44–47] Corticotropin-releasing factor (CRF) seems to play a central role in the behavioral and neuroendocrine responses to stress. There is convincing evidence

Table 2
Summary of reported urinary bladder abnormalities in cats with feline idiopathic cystitis

Reference	Finding	Significance
Altered tissue/urine concentration of inflammatory or bioactive molecules		
Lemberger et al,[37] 2011	Urine fibronectin content is increased in FIC cats vs control cats and those with urinary tract infection or urolithiasis	Urine fibronectin may serve as biomarker for the diagnosis of FIC
Lemberger et al,[38] 2011	Decreased Trefoil factor 2 was documented in cats with FIC vs healthy controls	Decreased Trefoil factor leads to impaired repairing abilities and may serve as a biomarker for the diagnosis of FIC
Treutlein et al,[41] 2012	Alterations were identified in expression level and pattern of numerous copurified proteins of fibronectin (C4a, galectin-7, I-FABP, thioredoxin, and p38 MAPK in urine and bladder tissue from FIC cats)	Changes indicate a role of these proteins in the pathogenesis of FIC and may provide a starting point for novel therapeutic approaches
Treutlein et al,[40] 2013	Urine total protein was transiently higher in obstructive FIC, whereas urine fibronectin and thioredoxin remained increased for 3 mo	Persistently increased fibronectin and thioredoxin may reflect ongoing structural or functional alterations in urinary bladders of cats with obstructive FIC
Neurologic abnormalities		
Buffington et al,[34] 2002	FIC bladders had significantly increased norepinephrine content and efflux in absence of alterations in acetylcholine. Adrenoceptor function was also altered in response to increased sympathetic stimulation	Other studies have identified increased sympathetic nervous system activity in cats with FIC. This study identifies the effect of increased sympathetic activity on bladder function in cats with FIC
Ikeda et al,[36] 2009	Mucosal layer of bladders in cats with FIC have increased spontaneous Ca^{2+} activity and are hypersensitive to low-dose muscarinic receptor agonists	Changes in expression or sensitivity of mucosal muscarinic receptors may contribute to FIC signs
Wu et al,[42] 2011	No evidence of overactive bladder was identified but there was significantly increased maximal urethral closure pressure and maximal urethral pressure in all portions of urethra in FIC cats	Medications for overactive bladder are not indicated for cats with FIC but α_1-adrenoceptor antagonists or skeletal muscle relaxants may be useful
Histologic changes in urinary bladder wall		
Hostutler et al,[35] 2005	Typical changes in the bladder include edema, hemorrhage, and dilation of blood vessels in the submucosa	Changes are nonspecific and not diagnostic for FIC
Sant et al,[39] 2007	Bladder mast cells are increased in FIC cats	Increased urothelial permeability with influx of potassium ions may lead to sensory afferent nerve upregulation and mast cell activation, which further stimulates afferent nerves in a vicious cycle

that an important aspect of both the onset and the exacerbation of IBS and IBD is local CRF-related peptide signaling, which results in altered permeability of the intestinal epithelial lining.[48] A similar mechanism may also be involved in the pathogenesis of FIC in cats. One theory postulates that chronic stress in susceptible cats results in an uncoupling of the normal stress response, producing an enhanced sympathetic nervous system outflow and suppressed adrenocortical responses, leading to increased sensory stimulation and altered urothelial permeability.[49] The altered hypothalamo-pituitary-adrenal (HPA) response in FIC cats is characterized by exaggerated catecholamine release and blunted cortisol response (**Fig. 2**). Support for this mechanism comes from studies that have documented the following alterations in the HPA axis and bladder in cats with FIC compared with healthy cats:

- Increased concentration of CRF in cerebrospinal fluid[50]
- Increased adrenocorticotrophic hormone (ACTH) response and decreased cortisol response after CRF administration[51]

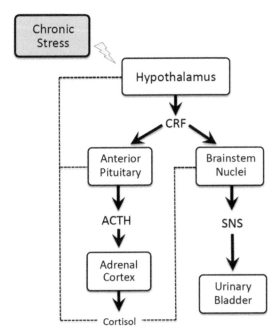

Fig. 2. Relationship between stress, the hypothalamic-pituitary-adrenal axis, and sympathetic nervous system (SNS) in cats with FIC. Perceived stress results in release of CRF from the hypothalamus. This causes the anterior pituitary to release ACTH and the brainstem nuclei activate the SNS, resulting in production of catecholamines (epinephrine and norepinephrine). In normal cats, corticosteroids have a negative feedback effect on the hypothalamus, anterior pituitary, and brainstem (*dotted line*). In cats with FIC, the excitatory SNS is inadequately restrained by cortisol and other adrenocortical steroids. The enhanced sympathetic activity is thought to increase tissue permeability in the urinary bladder, resulting in increased sensory afferent activity and the typical clinical signs of FIC. Feedback inhibition at the level of the anterior pituitary and hypothalamus also is reduced in cats with FIC, which tends to perpetuate CRF output. Solid line indicates stimulation; dotted line indicates inhibition. (*Adapted from* Westropp JL, Tony Buffington CA. FIC: current understanding of pathophysiology and management. Vet Clin North Am Small Anim Pract 2004;34(4):1043–55; with permission.)

- Smaller adrenal glands[52]
- Higher plasma catecholamine concentrations and increased urinary bladder permeability[53]

Given that systemic effects of stress are not limited to the urinary bladder, why do LUT signs predominate in cats with FIC? The anatomic proximity of the micturition and fear pathways, which overlap via connections from the amygdala to the periaqueductal gray, may be a factor. The periaqueductal gray is an anatomic and functional interface between the forebrain and lower brainstem; it has a major role in integrated behavioral responses to internal (eg, pain) or external (eg, threat) stressors. This connection may place the bladder at increased risk for activation during stress responses.[54] Documentation of involvement of other organ systems in cats with FIC also supports a role for neuroendocrine involvement. Indeed, cats often present with various comorbidities related to gastrointestinal, respiratory, dermatologic, and behavioral signs (nervousness/fearfulness).[4–6,47] Although much remains unknown, it is clear that the pathophysiology of FIC likely involves complex interactions between various body systems and is not just a "bladder disease."

DIAGNOSTIC APPROACH

On initial presentation, owners usually report acute onset of various combinations of signs related to LUT disease and/or urinary obstruction (periuria, pollakiuria, stranguria, dysuria, discolored urine due to hematuria). Physical examination of nonobstructed cats may include a small or minimally distended urinary bladder with thickened walls. Because these findings are nonspecific and FIC is a diagnosis of exclusion, other causes of LUT dysfunction must be eliminated (**Table 3**). At a

Table 3
Diagnostic evaluation of cats with nonobstructive lower urinary tract signs

Clinical Presentation	Relative Prevalence (%)	Most Common Primary Disease(s) to Exclude	Recommended Diagnostic Tests
Acute self-limiting episodes	80–90	Uroliths	Urinalysis Survey radiographs
Frequently recurring episodes	2–15	Uroliths Behavioral disorders Urinary tract infection	Urinalysis Survey radiographs Behavioral history[a] Quantitative urine culture
Chronic, persistent episodes	2–15	Uroliths Behavioral disorders Urinary tract infection Neoplasia Anatomic defects[b]	Urinalysis Survey radiographs Behavioral history[a] Quantitative urine culture Ultrasonographic examination Contrast cystourethrography

[a] For periuria, behavioral history should include information on the duration and location of inappropriate urination and material/substrate preferred by the cat (type of litter, rate of litter box cleaning, location and number of litter boxes). Household information should include number of cats and other pets and how they share the space, relationship with people, enrichment, and recent changes in environment.
[b] Anatomic defects reported in cats include urethral strictures, ectopic uterine horn entering the urinary bladder, patent urachus, urachal diverticula, ectopic urethra, and urethrorectal fistula.
Adapted from Lulich J, Osborne C, Kruger J. What constitutes a diagnosis of feline idiopathic cystitis? Proc ACVIM Forum 2010;630–1.

minimum, a urinalysis with sediment evaluation and survey abdominal radiographs should be performed on cats presenting with LUT signs. Because cats with FIC often have clinical signs outside the LUT that may be overlooked by both owners and clinicians, a complete history and physical examination of all organ systems as well as a detailed environmental history should be collected in all cats with LUT signs.[55]

EVIDENCE-BASED MANAGEMENT

In most cats with nonobstructive FIC, clinical signs resolve within 1 to 7 days without therapy.[23,56,57] However, up to 65% of cats with acute FIC will experience one or more recurrences of clinical signs within 1 to 2 years.[23,56,57] In a small percentage of cats (~15%), clinical signs persist for weeks to months or are frequently recurrent; these cats are classified as having chronic FIC. The generally self-limiting nature of clinical signs in most cats may explain why in the past decade greater than 80 agents or procedures have been recommended for cats with FIC.

Because most signs resolve in about a week, with or without therapy, almost any treatment may seem beneficial, emphasizing the critical need for applying principles of evidence-based medicine when selecting the best treatment options for cats with FIC. Veterinarians making therapeutic decisions should consider the quality of evidence supporting a recommendation to use (or not use) a particular treatment. Whenever possible, recommendations should be based on results of randomized and controlled scientific studies (ie, the highest quality of evidence), because this is the best predictor of results likely to occur in clinical patients.[58] In the absence of such studies, one should recognize inherent limitations of recommendations based on less secure forms of evidence. For dealing with such limitations, one suggested method is to assign a score defining the strength and quality of evidence, where grade I is the highest and grade IV is the lowest (**Box 1**).[58,59] The later discussion focuses on the evidence supporting commonly recommended treatments for cats with nonobstructive FIC. Although there are many recommended options, only a few have been carefully studied in cats with naturally occurring FIC.

Box 1
Description of grades use to classify evidence

Grade	Description of Evidence
I	At least one properly designed, randomized, controlled clinical study conducted in patients of the target species with naturally occurring disease living in pet owner's home
II	Evidence from properly designed, randomized, controlled studies in animals of the target species with naturally occurring disease living in a laboratory or colony environment
III	Appropriately controlled studies without randomization; appropriately designed case-control epidemiologic studies; animal models of disease in the target species; dramatic results from uncontrolled studies; case series
IV	Studies conducted in nontarget species; reports of expert panels; descriptive studies; case reports; pathophysiologic rationale; expert opinion

Abbreviations: I, highest quality; IV, lowest quality.

Adapted from Roudebush P, Allen TA, Dodd CE, et al. Application of evidence-based medicine to veterinary clinical nutrition. J Am Vet Med Assoc 2004;224:1766–71; and Roudebush P, Allen TA, Novotny BJ. Evidence-based clinical nutrition. small animal clinical nutrition. 5th edition. Topeka (KS): Mark Morris Institute; 2010. p. 23–30.

STRESS MANAGEMENT
Environmental Enrichment

Over the last 40 years, sociologic stress research in humans confirms that when stressors are methodically measured, their impacts on physical and mental health are substantial.[60] Preoperative stress and anxiety have been shown to predict postoperative pain in human orthopedic patients.[61] Studies in IC patients support an association between life stress and increased severity and frequency of clinical signs[62]; this is consistent with reports of stress-related exacerbations in other conditions that involve neurogenic inflammatory mechanisms (eg, rheumatoid arthritis, IBD, psoriasis).[45,63,64] Interestingly, placebo-treated IC patients attributed their statistically significant reduction in clinical signs, in part, to feeling decreased stress while in the study.[65] The authors recommended providing IC patients with advice and support, including nutritional recommendations and stress reduction, before starting medical therapy.

Because of documented abnormalities in the neuroendocrine system, treatment aimed at decreasing central noradrenergic drive (eg, stress) is also important for managing cats with FIC. Environmental enrichment is one method of decreasing stress, particularly for indoor-housed cats. In this context, the goal of environmental enrichment is to increase behavioral choices and draw out species-appropriate behaviors.[66] For indoor-housed cats with FIC, strategies include enhancing interactions with owners, minimizing conflict, providing all necessary resources, and making any changes gradually.[49]

In general, predictable routines and interactions with owners may help reduce stress in the cat. Some simple interventions that can improve intercat relations include providing an abundance of resources; placing a cat-safe belled collar on aggressor cat or cats, and partial or full segregation of the cats. For severe cases, consultation with a veterinary behaviorist for a comprehensive behavioral modification program that includes desensitization and counterconditioning should be considered. An abundance of feline resources, including toys and play activities and sites for watering, feeding, scratching, elimination, and resting/perching, should be spread throughout the home. A standard rule is to provide as many resources as there are cats plus an additional one. Litter box care and maintenance are also part of an enriched environment. In general, cats prefer clumping litter with sandlike texture in large uncovered boxes placed in quiet, easily accessible locations; however, preferences in individual cats may be highly variable.[67] As with other resources, there should be at least one litter box per cat, and one more litter box than the number of cats in the household is ideal. More detailed information on environmental enrichment is available.[68,69]

Supporting evidence

Although environmental enrichment has been recommended for cats with FIC and is thought to be beneficial, it has not been evaluated in a randomized controlled clinical trial. The best evidence supporting environmental enrichment comes from a controlled laboratory study of cats with naturally occurring disease (grade II), an uncontrolled, prospective clinical study in cats with FIC (grade III), pathophysiologic rationale, clinical experiences, and expert opinion (grade IV). A controlled laboratory study measured a variety of parameters in FIC-affected cats when exposed to stressful versus enriched environments.[53] Catecholamine concentrations and urinary bladder permeability decreased during the enrichment phase, suggesting environmental enrichment may have a beneficial effect for cats with FIC.[53] A prospective observational study (grade III) reported the effects of multimodal environmental modification in 46 client-owned cats with FIC.[5] There were significant reductions in LUT signs, fearfulness, and nervousness after treatment for 10 months. Veterinary specialists and behaviorists agree (grade IV) that housing cats indoors can be stressful when their environment lacks outlets for natural behaviors, such as scratching, chewing, elimination, resting/hiding, and hunting/playing.[70,71]

Recommendations

- Institute environmental enrichment and methods to reduce stress as part of the initial management of all cats with FIC.
- Consult additional resources for helpful information that can be used by veterinarians and cat owners.[68,70–75]

Feline Facial Pheromone

Pheromones are bioactive compounds emitted and detected by animals of the same species that influence social and reproductive behavior. Classically, pheromones are described as nonvolatile molecules that regulate innate social behavior by activating vomeronasal organ sensory neurons. Recent studies suggest this definition may be too restrictive. It appears that pheromones may activate vomeronasal or main olfactory epithelium neurons and may have their effects altered by context as opposed to being strictly innate.[76] Synthetic feline facial pheromone therapy has been recommended as a method to decrease signs of stress in cats with FIC.[77,78]

Supporting evidence

A recent systematic review of the scientific literature on the use of pheromones in cats with and without FIC concluded that, based on 7 published studies, there is insufficient evidence to support the use of feline facial pheromones to manage FIC, to decrease stress in hospitalized cats, or to calm cats in unfamiliar surroundings.[79] At this time, their use in cats with FIC is supported by grade IV evidence (pathophysiologic rationale).

Recommendations

- There is insufficient evidence to support the use of feline facial pheromones to manage FIC.
- It is possible feline facial pheromones may be helpful in some individual cats with FIC and could be used after recommending other treatments that are supported by higher grades of evidence.

Supplements/Therapeutic Foods for Stress

For centuries, practitioners of traditional Chinese medicine have recommended nutritional supplements as therapy for behavioral conditions such as anxiety or stress. Natural treatments, including amino acids, minerals, and fatty acids, have been shown to have beneficial effects on neurotransmitter concentrations and signs of anxiety in animal models and humans.[80] The neurotransmitter serotonin has remarkable modulatory effects in almost all central nervous system integrative functions, such as mood, anxiety, stress, aggression, feeding, cognition, and sexual behavior.[81] Increased concentrations of serotonin have been associated with decreased anxiety in people and animal models.[82] Cow's milk has long been considered to have natural "tranquilizing" properties. Milk protein hydrolysate is derived from milk (also known as hydrolyzed casein and α-casozepine) and has been associated with significant alleviation of stress in models of anxiety in rodents and people.[83] The exact mechanism of these anxiolytic effects is unknown but may be mediated through the γ-amino butyric acid/benzodiazepine receptor complex.[84]

Supporting evidence

Positive effects of various nutrients on anxiety and stress-related behaviors in mammals have been reported for L-tryptophan and milk protein hydrolysate. L-Tryptophan, a precursor for serotonin synthesis, has been evaluated as a method of managing stress-related behaviors in cats in one blinded placebo-controlled study (grade I).[85] In this 2-month study, the authors observed significant changes in a variety of behaviors, suggesting that L-tryptophan supplementation changed the frequency of stress-related behaviors, decreasing signs of anxiety. One multicenter grade I (placebo-controlled, blinded) study evaluated the anxiolytic effects of α-casozepine (Zylkene) in 34 cats (n = 17 placebo, n = 17 α-casozepine).[86] At the end of the study, 10 of the 14 cats judged to have a successful outcome were from the α-casozepine group. This study provides evidence for the efficacy of α-casozepine in the management of anxiety in cats, including socially stressful conditions. These studies provide grade I evidence for short-term relief of clinical signs; however, studies of greater duration would be helpful because of the waxing and waning nature of FIC episodes over time. Although evidence supports positive benefits of these compounds, daily administration of oral medications may be stressful for some cats. Providing a multipurpose therapeutic urinary food that contains specific nutrients with proven antianxiety benefits is a novel approach to stress management in cats with FIC.

Recommendations

- If oral administration does not increase stress, consider recommending L-tryptophan 12.5 mg/kg and or α-casozepine 15 mg/kg (Zylkene) in conjunction with implementing environmental enrichment in FIC cats with clinical signs of stress.
- Consider including a specific nutritional recommendation for a therapeutic urinary food containing nutrients with antianxiety benefits in conjunction with implementing environmental enrichment in FIC cats with clinical signs of stress.

NUTRITIONAL MANAGEMENT
Moist Food/Increased Water Intake

Increasing water intake by feeding moist food, increased sodium intake, and addition of broth or other methods may or may not be beneficial for cats with FIC. Of these methods, feeding moist food is the only method that has been evaluated in cats with FIC. Theoretically, diluting the urine via additional water intake could dilute potential noxious stimulants such as urea and potassium chloride. However, the exact role these noxious stimulants play in the pathogenesis of FIC remains unknown.

Supporting evidence

Two studies have documented some benefits associated with feeding moist foods to cats with FIC.[56,87] In a 1-year, nonrandomized prospective (grade III) study of 46 cats with FIC, feeding a moist therapeutic food (Waltham Veterinary Feline Control pHormula Diet in Gel) was associated with significant improvement compared with feeding a dry version of the food.[87] At the end of the 1-year study, recurrence of clinical signs in cats eating moist food was significantly less (11% of 18 cats) compared with cats eating dry food (39% of 28 cats) ($P = .04$). Compared with the dry food group, urine specific gravity was significantly less in cats eating moist food; throughout the 1-year study, mean urine specific gravity values ranged from 1.032 to 1.041 in cats eating moist food and from 1.051 to 1.052 in cats eating dry food ($P<.05$). In another study evaluating glucosamine in 40 cats with FIC, moist food was recommended for all cats in the treatment and control groups. Most owners (90%, or 36) increased amount of moist food given to their cats, and the majority (82.5%) began feeding moist food exclusively. Most cats in both groups improved significantly compared with their condition at baseline, and mean urine specific gravity was significantly lower at the 1-month recheck compared with baseline (1.036 ± 1.010 vs 1.050 ± 1.007) ($P<.01$).[56] The change in urine specific gravity coincided with the change to moist food and initial improvement in mean monthly clinical scores. In both studies described above, increased consumption of moist food was associated with less concentrated urine (specific gravity (SG) <1.040), which may have resulted in improved clinical signs; however, it is also possible that other factors associated with feeding moist food (eg, texture, taste, owner-cat interactions associated with delivery of moist food) may have served as a form of environmental enrichment and had a positive impact on the cats' well-being.

Increased dietary salt intake has also been proposed as a method of diluting urine, including cats consuming dry foods; however, its effects have not been studied in cats with FIC.[88] In healthy cats, increased sodium intake may or may not result in decreased urine specific gravity and/or increased urine volume.[89–93] In a 2-week study (grade II) of healthy cats, increased salt intake (1.2% sodium, dry matter basis) resulted in significantly decreased urine specific gravity compared with feeding 0.46% sodium, dry matter basis; however, urine volume did not increase in the high-salt group.[91] The mean daily urine specific gravity of cats fed higher sodium was not less than 1.045 at any time. In a 2-year study of healthy cats, mean urine specific gravity (spot measurements) was significantly lower at 3 months in cats fed higher sodium, but was not different at 6, 12, or 24 months.[92] In a controlled, 6-month study (grade II) of 24 normal cats randomized to receive either a high-sodium food (290 mg/100 kcal sodium) or a control food (140 mg/100 kcal sodium), there were no differences in mean urine specific gravity between groups at baseline, 3, or 6 months and mean values were not less than 1.040 at any point.[93] If the benefit of feeding increased sodium to cats with FIC depends on consistent lowering of urine specific gravity over the long term, it may not be an effective strategy. In addition, although there are no apparent contraindications for feeding high-sodium foods to healthy cats, there are differing opinions regarding the safety of increased sodium intake in cats with undetected kidney disease.[90–94] Consumption of moist food exclusively, regardless of sodium content, may be the most effective method for long-term urine dilution in cats, and this needs further study.[95]

Recommendations

- If transition to a new food does not increase stress for the cat or owner, make a specific nutritional recommendation for moist food (ie, which product, amount to feed, how often to feed). See later discussion for evidence supporting a therapeutic urinary food in cats with FIC signs.
- To minimize stress, transition to the new food gradually (weeks to months) and allow cats to self-select by offering the new food in a separate container beside the current food.

Therapeutic Urinary Food

Currently, there is no cure for FIC; therefore, goals for treatment are to improve quality of life for cats and owners by reducing duration and severity of clinical signs, the rate of recurrence of clinical signs, and the risk for urethral obstruction. Although there is no known benefit of urine acidification or controlling magnesium and phosphorus intake in cats with nonobstructive FIC, it may be important for preventing urethral obstruction, a potentially life-threatening complication in male cats. Over the last 30 years, struvite has consistently been the primary mineral component of the majority of urethral plugs submitted to the Minnesota Urolith Center.[96] In some cats with LUT signs, it can be challenging to definitively distinguish between FIC and struvite disease (urethral plugs or uroliths). Nutritional factors that may impact expression of LUT signs and help manage both FIC and struvite disease include the following:

- Decreasing urine concentrations of pro-inflammatory mediators and crystallo-genic minerals
- Decreasing retention of crystals in the urinary tract
- Increasing urine concentrations of anti-inflammatory/proresolving mediators and crystallization inhibitors
- Increasing solubility of crystalloids in urine

Urinary bladder inflammation is characteristic of LUT disorders, including FIC and urolithiasis. Long-chain ω-3 fatty acids, including eicosapentaenoic acid (EPA) and docosahexaenoic acid (DHA), and antioxidants such as vitamin E, are potent anti-inflammatory agents.[97,98] Dietary fatty acids are absorbed and incorporated into cell membranes, including those of the urinary bladder, where they may alter production of inflammatory mediators. Effects of ω-3 fatty acids alone have not been evaluated in cats with LUT disorders; however, they seem to have beneficial urinary effects in studies of other species. In a study evaluating the chemopreventive efficacy of EPA and DHA in a rat model of bladder cancer, ω-3 fatty acids inhibited development of premalignant and malignant lesions.[99] This effect was attributed to the anti-inflammatory, antioxidant, antiproliferative, and antiangiogenic properties of ω-3 fatty acids. Oxidative stress and increased free radical-induced peroxidation of cell membrane phospholipids may cause tissue injury by impairing cell membrane functions and inducing production of inflammatory cytokines.[98] Vitamin E and β-carotene, both potent antioxidants, have been shown to protect against cyclophosphamide-induced oxidative damage to bladder tissue in rats.[16] Commercially available multipurpose therapeutic urinary foods vary considerably in their ω-3 and antioxidant content.[100] Although the optimal therapeutic dose of ω-3 fatty acids and antioxidants for cats with FIC have not been determined, a recent study supports the long-term use of a multipurpose therapeutic urinary food with enhanced concentrations of these nutrients in cats with FIC.[101,102]

Supporting evidence

A recent prospective, randomized, double-masked (grade I) study evaluated the efficacy and safety of a multipurpose therapeutic urinary food, enriched with ω-3 fatty acids (EPA and DHA) and antioxidants (vitamin E and β-carotene), for the long-term management of acute FIC.[101–103] For the duration of the 12-month study, owners chose to offer either wet or dry food exclusively and then cats were randomly assigned to the test or control food groups. The test food was a commercially available multipurpose therapeutic urinary food (Hill's Prescription Diet c/d Multicare Feline), and the control food was custom manufactured and formulated to meet or exceed Association of American Feed Control Officials nutrient requirements for maintenance of adult cats. The mineral concentrations of the control food were designed to be similar to common grocery brands. Compared with the test food, the control food contained substantially lower concentrations of antioxidants and ω-3 fatty acids (EPA and DHA) (**Table 4**).

The primary endpoint was the frequency of recurrent episodes of LUT signs within 12 months. Twenty-five cats ranging in age from 1 to 9 years were included; 11 cats (5 males, 6 females) were fed the test food and 14 cats (11 males, 3 females) were fed the control food. Data were analyzed as a binomial proportion of the number of days that

Table 4
Selected nutrient values for test food compared with control food evaluated in a 1-year, randomized, controlled clinical study of cats with feline idiopathic cystitis

Nutrient Amounts (per 100 Kcal)	Test Food (Dry)	Test Food (Moist)	Control Food (Dry)	Control Food (Moist)
Protein (g)	9	10.7	8.7	11
Calcium (mg)	176	217	346	310
Phosphorous (mg)	182	209	291	289
Magnesium (mg)	17	19.5	29.4	25.4
Sodium (mg)	83	83	81	124
Vitamin E (IU)	24	30	1	3
Omega-3 EPA (mg)	53	65	4.6	10.5
Omega-3 DHA (mg)	36	44	2.7	10.5

Test food = Hill's Prescription Diet c/d Multicare Feline; Control food = custom manufactured maintenance food.

an event occurred or the number of episodes of LUT signs out of the total number of days a cat was in the study for a factorial arrangement of 2 foods and 2 formulations. Cats consuming the test food had a significantly lower proportion of total days with 2 or more clinical signs and total episodes of LUT signs ($P<.05$) with 4 of 11 (36%) test food group cats and 9 of 14 (64%) control food group cats exhibiting 2 or more clinical signs on at least one occasion during the 12-month study. The rate of recurrent episodes of LUT signs was 5 of 3904 days (1.28/1000 cat-days) in the test food group and 47 of 4215 days (11.15/1000 cat-days) in the control food group. This represents an 89% overall lower rate of recurrent episodes of LUT signs in cats fed the test food consistently compared with the control food (**Fig. 3**); this is the first study to definitively show that foods of different nutritional profiles impact the expression of LUT signs in cats with acute FIC.

Recommendations

- Make a specific nutritional recommendation for a multipurpose therapeutic urinary food (Hill's Prescription Diet c/d Multicare) to reduce rate of recurrent episodes of LUT signs in cats with FIC.
- Consider recommending therapeutic foods for struvite management when struvite disease cannot be excluded in cats with suspected FIC, especially those prone to urethral obstruction.

PHARMACOLOGIC THERAPY
Glycosaminoglycans

Treatment with GAGs (eg, pentosan polysulfate [PPS], glucosamine, chondroitin sulfate) has been suggested for cats with FIC because defects in the GAG layer covering the urinary bladder epithelium may play a role in the pathogenesis of the disease. Intravesical application of these agents seems to be useful in women with IC, a condition similar to FIC; however, a recent review of the literature concluded that additional large-scale trials are needed to confirm the benefit of this therapy.[104] Early studies

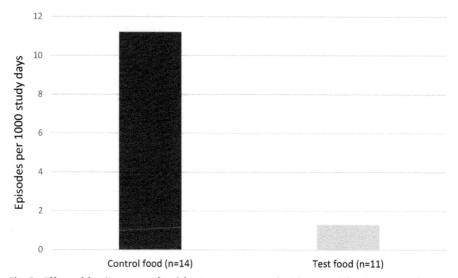

Fig. 3. Effect of feeding a test food for 1 year compared with control food on rate of recurrence of LUT signs in cats with FIC. Cats fed test food (Hill's Prescription Diet c/d Multicare) had a significantly lower proportion of total days with episodes of FIC signs (P<.05) compared with cats fed a control food.

suggested a positive effect of oral PPS in a proportion of human patients with IC.[105] However, a recent randomized, controlled clinical study in 368 adults with IC revealed no treatment effect versus placebo over 24 weeks at the currently established daily dose.[106] A similar trend has been reported in studies of cats with FIC.

Supporting evidence

A randomized, double-blind, placebo-controlled study was conducted to determine whether administration of glucosamine (Cystease, 125 mg administered per mouth once daily for 6 months; Ceva Animal Health) would reduce the severity or recurrence rate of clinical signs in cats with FIC compared with placebo.[56] Owner assessments suggested that glucosamine-treated cats achieved a slightly greater improvement by the end of the study (mean health score: 4.4 ± 0.7) compared with the placebo group (mean health score: 3.9 ± 1.6); however, this difference was not statistically significant (P>.05). There were no statistically significant differences in clinical signs between groups during treatment or at re-evaluation. A more recent randomized controlled study (grade I) confirmed that FIC cats receiving once daily oral administration of 250 mg N-acetyl-D-glucosamine (Cystaid) had increased the mean plasma GAG concentrations compared with placebo-treated cats (P<.05).[30] However, in the treated group, urine GAG-to-creatinine concentrations did not differ significantly from baseline or between the treated and placebo groups. Detailed information on severity and recurrence of clinical signs was not collected.

A randomized, double-blind, placebo-controlled study (grade I) was conducted to assess efficacy of subcutaneous injections of PPS (n = 9) versus placebo (n = 9) in cats with acute FIC.[107] During the year-long study, there was no statistically significant difference between cats treated with PPS and the placebo group, in either short-term or long-term follow-up. The authors concluded that PPS cannot be recommended for use in cats with FIC. However, only 6 cats (33%) had a recurrent episode and only one cat had greater than one recurrence. A similar (grade I) study compared placebo with 3 oral doses of PPS in 107 cats with at least 2 episodes of LUT signs within the previous 6 months.[108] Clinical improvement occurred in all cats, regardless of the dose of PPS administration or changes in cystoscopic appearance of the bladder. These results indicate that PPS is equivalent to placebo for treatment of FIC.

Recommendations

- Currently, there is insufficient evidence to recommend oral or subcutaneous GAG therapy in cats with FIC.
- It is possible that GAGs could be helpful in individual cats; however, at this time its use is based on grade IV evidence (pathophysiologic rationale).

Amitriptyline

Amitriptyline (Elavil) is a tricyclic antidepressant with anticholinergic, antihistaminic, sympatholytic, analgesic, and anti-inflammatory properties that has been used in cats with FIC and in women with IC. A recent meta-analysis of randomized controlled trials in humans showed that amitriptyline had some beneficial effects in women with IC; however, the authors emphasized that only limited evidence exists for treatments recommended for painful bladder syndrome/IC, and more well-controlled studies are needed.[109]

Supporting evidence

In an uncontrolled (grade III) study of cats with severe recurrent FIC that failed to respond to other treatments, administration of amitriptyline for 12 months was associated with decreased clinical signs in 9 (60%) of 15 cats during the last 6 months of treatment.[110] A randomized controlled clinical trial (grade I) of amitriptyline treatment for 7 days revealed no significant difference in the rate of recovery from pollakiuria or hematuria; overall, clinical signs recurred significantly faster and more frequently in cats treated with amitriptyline compared with control cats.[57] In a similar grade I study, amitriptyline combined with amoxicillin was no more effective than placebo and amoxicillin when given for 7 days to cats with FIC.[111] Based on current information, amitriptyline does not seem to be beneficial for short-term management of cats with FIC. There is grade III evidence that longer use (minimum of weeks to months) may be helpful.

Recommendations

- There is insufficient evidence to recommend short-term treatment with amitriptyline.
- Consider long-term treatment with amitriptyline (5–10 mg per cat by mouth once daily) if cats with FIC continue to have recurrent episodes despite the use of treatments with a higher grade of evidence (ie, multipurpose therapeutic urinary food, feeding moist food, and environmental enrichment).

Anti-inflammatory Agents and Analgesics

In 2011, the American Urological Association provided guidelines for the diagnosis and treatment of IC/bladder pain syndrome in humans. Interestingly, the first-line treatments recommended for all patients include patient education, self-care practices, behavior modifications, stress management, and coping techniques.[112] However, because pain seems to be a prominent result of FIC, analgesics should be administered to help control these clinical signs. There have been no clinical trials evaluating opioid analgesics (eg, butorphanol) or nonsteroidal anti-inflammatory drugs (NSAIDs), such as meloxicam, piroxicam, or robenacoxib, in cats with FIC.

Supporting evidence

Prednisolone (1 mg/kg administered by mouth twice daily for 10 days) was evaluated in a double-blind randomized controlled clinical trial of 12 cats with FIC and was found to be no more effective than placebo for reducing severity or duration of clinical signs in affected cats.[113] The best evidence supporting use of analgesics and NSAIDs comes from expert opinion and pathophysiologic rationale (grade IV).

Recommendations

- In addition to initiating stress reduction, environmental enrichment, and a specific nutritional recommendation, provide analgesia with narcotics such as buprenorphine (0.01 mg/kg orally every 8–12 hours), butorphanol (0.2 mg/kg subcutaneously or orally every 8–12 hours), or a fentanyl patch, depending on severity of pain/discomfort.
- NSAIDs should be used with caution in dehydrated patients because of the risk of reduced blood flow to the kidneys and potential for acute kidney injury. It is appropriate to contact the manufacturer for guidance when recommending a particular NSAID for individual patients.

SUMMARY

Two obstacles stand in the way of a cure for FIC: lack of an identifiable cause and a paucity of randomized controlled studies evaluating different treatment options. The same issues confound management of IC in human patients. As a result, current best evidence suggests a multimodal approach to patient management provides the best outcome for humans with IC.[114] Based on the current best evidence for cats with acute nonobstructive FIC, a multimodal approach is also advised; this includes a specific nutritional recommendation for a multipurpose therapeutic urinary food proven to reduce rate of recurrent episodes of FIC signs, environmental enrichment, and feeding moist food. Short-term analgesics are indicated to control signs of pain. The self-limiting nature of FIC and importance of environmental factors on recurrence of clinical signs emphasize the need for controlled, prospective, double-blinded clinical studies to determine the best management options for this complex condition.

REFERENCES

1. Osborne CA, Kruger JM, Lulich JP. Feline lower urinary tract disorders. Definition of terms and concepts. Vet Clin North Am Small Anim Pract 1996;26: 169–79.
2. Buffington CA, Chew DJ, DiBartola SP. Interstitial cystitis in cats. Vet Clin North Am Small Anim Pract 1996;26:317–26.
3. Chew D, Buffington C. Pandora syndrome: it's more than just the bladder. In: Proc Am Assoc Fel Pract Conf. 2013.
4. Buffington CA. Idiopathic cystitis in domestic cats–beyond the lower urinary tract. J Vet Intern Med 2011;25:784–96.
5. Buffington CA, Westropp JL, Chew DJ, et al. Clinical evaluation of multimodal environmental modification (MEMO) in the management of cats with idiopathic cystitis. J Feline Med Surg 2006;8:261–8.

6. Buffington CA, Westropp JL, Chew DJ, et al. Risk factors associated with clinical signs of lower urinary tract disease in indoor-housed cats. J Am Vet Med Assoc 2006;228:722–5.

7. Buffington CA. Comorbidity of interstitial cystitis with other unexplained clinical conditions. J Urol 2004;172:1242–8.

8. Buffington CA. External and internal influences on disease risk in cats. J Am Vet Med Assoc 2002;220:994–1002.

9. Freeman LM, Brown DJ, Smith FW, et al. Magnesium status and the effect of magnesium supplementation in feline hypertrophic cardiomyopathy. Can J Vet Res 1997;61:227–31.

10. Buffington CA, Chew DJ, Kendall MS, et al. Clinical evaluation of cats with non-obstructive urinary tract diseases. J Am Vet Med Assoc 1997;210:46–50.

11. Dorsch R, Remer C, Sauter-Louis C, et al. Feline lower urinary tract disease in a German cat population. A retrospective analysis of demographic data, causes and clinical signs. Tierarztl Prax Ausg K Kleintiere Heimtiere 2014;42:231–9.

12. Gerber B, Boretti FS, Kley S, et al. Evaluation of clinical signs and causes of lower urinary tract disease in European cats. J Small Anim Pract 2005;46:571–7.

13. Kruger JM, Osborne CA, Goyal SM, et al. Clinical evaluation of cats with lower urinary tract disease. J Am Vet Med Assoc 1991;199:211–6.

14. Lekcharosensuk C, Osborne CA, Lulich JP. Epidemiologic study of risk factors for lower urinary tract diseases in cats. J Am Vet Med Assoc 2001;218:1429–35.

15. Lund HS, Krontveit RI, Halvorsen I, et al. Evaluation of urinalyses from untreated adult cats with lower urinary tract disease and healthy control cats: predictive abilities and clinical relevance. J Feline Med Surg 2013;15:1086–97.

16. Saevik BK, Trangerud C, Ottesen N, et al. Causes of lower urinary tract disease in Norwegian cats. J Feline Med Surg 2011;13:410–7.

17. Pusoonthornthum R, Pusoonthornthum P, Osborne C. Risk factors for feline lower urinary tract diseases in Thailand. Thai Journal Veterinary Medicine 2012;42: 517–22.

18. Lulich J, Osborne C, Kruger J. What constitutes a diagnosis of feline idiopathic cystitis? Proc ACVIM Forum 2010. 630–31.

19. Jones BR, Sanson RL, Morris RS. Elucidating the risk factors of feline lower urinary tract disease. N Z Vet J 1997;45:100–8.

20. Lund EM, Armstrong PJ, Kirk CA, et al. Prevalence and risk factors for obesity in adult cats from private veterinary US practices. Intern J Appl Res Vet Med 2005; 3:88–96.

21. Egenvall A, Bonnett BN, Haggstrom J, et al. Morbidity of insured Swedish cats during 1999-2006 by age, breed, sex, and diagnosis. J Feline Med Surg 2010; 12:948–59.

22. Cameron ME, Casey RA, Bradshaw JW, et al. A study of environmental and behavioural factors that may be associated with feline idiopathic cystitis. J Small Anim Pract 2004;45:144–7.

23. Defauw PA, Van de Maele I, Duchateau L, et al. Risk factors and clinical presentation of cats with feline idiopathic cystitis. J Feline Med Surg 2011;13:967–75.

24. Heidenberger E. Housing conditions and behavioural problems of indoor cats as assessed by their owners. Appl Anim Behav Sci 1997;52:345–64.

25. Lilly JD, Parsons CL. Bladder surface glycosaminoglycans is a human epithelial permeability barrier. Surg Gynecol Obstet 1990;171:493–6.

26. Parsons CL. Interstitial cystitis and lower urinary tract symptoms in males and females-the combined role of potassium and epithelial dysfunction. Rev Urol 2002;4(Suppl 1):S49–55.

27. Parsons CL. The role of the urinary epithelium in the pathogenesis of interstitial cystitis/prostatitis/urethritis. Urology 2007;69:9–16.
28. Parsons CL, Lilly JD, Stein P. Epithelial dysfunction in nonbacterial cystitis (interstitial cystitis). J Urol 1991;145:732–5.
29. Buffington CA, Blaisdell JL, Binns SP Jr, et al. Decreased urine glycosaminoglycan excretion in cats with interstitial cystitis. J Urol 1996;155:1801–4.
30. Panchaphanpong J, Asawakarn T, Pusoonthornthum R. Effects of oral administration of N-acetyl-D-glucosamine on plasma and urine concentrations of glycosaminoglycans in cats with idiopathic cystitis. Am J Vet Res 2011;72:843–50.
31. Pereira DA, Aguiar JA, Hagiwara MK, et al. Changes in cat urinary glycosaminoglycans with age and in feline urologic syndrome. Biochim Biophys Acta 2004;1672:1–11.
32. Lavelle JP, Meyers SA, Ruiz WG, et al. Urothelial pathophysiological changes in feline interstitial cystitis: a human model. Am J Physiol Renal Physiol 2000;278:F540–53.
33. Birder LA, Wolf-Johnston A, Buffington CA, et al. Altered inducible nitric oxide synthase expression and nitric oxide production in the bladder of cats with feline interstitial cystitis. J Urol 2005;173:625–9.
34. Buffington CA, Teng B, Somogyi GT. Norepinephrine content and adrenoceptor function in the bladder of cats with feline interstitial cystitis. J Urol 2002;167:1876–80.
35. Hostutler RA, Chew DJ, DiBartola SP. Recent concepts in feline lower urinary tract disease. Vet Clin North Am Small Anim Pract 2005;35:147–70, vii.
36. Ikeda Y, Birder L, Buffington C, et al. Mucosal muscarinic receptors enhance bladder activity in cats with feline interstitial cystitis. J Urol 2009;181:1415–22.
37. Lemberger SI, Deeg CA, Hauck SM, et al. Comparison of urine protein profiles in cats without urinary tract disease and cats with idiopathic cystitis, bacterial urinary tract infection, or urolithiasis. Am J Vet Res 2011;72:1407–15.
38. Lemberger SI, Dorsch R, Hauck SM, et al. Decrease of Trefoil factor 2 in cats with feline idiopathic cystitis. BJU Int 2011;107:670–7.
39. Sant GR, Kempuraj D, Marchand JE, et al. The mast cell in interstitial cystitis: role in pathophysiology and pathogenesis. Urology 2007;69:34–40.
40. Treutlein G, Deeg CA, Hauck SM, et al. Follow-up protein profiles in urine samples during the course of obstructive feline idiopathic cystitis. Vet J 2013;198:625–30.
41. Treutlein G, Dorsch R, Euler KN, et al. Novel potential interacting partners of fibronectin in spontaneous animal model of interstitial cystitis. PLoS One 2012;7:e51391.
42. Wu CH, Buffington CA, Fraser MO, et al. Urodynamic evaluation of female cats with idiopathic cystitis. Am J Vet Res 2011;72:578–82.
43. Szabo S, Tache Y, Somogyi A. The legacy of Hans Selye and the origins of stress research: a retrospective 75 years after his landmark brief "letter" to the editor of nature. Stress 2012;15:472–8.
44. Qin HY, Cheng CW, Tang XD, et al. Impact of psychological stress on irritable bowel syndrome. World J Gastroenterol 2014;20:14126–31.
45. Martin TD, Chan SS, Hart AR. Environmental factors in the relapse and recurrence of inflammatory bowel disease: a review of the literature. Dig Dis Sci 2014. [Epub ahead of print].
46. Lutgendorf SK, Kreder KJ, Rothrock NE, et al. Stress and symptomatology in patients with interstitial cystitis: a laboratory stress model. J Urol 2000;164:1265–9.

47. Stella JL, Lord LK, Buffington CA. Sickness behaviors in response to unusual external events in healthy cats and cats with feline interstitial cystitis. J Am Vet Med Assoc 2011;238:67–73.
48. Larauche M, Kiank C, Tache Y. Corticotropin releasing factor signaling in colon and ileum: regulation by stress and pathophysiological implications. J Physiol Pharmacol 2009;60(Suppl 7):33–46.
49. Westropp JL, Tony Buffington CA. Feline idiopathic cystitis: current understanding of pathophysiology and management. Vet Clin North Am Small Anim Pract 2004;34:1043–55.
50. Westropp JL, Buffington CA. Cerebrospinal fluid corticotrophin releasing factor and catecholamine concentrations in healthy cats and cats with interstitial cystitis. In: Proceedings Research Insights into Interstitial Cystitis. 2003.
51. Westropp JL, Buffington CA. Effect of a corticotropin releasing factor antagonist on hypothalamic-pituitary-adrenal activation in response to chronic renal failure in cats with interstitial cystitis. In: Proceedings Research Insights into Interstitial Cystitis. 2003.
52. Westropp JL, Welk KA, Buffington CA. Small adrenal glands in cats with feline interstitial cystitis. J Urol 2003;170:2494–7.
53. Westropp JL, Kass PH, Buffington CA. Evaluation of the effects of stress in cats with idiopathic cystitis. Am J Vet Res 2006;67:731–6.
54. Brodal P. The Central nervous system. 4th edition. Oxford University Press, USA; 2010.
55. Chew DJ, Buffington CA. Diagnostic approach to cats with lower urinary tract signs. Hill's Global Symposium on feline lower urinary tract health. Prague, Czech Republic, April 23-24, 2014. p. 23–30.
56. Gunn-Moore DA, Shenoy CM. Oral glucosamine and the management of feline idiopathic cystitis. J Feline Med Surg 2004;6:219–25.
57. Kruger JM, Conway TS, Kaneene JB, et al. Randomized controlled trial of the efficacy of short-term amitriptyline administration for treatment of acute, nonobstructive, idiopathic lower urinary tract disease in cats. J Am Vet Med Assoc 2003;222:749–58.
58. Roudebush P, Allen TA, Dodd CE, et al. Application of evidence-based medicine to veterinary clinical nutrition. J Am Vet Med Assoc 2004;224:1766–71.
59. Roudebush P, Allen TA, Novotny BJ. Evidence-based clinical nutrition. Small animal clinical nutrition. 5th edition. Topeka (KS): Mark Morris Institute; 2010. p. 23–30.
60. Thoits PA. Stress and health: major findings and policy implications. J Health Soc Behav 2010;51(Suppl):S41–53.
61. Robleda G, Sillero-Sillero A, Puig T, et al. Influence of preoperative emotional state on postoperative pain following orthopedic and trauma surgery. Rev Lat Am Enfermagem 2014;22:785–91.
62. Rothrock NE, Lutgendorf SK, Kreder KJ, et al. Stress and symptoms in patients with interstitial cystitis: a life stress model. Urology 2001;57:422–7.
63. Overman CL, Bossema ER, van Middendorp H, et al. The prospective association between psychological distress and disease activity in rheumatoid arthritis: a multilevel regression analysis. Ann Rheum Dis 2012;71:192–7.
64. Hunter HJ, Griffiths CE, Kleyn CE. Does psychosocial stress play a role in the exacerbation of psoriasis? Br J Dermatol 2013;169:965–74.
65. Bosch PC. Examination of the significant placebo effect in the treatment of interstitial cystitis/bladder pain syndrome. Urology 2014;84:321–6.
66. Laule GE. Positive reinforcement training and environmental enrichment: enhancing animal well-being. J Am Vet Med Assoc 2003;223:969–73.

67. Neilson JC. The latest scoop on litter. Vet Med 2009;140–4.
68. Feline house-soiling: useful information for cat owners. J Feline Med Surg 2014; 16:770–1.
69. Neilson JC. Feline house soiling: elimination and marking behaviors. Vet Clin North Am Small Anim Pract 2003;33:287–301.
70. Herron ME, Buffington CA. Environmental enrichment for indoor cats: implementing enrichment. Compend Contin Educ Vet 2012;34:E3.
71. Radosta L. Environmental enrichment for cats. Clinician's Brief 2014;13–5.
72. Buffington CA. Keeping cats indoors. Indoorpetosuedu. Columbus (OH): The Ohio State University Veterinary Medical Center; 2013.
73. Buffington CA. The indoor pet initiative. 2013. Available at: www.indoorpet.osu. edu. Accessed March 12, 2015.
74. Herron ME, Buffington CA. Environmental enrichment for indoor cats. Compend Contin Educ Vet 2010;32:E4.
75. ISFM A. Your cat's environmental needs. 2013. Available at: www.catvets.com. Accessed March 12, 2015.
76. Stowers L, Marton TF. What is a pheromone? Mammalian pheromones reconsidered. Neuron 2005;46:699–702.
77. Griffith CA, Steigerwald ES, Buffington CA. Effects of a synthetic facial pheromone on behavior of cats. J Am Vet Med Assoc 2000;217:1154–6.
78. Gunn-Moore DA, Cameron ME. A pilot study using synthetic feline facial pheromone for the management of feline idiopathic cystitis. J Feline Med Surg 2004;6: 133–8.
79. Frank D, Beauchamp G, Palestrini C. Systematic review of the use of pheromones for treatment of undesirable behavior in cats and dogs. J Am Vet Med Assoc 2010;236:1308–16.
80. Alramadhan E, Hanna MS, Hanna MS, et al. Dietary and botanical anxiolytics. Med Sci Monit 2012;18:Ra40–8.
81. Olivier B. Serotonin: a never-ending story. Eur J Pharmacol 2014. [Epub ahead of print].
82. Zhou J, Cao X, Mar AC, et al. Activation of postsynaptic 5-HT1A receptors improve stress adaptation. Psychopharmacology (Berl) 2014;231:2067–75.
83. Meisel H. Multifunctional peptides encrypted in milk proteins. Biofactors 2004; 21:55–61.
84. Miclo L, Perrin E, Driou A, et al. Characterization of alpha-casozepine, a tryptic peptide from bovine alpha(s1)-casein with benzodiazepine-like activity. FASEB J 2001;15:1780–2.
85. Pereira GG, Fragoso S, Pires E. Effect of dietary intake of L-tryptophan supplementation on multihoused cats presenting stress related behaviours. Birmingham (United Kingdom): BSAVA; 2010.
86. Beata C, Beaumont-Graff E, Coll V, et al. Effect of alpha-casozepine (Zylkene) on anxiety in cats. J Vet Behav 2007;2:40–6.
87. Markwell PJ, Buffington CA, Chew DJ, et al. Clinical evaluation of commercially available urinary acidification diets in the management of idiopathic cystitis in cats. J Am Vet Med Assoc 1999;214:361–5.
88. Markwell PJ, Buffington CT, Smith BH. The effect of diet on lower urinary tract diseases in cats. J Nutr 1998;128:2753S–7S.
89. Hawthorne AJ, Markwell PJ. Dietary sodium promotes increased water intake and urine volume in cats. J Nutr 2004;134:2128S–9S.
90. Kirk CA, Jewell DE, Lowry SR. Effects of sodium chloride on selected parameters in cats. Vet Ther 2006;7:333–46.

91. Luckschander N, Iben C, Hosgood G, et al. Dietary NaCl does not affect blood pressure in healthy cats. J Vet Intern Med 2004;18:463–7.
92. Reynolds BS, Chetboul V, Nguyen P, et al. Effects of dietary salt intake on renal function: a 2-year study in healthy aged cats. J Vet Intern Med 2013;27:507–15.
93. Xu H, Laflamme DP, Long GL. Effects of dietary sodium chloride on health parameters in mature cats. J Feline Med Surg 2009;11:435–41.
94. Buranakarl C, Mathur S, Brown SA. Effects of dietary sodium chloride intake on renal function and blood pressure in cats with normal and reduced renal function. Am J Vet Res 2004;65:620–7.
95. Burger IH, Smith PM. Effects of diet on the urine characteristics of the cat. Nutrition, Malnutrition and Dietetics in the Dog and Cat Proceedings of an International Symposium. London. 1987. p. 71–3.
96. Osborne CA, Lulich JP, Kruger JM, et al. Analysis of 451,891 canine uroliths, feline uroliths, and feline urethral plugs from 1981 to 2007: perspectives from the Minnesota Urolith Center. Vet Clin North Am Small Anim Pract 2009;39:183–97.
97. Calder PC. n-3 polyunsaturated fatty acids, inflammation, and inflammatory diseases. Am J Clin Nutr 2006;83:1505S–19S.
98. Singh U, Devaraj S, Jialal I. Vitamin E, oxidative stress, and inflammation. Annu Rev Nutr 2005;25:151–74.
99. Parada B, Reis F, Cerejo R, et al. Omega-3 fatty acids inhibit tumor growth in a rat model of bladder cancer. Biomed Res Int 2013;2013:368178.
100. Forrester SD, Kruger JM, Allen TW. Feline lower urinary tract diseases. Small Animal Clinical Nutrition 2010;5:925–76.
101. Kruger JM, Lulich J, Merrills J, et al. A year-long prospective, randomized, double-masked study of nutrition on feline idiopathic cystitis. In: Proceedings American College of Veterinary Internal Medicine Annual Forum. 2013.
102. Lulich J, Kruger J, MacLeay J, et al. A randomized, controlled clinical trial evaluating the effect of a therapeutic urinary food for feline idiopathic cystitis. Hill's Global Symposium on Feline Lower Urinary Tract Health. Prague, Czech Republic. April 23-24, 2014. p. 55–9.
103. Kruger J, Lulich J, MacLeay J, et al. A randomized, double-masked, multicenter, clinical trial of two foods for long-term management of acute nonobstructive feline idiopathic cystitis (FIC). J Am Vet Med Assoc, in press.
104. Madersbacher H, van Ophoven A, van Kerrebroeck PE. GAG layer replenishment therapy for chronic forms of cystitis with intravesical glycosaminoglycans–a review. Neurourol Urodyn 2013;32:9–18.
105. Anderson VR, Perry CM. Pentosan polysulfate: a review of its use in the relief of bladder pain or discomfort in interstitial cystitis. Drugs 2006;66:821–35.
106. Nickel JC, Herschorn S, Whitmore KE, et al. Pentosan polysulfate sodium for treatment of interstitial cystitis-bladder pain syndrome: insights from a randomized, double-blind, placebo controlled study. J Urol 2014;193(3):857–62.
107. Wallius BM, Tidholm AE. Use of pentosan polysulphate in cats with idiopathic, non-obstructive lower urinary tract disease: a double-blind, randomised, placebo-controlled trial. J Feline Med Surg 2009;11:409–12.
108. Buffington T, Chew D, Kruger J, et al. Evaluation of pentosan polysulfate sodium in the treatment of feline interstitial cystitis—a randomized, placebo-controlled clinical trial. J Urol 2011;185:e382.
109. Giannantoni A, Bini V, Dmochowski R, et al. Contemporary management of the painful bladder: a systematic review. Eur Urol 2012;61:29–53.
110. Chew DJ, Buffington CA, Kendall MS, et al. Amitriptyline treatment for severe recurrent idiopathic cystitis in cats. J Am Vet Med Assoc 1998;213:1282–6.

111. Kraijer M, Fink-Gremmels J, Nickel RF. The short-term clinical efficacy of amitriptyline in the management of idiopathic feline lower urinary tract disease: a controlled clinical study. J Feline Med Surg 2003;5:191–6.
112. Bosch PC, Bosch DC. Treating interstitial cystitis/bladder pain syndrome as a chronic disease. Rev Urol 2014;16:83–7.
113. Osborne CA, Kruger JM, Lulich JP, et al. Prednisolone therapy of idiopathic feline lower urinary tract disease: a double-blind clinical study. Vet Clin North Am Small Anim Pract 1996;26:563–9.
114. Rourke W, Khan SA, Ahmed K, et al. Painful bladder syndrome/interstitial cystitis: aetiology, evaluation and management. Arch Ital Urol Androl 2014;86: 126–31.

Lower Urinary Tract Cancer

Claire M. Cannon[a], Sara D. Allstadt, DVM[b],*

KEYWORDS

- Transitional cell carcinoma • Prostate tumor • Chemotherapy • Radiation therapy

KEY POINTS

- Transitional cell carcinoma (TCC) is the most common urinary tract tumor in both cats and dogs.
- The most common location in the bladder for canine TCC is the trigone, making local control challenging. Local control is also challenging for canine prostate tumors.
- Systemic therapy is often the treatment of choice for urinary tract tumors and may be used in combination with other local therapies.
- Median survival time (MST) for dogs with TCC treated with nonsteroidal anti-inflammatory drugs (NSAIDS) alone is 4 to 6 months and with NSAIDs plus chemotherapy is 9 to 11 months.
- MST for cats with TCC treated with surgery, chemotherapy, NSAIDs, or a combination of these modalities is approximately 8.5 to 12 months.

CANINE URINARY BLADDER TUMORS

Urinary bladder tumors account for only about 2% of all canine tumors. Of these, transitional cell carcinoma (TCC) is the most common, affecting approximately 20,000 dogs each year.[1–4] Canine TCC develops most often in the trigone region of the bladder and commonly also involves the urethra or prostate. Interestingly, canine TCC closely resembles high-grade, muscle-invasive TCC in humans, making it a relevant animal model for research and translational study.[1,3]

Patient Evaluation Overview

A number of risk factors associated with an increased risk for development canine urinary bladder TCC have been noted (**Table 1**). In addition to the inherent risk factors outlined in **Table 1**, obesity and exposure to certain chemicals (older flea control

The authors have nothing to disclose.
[a] Department of Small Animal Clinical Sciences, College of Veterinary Medicine, University of Tennessee, 2407 River Drive, Knoxville, TN 37996, USA; [b] BluePearl Veterinary Partners, 13160 Magisterial Drive, Louisville, KY 40223, USA
* Corresponding author.
E-mail address: sara.allstadt@gmail.com

| Table 1 |
| Inherent risk factors for canine urinary bladder TCC |

Factor	Odds Ratio
Sex (female:male)	1.71–1.95:1
Breed	
Scottish Terrier	18.09
Shetland Sheepdog	4.46
Beagle	4.15
Wire-Haired Fox Terrier	3.20
West Highland White Terrier	3.03

Data from Refs.[2–9]

products, herbicides, and pesticides) are also considered to increase the risk of TCC; newer topical flea/tick control products, specifically those containing fipronil, are not of concern.[2–9] Therefore, dogs at highest risk are obese female dogs exposed to insecticides (odds ratio, 28). To date, no studies evaluating prevention in high-risk breeds have been performed, but given the data available, keeping pets at a lean body weight, limiting exposure to herbicides and pesticides, and feeding vegetables at least three times per week seem to be appropriate as preventive measures.[2–9]

Clinical Signs

Clinical signs (eg, hematuria, stranguria, pollakiuria, and dysuria) mimic other lower urinary tract diseases, and many dogs have concurrent urinary tract infections (UTIs), which may initially delay diagnosis. The secondary UTI is often resolved with appropriate antibiotic therapy and may result in temporary alleviation of the clinical signs, but signs recur. Thus, the presentation of a middle-aged dog with its first UTI should prompt imaging of the bladder to rule out bladder stones and/or a bladder mass in addition to ruling out other medical conditions that may predispose to a UTI (such as diabetes or hyperadrenocorticism). Physical examination may reveal a thickened urethra or trigonal region or an irregular prostate, which may be painful on digital rectal examination. Some cases may reveal no abnormalities on physical examination.[5] Only about 1 in 6 cases of urinary bladder TCC will have metastasis documented at the time of diagnosis, usually to the lymph nodes and/or lungs.[2,3,5,10,11] Mortality associated with TCC most commonly occurs owing to urinary tract obstruction or clinical signs associated with the primary tumor, rather than metastasis, owing to the challenges with local control.

Diagnostic Tests

Imaging

A urethral or bladder mass on ultrasound is suggestive for TCC or other neoplasia, but polyps and polypoid or other chronic cystitis can mimic neoplastic conditions, so ultimately cytology or histopathology is required. Thoracic and abdominal imaging with both radiography and ultrasonography in patients with known or suspected TCC is recommended to screen for metastatic disease, with common locations including lymph nodes, lungs, and liver. Less frequently, TCC may metastasize to other sites, including bone. Recently, CT has been shown to be the optimal way to serially image and monitor bladder tumors.[12] Dogs with higher stage tumors (eg, those with larger tumors or with metastasis) have shorter expected survival times.[7]

Antigen tests

Urine bladder tumor antigen tests have been reported to be 88% sensitive for detection of TCC, but a high number of false-positive results limit their usefulness.[13,14] These tests are useful only in a clinically normal dog with no known urinary tract abnormalities (such as screening for at-risk breeds); if the test is negative, there is a very low probability of TCC.

Definitive diagnosis

Options for obtaining a sample of a bladder mass include biopsy via cystoscopy, cystotomy, traumatic catheterization, or fine needle aspiration (FNA). Evaluation of sediment cytology samples is often misleading because urinary bladder epithelial cells may mimic a neoplastic population when cystitis is present. Bladder mass FNA is controversial because seeding of these tumors along the needle tract has been reported.[15,16] However, FNA may be considered in cases in which the tumor is large and nonresectable, after counseling of the owners on the risks and careful consideration of the all of the options available for diagnosis. A complete blood count and full serum chemistry profile with electrolytes to evaluate overall health and biochemical function is recommended along with urinalysis and urine culture. Azotemia may be present in patients with any degree of urinary tract obstruction.

Treatment Options

Surgery

Complete excision of TCC is often not feasible in dogs owing to urethral, prostatic or ureteral involvement, as well as the morbidity associated with complete cystectomy. In dogs where excision is feasible (eg, apically located tumors), surgery may prolong survival.[17,18] Robat and colleagues[18] reported a significantly increased overall median survival time (MST) in dogs who underwent chemotherapy plus cytoreductive surgery compared with dogs who received chemotherapy alone (217 vs 133 days, respectively; $P = .02$). Molnar and colleagues[17] found a significant survival benefit in a small number of dogs who underwent both surgery and chemotherapy compared with dogs who received chemotherapy alone (475 vs 31 days, respectively; $P<.001$). A "field effect" has been proposed for TCC because the entire bladder epithelium is exposed to carcinogens in the urine, and thus multifocal malignant changes are likely present. Therefore, recurrence either at the site of original surgery owing to inability to take wide margins, or at distant sites in the bladder owing to the field effect, is common. Nonetheless, given the available data, consideration should be given to surgery followed by chemotherapy when excision is possible.

Stenting

Urethral or ureteral stents can be used in dogs with evidence of obstruction and are often placed by fluoroscopic or ultrasonographic guidance.[19,20] Female dogs are commonly incontinent after urethral stent placement, which raises concerns for potential owner exposure in dogs that go on to receive chemotherapy. Approximately 39% of dogs (male and female) are incontinent after stent placement, and other complications include reobstruction (22%), stent migration, and bladder atony.[19] Other options for relief of ureteral or urethral obstruction include urinary diversion via subcutaneous ureteral bypass devices. It is unknown at the time of this writing how these new procedures may affect survival times, but because obstruction is often the factor leading to euthanasia in patients with TCC, any method that can manage obstruction would likely prolong survival. Laser ablation has also been described recently and may provide relief of clinical signs but has not yet been thoroughly studied or shown to alter overall survival greatly.[21,22]

Chemotherapy

Systemic chemotherapy is often the standard-of-care treatment for TCC owing to the lack of good options for local control. Typical approaches include treatment with nonsteroidal antiinflammatory drugs (NSAIDs) alone or in combination with systemic chemotherapy agents. Piroxicam is commonly favored as the first-line NSAID, although treatment with other NSAIDs such as deracoxib and firocoxib has also been reported.[23-25] Complete responses have been reported in a small number of cases treated with piroxicam alone, with an MST of 5.9 months.[24] The MST in a single report of 26 deracoxib-treated dogs was longer; however, those dogs received other chemotherapy agents after deracoxib.[25] Piroxicam has been noted to cause both nephrotoxicosis as well as gastrointestinal upset; thus, routine monitoring of the dog's renal function and gastrointestinal signs is indicated when administering piroxicam. Misoprostol can be used to prevent NSAID-induced ulceration; however, in the authors' experience, many dogs experience gastrointestinal cramping and upset from this drug. Misoprostol is also an abortifacient and, thus, women of child-bearing age should not be exposed to this drug. Drugs such as omeprazole or famotidine could be considered to reduce the risk of gastrointestinal side effects from NSAIDs; although there is no published evidence in companion animals, there is evidence in humans that this approach can reduce the risk of NSAID-induced gastric or duodenal ulceration.[26-28] Routine biochemical monitoring for renal and liver function and evidence of gastrointestinal ulceration is recommended for all dogs on NSAIDs, especially those considered at risk of urinary tract obstruction.

Cytotoxic agents with reported activity include mitoxantrone, carboplatin, cisplatin, doxorubicin, vinblastine, gemcitabine, vinorelbine, metronomic chlorambucil, and intravesical mitomycin C.[18,29-39] Mitoxantrone, carboplatin, and vinblastine in combination with NSAIDs are common first-line agents with reported response rates ranging from 35% to 38%.[29,31,35] Although favorable tumor responses to cisplatin and piroxicam are also noted, this combination is not recommended because of high nephrotoxicity.[32,33] A summary of study results for treatments for canine TCC is shown in **Table 2**. Overall, it seems there are similar outcomes for many drugs, and thus the advantages and disadvantages of each—cost, time, toxicity, and systemic health of the pet, including renal and hepatic function—should be taken into consideration when choosing a treatment regimen.

Radiation therapy

Early reports of radiation therapy for TCC in dogs were discouraging owing to side effects; however, more recently published protocols have been well-tolerated. Invasive TCC in humans is often treated with radiation therapy, either alone or in combination with surgery and/or chemotherapy, and radiation has been shown to be the most important component of therapy for this disease in humans.[40-44] To date, radiation therapy has not been extensively studied in dogs. High dose per fraction (21.88–27.00 Gy) intraoperative radiotherapy had a high risk of complications in one study, with 46% of dogs experiencing increased frequency of urination, 46% urinary incontinence, 38% cystitis, and 15% stranguria.[45] Despite this, MST was 16.8 months, implying that radiation therapy may have a role in treatment of canine TCC.

In 2004, Poirier and colleagues[46] investigated the use of piroxicam, mitoxantrone, and a coarse-fractionated protocol of radiation therapy (6 weekly fractions of 5.75 Gy) in 10 dogs with TCC, but did not find a superior response rate when compared with another study of mitoxantrone and piroxicam alone (response rate of 22% vs 34.5%; respectively).[29] Despite the lower objective response rate, 90% of patients had amelioration of clinical signs, and late side effects occurred in 3

Table 2
Summary of study results for treatments for canine urinary bladder TCC

Modality	Availability	Side Effects	Outcome	Recommended?
NSAIDs[23-25]	GP	Nephrotoxicity, hepatotoxicity	MST, ~4–6 mo	Yes, unless other contraindications (eg, renal failure)
Cytotoxic chemotherapy[23–25,29–39]	Specialist recommended/ some GPs may be trained in chemotherapy	Different drugs carry different risks and side effects: bone marrow suppression, GI upset, other; in general, ~80%–85% of dogs tolerate chemotherapy with a good quality of life	MST, ~8–11 mo	Yes, unless other contraindications (eg, biochemical abnormalities, MDR1 mutations)
Surgery[17,19]	Specialist, some GPs	General risks of surgery and anesthesia; TCC is highly prone to transplantation so care should be taken to reduce that risk	In combination with chemotherapy: MST, 7.1–15.5 m; more study needed to define outcome	Careful case selection recommended; apically located tumors are likely best candidates for surgical resection
Radiation therapy— palliative[29,46]	Specialist	Pollakuria, urinary incontinence, cystitis, and stranguria	Improved clinical signs in 90% of cases in 1 report	Consider in advanced cases
Radiation therapy— IMRT[47]	Specialist	Acute: hematuria and stranguria; late: strictures (rectal, ureteral, and urethral)	Limited data (single report) in combination with chemotherapy MST, 21.4 mo	Consider if no distant metastatic disease and committed owners; considerable time and financial commitment
Stenting[19,20]	Specialist	Incontinence (39%); reobstruction (22%), stent migration, and bladder atony; if incontinent, raises concerns for home and owner exposure to chemotherapy if chemotherapy is pursued after stent placement	Resolves obstruction; survival times not well-described, but expected to increase outcomes; about 20% reobstruct	Consider if obstructed; careful owner counseling recommended before pursuing stenting in case of incontinence after the procedure
Laser ablation[21,22]	Specialist	Stranguria, hematuria, stenosis, seeding of TCC, urethral and bladder perforation, bacterial cystitis	More study needed but reported MST 9.8–13.4 mo in combination with other therapies	Consider if obstructed; cases should be carefully selected

Abbreviations: GI, gastrointestinal; GP, general practitioner; IMRT, intensity-modulated radiation therapy; MST, median survival time; NSAID, nonsteroidal anti-inflammatory drug; TCC, transitional cell carcinoma.

dogs. More recently, image-guided, intensity-modulated radiation therapy (IMRT) has been studied in dogs with genitourinary tract tumors (bladder, urethra, and prostate).[47] In 21 dogs treated with IMRT (54–58 Gy delivered in 20 fractions on a Monday to Friday basis) and chemotherapy, MST was 654 days.[47] Two patients developed acute urinary complications, including hematuria and stranguria (1 each). Four patients developed urethral, ureteral, or rectal strictures as late complications; all were successfully palliated with either stenting or surgery.[47]

Evaluation of Outcome and Long-Term Recommendations

Overall, canine TCC carries a poor prognosis, and the majority of dogs succumb to this disease. However, the quality of life for most dogs receiving chemotherapy is excellent, and new therapies are being evaluated constantly. Dogs with larger tumors invading locoregionally or with evidence of metastasis (ie, more advanced stage) have a less favorable prognosis with shorter survival times or shorter time to obstruction.[2,7,47] Dogs at an increased risk for metastasis include younger dogs (increased risk of lymph node metastasis), dogs with prostate involvement (increased risk of distant metastasis), and dogs with larger tumors (increased risk for both nodal and distant metastasis).[2,47]

Many publications describe heavily pretreated dogs or dogs that go on to receive other treatments, which makes survival data for dogs with this tumor challenging to summarize. However, the following deductions may be made from the published data (**Table 2**):

- With NSAID therapy alone, expected MST is about 4 to 6 months.
- Addition of chemotherapy to NSAID therapy is expected to increase MST to approximately 9 to 11 months.
- Surgery, stenting, and radiation therapy all warrant consideration in appropriate cases and may improve survival.

CANINE PROSTATE TUMORS

Canine prostate tumors are uncommon, occurring in less than 1% of dogs.[48] The majority are carcinomas and may arise from the glandular epithelium, prostatic ducts, or prostatic urethra. Other reported prostate tumors in dogs include lymphoma,[49,50] hemangiosarcoma,[51,52] and leiomyosarcoma.[53]

Patient Evaluation Overview

Risk factors

Older, neutered male dogs are predisposed (**Box 1**). Many predisposed breeds are also predisposed to urinary bladder TCC, which may reflect the fact that many prostate tumors are TCCs arising from the prostatic urethra.

Clinical signs are indistinguishable from other causes of prostatic disease and most commonly include tenesmus, constipation, dyschezia, hematuria, stranguria, and dysuria, as well as systemic signs such as lethargy, weight loss, and anorexia. Patients may also present with lameness or skeletal pain owing to bony reaction or metastatic disease, and signs of skeletal metastasis may be the only presenting sign in some cases.[54–58]

Physical Examination

Prostatomegaly (typically asymmetric) is the most common abnormality, although it may not be present in all dogs.[56] No other consistent physical examination abnormalities have been reported, but may include abdominal pain, a palpable abdominal

---

Box 1
Potential risk factors for canine prostate tumors

Age[54,55,99,100]:

- Older dogs (median, 9–10 years)

Neuter status[48,99–101]:

- Neutered dogs at increased risk (OR 2–8 times compared with intact dogs, depending on type of tumor; most effect in TCC and least in adenocarcinoma)

Breed[48,102]:

- Mixed-breed
- Shetland Sheepdog
- Scottish Terrier
- Beagle
- German Shorthaired Pointer
- Airedale
- Norwegian Elkhounds
- Bouvier des Flandres

Abbreviations: OR, odds ratio; TCC, transitional cell carcinoma.

---

mass, pyrexia, depression, and musculoskeletal pain; special attention should be paid to signs of pain or lameness given the high propensity for bony metastasis. Prostatomegaly and associated clinical signs in an older neutered male dog should raise a strong suspicion for prostate cancer.

Diagnostic Tests

Radiography
Prostatomegaly and mineralization are associated strongly with neoplasia in neutered dogs. More caution is needed in interpretation in intact dogs (also seen with benign prostatic hyperplasia, prostatitis, and prostatic cysts).[59,60] Other abnormalities noted with prostatic neoplasia include bony reaction, especially of the pelvis or lumbar vertebrae, and lymphadenopathy.[59,60] Thoracic radiographs should be performed in every case of prostatic neoplasia because the lungs are common sites of metastasis.[55,56,58] Skeletal metastases are common (especially affecting the axial skeleton) and most, but not all, dogs with skeletal metastases also had visceral metastases in 1 study.[55] Skeletal survey radiographs could be considered if aggressive therapy is an option (eg, definitive radiation therapy), but at the very least, radiographs of affected areas for dogs displaying signs of musculoskeletal pain or myelopathy should be performed.

Abdominal ultrasound
Disruption of the prostatic capsule, focal to multifocal areas of increased echogenicity/mineralization in the prostate, and enlarged lymph nodes are associated with neoplasia.[59,61] A complete abdominal ultrasound should be performed to evaluate for metastasis—local lymph nodes are the most common sites, but others include the liver, kidneys, distant lymph nodes, large intestines, heart, adrenal glands, brain, and spleen. Diffuse peritoneal metastasis/carcinomatosis is also reported.[55,56,62]

Definitive diagnosis

Cytology samples may be obtained via prostatic wash or FNA. Occasionally, neoplastic cells may be detected in the urine.[56] Biopsies for histopathology may be obtained via ultrasound-guided needle core biopsy or laparotomy. Given that there are currently no proven prognostic or therapeutic differences between different types of carcinoma (eg, ductal vs glandular origin vs TCC of prostatic urethra), the authors do not recommend additional procedures for histopathology in cases where cytology confirms carcinoma. In cases of suspected prostate cancer, the risk of seeding cancer cells along a needle tract should be considered before aspiration or biopsy,[15,63] and this is of particular concern when owners may consider aggressive therapy (eg, IMRT); noninvasive options such as prostatic wash are preferable in these situations. Urine culture should be performed in all patients because secondary infections are common.[56]

Treatment Options

Non-steroidal anti-inflammatory drugs

Canine prostate tumors frequently express cyclooxygenase (COX)-1 and COX-2,[64–66] and the use of NSAIDs (piroxicam or carprofen) has shown a significant improvement in survival in dogs with prostate tumors (most of which were of urothelial origin; **Table 3**).[66] Cytotoxic chemotherapy has not been evaluated specifically in canine prostate tumors, but its utility in canine bladder TCC suggests that it could be considered, and anecdotally it is recommended commonly. There is some in vitro evidence for the effectiveness of paclitaxel,[67] and this may bear further clinical investigation given the recent approval of Paccal Vet-CA1. However, the current conditional approval means that this drug cannot be used routinely for canine prostate cancer (not a labeled indication).

Radiation Therapy

The previously mentioned study of IMRT showed promising outcomes for dogs with prostatic neoplasia. However, this modality is not suitable for dogs with distant metastatic disease, and owners should be counseled about risks of side effects, as discussed.[47] Palliative radiation therapy may be used to relieve severe clinical signs, urethral obstruction, or pain from bone metastases. The risk of late side effects to the gastrointestinal and urinary tract is theoretically considerable with palliative protocols, but clinically not of great concern because of the palliative intent—most patients do not live long enough to experience late side effects.

Other

Urethral stenting can palliate dogs with obstruction, and although incontinence is common, most dogs were judged to have good outcomes in 1 study.[20] Based on the available literature, NSAIDs should be recommended in all patients, and IMRT should be offered to suitable candidates; cytotoxic chemotherapy should be considered, but evidence as to its true efficacy is lacking. Surgery is not recommended owing to a high incidence of complications and lack of improvement in outcomes over NSAIDs alone, and other investigational treatments such as photodynamic therapy have likewise shown no additional benefit.

Evaluation of Outcome and Long-term Recommendations

Canine prostate cancer has a poor to grave prognosis given the difficulty in controlling the local disease and the high risk of metastasis. With treatment, reported MST range from approximately 3 to 4 months to up to 1.8 years for dogs with disease

Table 3
Treatment options in canine prostate cancer

Modality	Availability	Side Effects	Outcomes	Recommended?
NSAIDs[66]	GP	Renal, GI	MST, 6.9 vs 0.7 mo for untreated	Yes, unless other contraindications
Cytotoxic chemotherapy	Specialist/some GPs	Bone marrow suppression, GI upset, other	Unknown in primary prostate tumors	Consider owing to high metastatic potential, although unknown benefit; indicated in lymphoma
Radiation therapy, palliative	Specialist	Acute: colitis most common; late: usually not clinically relevant owing to short survival	Anecdotal palliation of clinical signs, no large studies	Consider if obstruction, clinical signs not responding to other therapy, bone metastasis
Radiation therapy, definitive IMRT (± chemotherapy)[47]	Specialist	Colitis, skin effects most common—generally mild, severe late side effects possible but rare	Potential clinical benefit in 90%; median event-free survival (local recurrence or metastasis), 10 mo	Consider if no distant metastatic disease and committed owners, considerable time and financial commitment
Urethral stent[20]	Specialist	Incontinence, stranguria	5/7 dogs judged to have good to excellent outcome	Consider if obstructed, palliative only
Photodynamic therapy (± surgery, NSAIDs)[94,95]	Specialist/investigational	Not identified	No apparent benefit overall, one report of potential long-term response	Not recommended
Total prostatectomy[96]	Specialist	Incontinence, hematuria, detrusor atony, others	Complications life-limiting in many dogs	Not recommended
Subcapsular prostatectomy (laser or surgical) ± NSAIDs, adjuvant therapy[97,98]	Specialist	Complications requiring euthanasia possible (≤26%), otherwise mild, eg, incontinence	Improvement in clinical signs in most, but MST ~3–6 mo	Not recommended

Abbreviations: GI, gastrointestinal; GP, general practitioner; IMRT, image-guided, intensity-modulated radiation therapy; MST, median survival time; NSAID, nonsteroidal anti-inflammatory drug; TCC, transitional cell carcinoma.

confined to the prostate treated with IMRT.[47] Therapy is generally aimed at relieving clinical signs and improving comfort with long-term tumor control not expected in most cases.

FELINE LOWER URINARY TRACT TUMORS

Lower urinary tract tumors in cats are very uncommon and mostly affect the urinary bladder, with primary urethral and prostatic tumors being exceedingly rare.[68–74] Like dogs, the most common lower urinary tract tumor is TCC.[75–80] Others include various sarcomas,[75,81,82] leiomyomas,[83] lipomas,[84] and lymphoma, either as part of multicentric disease or localized to the urinary bladder.[75,77,78,85,86]

Patient Evaluation Overview

Signalment

Older cats (median age, 10–15 years) are predisposed to urinary bladder tumors in general, but lymphoma may be seen in cats as young as 1 year of age.[75,76,78–80] A male predisposition has been seen in some studies but not others,[76,78,80] and there is no known breed predilection. Interestingly, a genetic predisposition is possible with 2 case series describing urinary bladder TCC in related captive fishing cats, though there are no similar reports in related domestic cats.[87,88]

Clinical signs

Clinical signs are consistent with lower urinary tract disease (**Box 2**), and systemic signs are also common.[69,79,83–86] Rarely, TCC is diagnosed in cats presenting for non–urinary-tract–related signs.[76,78,80] Because the median age of cats with urinary bladder neoplasia is significantly older than cats with idiopathic lower urinary tract disease,[89] lower urinary tract signs in any older cat should raise the suspicion for neoplasia; cats with severe clinical signs (eg, marked hematuria) or cats with chronic intermittent lower urinary tract signs also bear further investigation for an underlying cause. Some cats with urinary bladder neoplasia have a history of suspected or confirmed idiopathic cystitis for months to years,[78,80,83] and chronic inflammation may have promoted tumor development in these cases (although an association has not been demonstrated).

Physical Examination

There are no findings that are specific for urinary bladder neoplasia, although a distended bladder or abdominal mass effect may be palpable. An enlarged, irregular

---

Box 2
Clinical signs of lower urinary tract neoplasia in cats

- Hematuria (may be profound)
- Stranguria/dysuria/pollakiuria
- Incontinence
- Inappropriate elimination
- Urethral obstruction
- Systemic signs (eg, anorexia, weight loss, lethargy)

Modified from Refs.[76,78–80,86]

prostate on rectal examination is very suspicious for prostatic neoplasia; other prostatic disease is even less common than prostatic neoplasia in cats.

Diagnostic Tests

Diagnostic tests are aimed at diagnosing the primary tumor and screening for metastasis. Although metastasis is not common (0%–27%) at diagnosis in TCC,[76,80] widespread disease can occur (lymph nodes and lungs are common sites), and complete abdominal ultrasound and thoracic radiographs should be performed.[76–78,86,90]

Imaging

Reported abnormalities on abdominal radiographs (plain or contrast studies) include bladder distension, thickened or calcified bladder wall, and presence of a mass.[78] Ultrasound has mostly superseded radiography for detection of lower urinary tract neoplasia. A mass is identifiable in most cases, but the bladder wall may seem to be thickened diffusely.[80] In contrast with dogs, TCC occurs in cats most commonly in nontrigonal regions of the bladder wall.[76,78–80] Cats with tumors causing urethral or ureteral obstruction may have ultrasonographic evidence of hydronephrosis.

Definitive diagnosis has been achieved via urine cytology,[76,80,86] cytology of catheter suction biopsies/traumatic catheterization,[76,80] FNA,[76,91] and histopathology, usually via laparotomy and cystotomy for biopsy or partial cystectomy.[78–80] Although not reported in cats, there may be a risk of tumor seeding to the abdominal wall along needle tracts, and less invasive methods (eg, traumatic catheterization) should be considered first, especially for surgical candidates.

Common abnormalities on routine laboratory tests (complete blood count, chemistry panel, and urinalysis) include anemia and azotemia, either owing to preexisting chronic kidney disease or obstruction caused by the tumor.[75,76,78] In cats with urinary bladder lymphoma, feline leukemia virus (with or without feline immunodeficiency virus) testing should be performed.[85] There is 1 report of suspected paraneoplastic hypereosinophilia in a cat with urinary bladder TCC and widespread metastasis.[90] Hematuria and pyuria are common, and neoplastic cells in the urine have been identified in rare cases,[76,80] but atypical transitional cells in urine, as discussed in canine TCC, should always be interpreted with caution. Urine culture is recommended in all cases of suspected urinary tract neoplasia because secondary infections are common.[76,78]

Treatment Options

Urinary bladder TCCs in cats frequently express COX-1 and COX-2,[80,88] so NSAIDs are a rational therapeutic choice. Surgical excision is commonly performed for TCC and may also be effective for other urinary bladder tumors and some prostate tumors.[72,73] Urethral stents or cystostomy tubes may be used to palliate patients with urethral obstruction.[80,92,93] **Table 4** for details about these options.

Evaluation of Outcome and Long-term Recommendations

Many cats with urinary bladder TCC are euthanized at diagnosis owing to debilitation, urethral obstruction, or evidence of metastatic disease. Ultimately, most cats with urinary bladder TCC will die owing to local or metastatic disease. Local recurrence is common after surgical excision, but because prolonged tumor control may be seen in some cases and surgery may improve survival, surgery is recommended for accessible (nontrigonal), nonmetastatic TCC.[76,80] Median survival time for cats treated with surgery, chemotherapy, NSAIDs, or a combination of these modalities is approximately 8.5 to 12 months.[76,80] Given the paucity of the literature, it is impossible to

Table 4
Treatment options for cats with urinary bladder neoplasia

Modality	Availability	Side Effects	Recommended?
Surgery (partial cystectomy)[72,73,76,80]	GP	Decreased bladder capacity	Yes, for tumors other than lymphoma in accessible (nontrigonal) locations, without metastatic disease
NSAIDs: Meloxicam (0.1 mg/kg PO SID initially, then 0.05 mg/kg SID) or piroxicam (0.3 mg/kg PO SID 2–3 times per week). Although not evaluated, robenacoxib should be considered owing to its favorable safety profile. All off-label.[76,80]	GP	Renal failure, GI (diarrhea, melena)	Yes, in TCC–can palliate clinical signs (potentially for months) used alone, consider adjunctively after surgery. Preexisting chronic kidney disease does not necessarily preclude NSAID use, but renal function must be closely monitored in all patients.[80]
Cytotoxic chemotherapy	Specialist/some GPs	Bone marrow suppression, GI upset, other	Indicated in lymphoma, not strongly recommended for TCC
Urethral stent[92]	Specialist	Infections and incontinence– $\leq 50\%$[92]	Consider if obstructed–palliative only

Abbreviations: GI, gastrointestinal; GP, general practitioner; NSAID, nonsteroidal anti-inflammatory drug; PO, orally; SID, once a day; TCC, transitional cell carcinoma.

prognosticate for other bladder tumor types or for primary prostate tumors, but surgery should be considered where appropriate because prolonged, good outcomes have been reported in some cases.

ACKNOWLEDGMENTS

The authors thank Misty Bailey for her editorial assistance.

REFERENCES

1. Knapp DW, Ramos-Vara JA, Moore GE, et al. Urinary bladder cancer in dogs, a naturally occurring model for cancer biology and drug development. ILAR J 2014;55:100–18.
2. Knapp DW, Glickman NW, Denicola DB, et al. Naturally-occurring canine transitional cell carcinoma of the urinary bladder: a relevant model of human invasive bladder cancer. Urol Oncol 2000;5:47–59.
3. Knapp DW. Animal models of naturally occurring canine urinary bladder cancer. In: Lerner SP, Schoenberg MP, Sternberg C, editors. Textbook of bladder cancer. (United Kingdom): Taylor and Francis; 2006. p. 171–5.

4. Mutsaers AJ, Widmer WR, Knapp DW. Canine transitional cell carcinoma. J Vet Intern Med 2003;17(2):136–44.
5. Norris AM, Laing EJ, Valli VE, et al. Canine bladder and urethral tumors: a retrospective study of 115 cases (1980-1985). J Vet Intern Med 1992;6:149–53.
6. Hayes HM Jr. Canine bladder cancer: epidemiologic features. Am J Epidemiol 1976;104:673–7.
7. Knapp DW, McMillan SK. Tumors of the urinary system. In: Withrow SJ, Vail DM, Page RL, editors. Withrow and MacEwen's small animal clinical oncology. 5th edition. St Louis (MO): Saunders Elsevier; 2013. p. 572–82.
8. Glickman LT, Raghavan M, Knapp DW, et al. Herbicide exposure and the risk of transitional cell carcinoma of the urinary bladder in Scottish Terriers. J Am Vet Med Assoc 2004;224:1290–7.
9. Raghavan M, Knapp DW, Bonney PL, et al. Evaluation of the effect of dietary vegetable consumption on reducing risk of transitional cell carcinoma of the urinary bladder in Scottish Terriers. J Am Vet Med Assoc 2005;227:94–100.
10. Tarvin G, Patnaik A, Greene R. Primary urethral tumors in dogs. J Am Vet Med Assoc 1978;172:931–3.
11. Santos M, Dias Pereira P, Montenegro L, et al. Recurrent and metastatic canine urethral transitional cell carcinoma without bladder involvement. Vet Rec 2007; 160:557–8.
12. Nieset JR, Harmon JF, Larue SM. Use of cone-beam computed tomography to characterize daily urinary bladder variations during fractionated radiotherapy for canine bladder cancer. Vet Radiol Ultrasound 2011;52:580–8.
13. Borjesson DL, Christopher MM, Ling GV. Detection of canine transitional cell carcinoma using a bladder tumor antigen urine dipstick test. Vet Clin Pathol 1999; 28:33–8.
14. Henry CJ, Tyler JW, McEntee MC, et al. Evaluation of a bladder tumor antigen test as a screening test for transitional cell carcinoma of the lower urinary tract in dogs. Am J Vet Res 2003;64:1017–20.
15. Nyland TG, Wallack ST, Wisner ER. Needle-tract implantation following us-guided fine-needle aspiration biopsy of transitional cell carcinoma of the bladder, urethra, and prostate. Vet Radiol Ultrasound 2002;43:50–3.
16. Vignoli M, Rossi F, Chierici C, et al. Needle tract implantation after fine needle aspiration biopsy (FNAB) of transitional cell carcinoma of the urinary bladder and adenocarcinoma of the lung. Schweiz Arch Tierheilkd 2007; 149:314–8.
17. Molnar T, Vajdovich P. Clinical factors determining the efficacy of urinary bladder tumour treatments in dogs: surgery, chemotherapy or both? Acta Vet Hung 2012;60:55–68.
18. Robat C, Burton J, Thamm D, et al. Retrospective evaluation of doxorubicin-piroxicam combination for the treatment of transitional cell carcinoma in dogs. J Small Anim Pract 2013;54:67–74.
19. Blackburn AL, Berent AC, Weisse CW, et al. Evaluation of outcome following urethral stent placement for the treatment of obstructive carcinoma of the urethra in dogs: 42 cases (2004-2008). J Am Vet Med Assoc 2013;242:59–68.
20. Weisse C, Berent A, Todd K, et al. Evaluation of palliative stenting for management of malignant urethral obstructions in dogs. J Am Vet Med Assoc 2006;229: 226–34.
21. Cerf DJ, Lindquist EC. Palliative ultrasound-guided endoscopic diode laser ablation of transitional cell carcinomas of the lower urinary tract in dogs. J Am Vet Med Assoc 2012;240:51–60.

22. Upton ML, Tangner CH, Payton ME. Evaluation of carbon dioxide laser ablation combined with mitoxantrone and piroxicam treatment in dogs with transitional cell carcinoma. J Am Vet Med Assoc 2006;228:549–52.

23. Knapp DW, Henry CJ, Widmer WR, et al. Randomized trial of cisplatin versus firocoxib versus cisplatin/firocoxib in dogs with transitional cell carcinoma of the urinary bladder. J Vet Intern Med 2013;27:126–33.

24. Knapp DW, Richardson RC, Chan TC, et al. Piroxicam therapy in 34 dogs with transitional cell carcinoma of the urinary bladder. J Vet Intern Med 1994; 8:273–8.

25. McMillan SK, Boria P, Moore GE, et al. Antitumor effects of deracoxib treatment in 26 dogs with transitional cell carcinoma of the urinary bladder. J Am Vet Med Assoc 2011;239:1084–9.

26. Desai JC, Sanyai SM, Goo T, et al. Primary prevention of adverse gastroduodenal effects from short-term use of non-steroidal anti-inflammatory drugs by omeprazole 20mg in healthy subjects: a randomized, double-blind, placebo controlled study. Dig Dis Sci 2008;53:2059–65.

27. Graham DY, Agrawal NM, Campbell DR, et al. Ulcer prevention in long-term users of nonsteroidal anti-inflammatory drugs: results of a double-blind, randomized, multicenter active- and placebo-controlled study of misoprostol vs lansoprazole. Arch Intern Med 2002;162:169–75.

28. Cullen D, Bardhan KD, Eisner M, et al. Primary gastroduodenal prophylaxis with omemprazole for non-steroidal anti-inflammatory drug users. Aliment Pharmacol Ther 1998;12:135–40.

29. Henry CJ, McCaw DL, Turnquist SE, et al. Clinical evaluation of mitoxantrone and piroxicam in a canine model of human invasive urinary bladder carcinoma. Clin Cancer Res 2003;9:906–11.

30. Chun R, Knapp DW, Widmer WR, et al. Phase II clinical trial of carboplatin in canine transitional cell carcinoma of the urinary bladder. J Vet Intern Med 1997;11:279–83.

31. Boria PA, Glickman NW, Schmidt BR, et al. Carboplatin and piroxicam therapy in 31 dogs with transitional cell carcinoma of the urinary bladder. Vet Comp Oncol 2005;3:73–80.

32. Chun R, Knapp DW, Widmer WR, et al. Cisplatin treatment of transitional cell carcinoma of the urinary bladder in dogs: 18 cases (1983-1993). J Am Vet Med Assoc 1996;209:1588–91.

33. Knapp DW, Glickman NW, Widmer WR, et al. Cisplatin versus cisplatin combined with piroxicam in a canine model of human invasive urinary bladder cancer. Cancer Chemother Pharmacol 2000;46:221–6.

34. Greene SN, Lucroy MD, Greenberg CB, et al. Evaluation of cisplatin administered with piroxicam in dogs with transitional cell carcinoma of the urinary bladder. J Am Vet Med Assoc 2007;231:1056–60.

35. Arnold EJ, Childress MO, Fourez LM, et al. Clinical trial of vinblastine in dogs with transitional cell carcinoma of the urinary bladder. J Vet Intern Med 2011; 25:1385–90.

36. Marconato L, Zini E, Lindner D, et al. Toxic effects and antitumor response of gemcitabine in combination with piroxicam treatment in dogs with transitional cell carcinoma of the urinary bladder. J Am Vet Med Assoc 2011;238: 1004–10.

37. Kaye ME, Thamm DH, Weishaar K, et al. Vinorelbine rescue therapy for dogs with primary urinary bladder carcinoma. Vet Comp Oncol 2013. http://dx.doi.org/10.1111/vco.12065.

38. Schrempp DR, Childress MO, Stewart JC, et al. Metronomic administration of chlorambucil for treatment of dogs with urinary bladder transitional cell carcinoma. J Am Vet Med Assoc 2013;242:1534–8.
39. Abbo AH, Jones DR, Masters AR, et al. Phase I clinical trial and pharmacokinetics of intravesical mitomycin C in dogs with localized transitional cell carcinoma of the urinary bladder. J Vet Intern Med 2010;24:1124–30.
40. Foroudi F, Pham D, Bressel M, et al. Bladder cancer radiotherapy margins: a comparison of daily alignment using skin, bone or soft tissue. Clin Oncol 2012;24:673–81.
41. Ichinohe K, Ijima M, Usami T, et al. Complete remission of primary retroperitoneal transitional cell carcinoma after radiotherapy and oral chemotherapy: a case report. Ann R Coll Surg Engl 2013;95:e52–4.
42. Jang NY, Kim IA, Byun SS, et al. Patterns of failure and prognostic factors for locoregional recurrence after radical surgery in upper urinary tract transitional cell carcinoma: implications for adjuvant radiotherapy. Urol Int 2013;90:202–6.
43. Mitin T, Hunt D, Shipley WU, et al. Transurethral surgery and twice-daily radiation plus paclitaxel-cisplatin or fluorouracil-cisplatin with selective bladder preservation and adjuvant chemotherapy for patients with muscle invasive bladder cancer (RTOG 0233): a randomised multicentre phase 2 trial. Lancet Oncol 2013;14:863–72.
44. Zapatero A, Martin De Vidales C, Arellano R, et al. Long-term results of two prospective bladder-sparing trimodality approaches for invasive bladder cancer: neoadjuvant chemotherapy and concurrent radio-chemotherapy. Urology 2012;80:1056–62.
45. Walker MB, Breider M. Intraoperative radiotherapy of canine bladder cancer. Vet Radiol 1987;28:200–4.
46. Poirier VJ, Forrest LJ, Adams WM, et al. Piroxicam, mitoxantrone, and coarse fraction radiotherapy for the treatment of transitional cell carcinoma of the bladder in 10 dogs: a pilot study. J Am Anim Hosp Assoc 2004;40:131–6.
47. Nolan MW, Kogan L, Griffin LR, et al. Intensity-modulated and image-guided radiation therapy for treatment of genitourinary carcinomas in dogs. J Vet Intern Med 2012;26:987–95.
48. Bryan JN, Keeler MR, Henry CJ, et al. A population study of neutering status as a risk factor for canine prostate cancer. Prostate 2007;67:1174–81.
49. Assin R, Baldi A, Citro G, et al. Prostate as sole unusual recurrence site of lymphoma in a dog. In Vivo 2008;22:755–7.
50. Winter MD, Locke JE, Penninck DG. Imaging diagnosis–urinary obstruction secondary to prostatic lymphoma in a young dog. Vet Radiol Ultrasound 2006;47:597–601.
51. Della Santa D, Dandrieux J, Psalla D, et al. Primary prostatic haemangiosarcoma causing severe haematuria in a dog. J Small Anim Pract 2008;49:249–51.
52. Hayden DW, Bartges JW, Bell FW, et al. Prostatic hemangiosarcoma in a dog: clinical and pathologic findings. J Vet Diagn Invest 1992;4:209–11.
53. Hayden DW, Klausner JS, Waters DJ. Prostatic leiomyosarcoma in a dog. J Vet Diag Invest 1999;11:283–6.
54. Krawiec DR, Heflin D. Study of prostatic disease in dogs: 177 cases (1981-1986). J Am Vet Med Assoc 1992;200:1119–22.
55. Cornell KK, Bostwick DG, Cooley DM, et al. Clinical and pathologic aspects of spontaneous canine prostate carcinoma: a retrospective analysis of 76 cases. Prostate 2000;45:173–83.

56. Bell FW, Klausner JS, Hayden DW, et al. Clinical and pathologic features of prostatic adenocarcinoma in sexually intact and castrated dogs: 31 cases (1970-1987). J Am Vet Med Assoc 1991;199:1623–30.
57. Malek S, Murphy KA, Nykamp SG, et al. Metastatic transitional cell carcinoma in proximal humerus of a dog. Can Vet J 2011;52:1013–7.
58. Cooley DM, Waters DJ. Skeletal metastasis as the initial clinical manifestation of metastatic carcinoma in 19 dogs. J Vet Intern Med 1998;12:288–93.
59. Bradbury CA, Westropp JL, Pollard RE. Relationship between prostatomegaly, prostatic mineralization, and cytologic diagnosis. Vet Radiol Ultrasound 2009; 50:167–71.
60. Feeney DA, Johnston GR, Klausner JS, et al. Canine prostatic disease–comparison of radiographic appearance with morphologic and microbiologic findings: 30 cases (1981-1985). J Am Vet Med Assoc 1987;190:1018–26.
61. Feeney DA, Johnston GR, Klausner JS, et al. Canine prostatic disease–comparison of ultrasonographic appearance with morphologic and microbiologic findings: 30 cases (1981-1985). J Am Vet Med Assoc 1987;190:1027–34.
62. Swinney GR. Prostatic neoplasia in five dogs. Aust Vet J 1998;76:669–74.
63. Higuchi T, Burcham GN, Childress MO, et al. Characterization and treatment of transitional cell carcinoma of the abdominal wall in dogs: 24 cases (1985-2010). J Am Vet Med Assoc 2013;242:499–506.
64. Mohammed SI, Khan KN, Sellers RS, et al. Expression of cyclooxygenase-1 and 2 in naturally-occurring canine cancer. Prostaglandins Leukot Essent Fatty Acids 2004;70:479–83.
65. L'Eplattenier HF, Lai CL, van den Ham R, et al. Regulation of COX-2 expression in canine prostate carcinoma: increased COX-2 expression is not related to inflammation. J Vet Intern Med 2007;21:776–82.
66. Sorenmo KU, Goldschmidt MH, Shofer FS, et al. Evaluation of cyclooxygenase-1 and cyclooxygenase-2 expression and the effect of cyclooxygenase inhibitors in canine prostatic carcinoma. Vet Comp Oncol 2004;2:13–23.
67. Axiak-Bechtel SM, Kumar SR, Dank KK, et al. Nanoparticulate paclitaxel demonstrates antitumor activity in PC3 and Ace-1 aggressive prostate cancer cell lines. Invest New Drugs 2013;31:1609–15.
68. Osborne CA, Low DG, Perman V, et al. Neoplasms of the canine and feline urinary bladder: incidence, etiologic factors, occurrence and pathologic features. Am J Vet Res 1968;29:2041–55.
69. Barrett RE, Nobel TA. Transitional cell carcinoma of the urethra in a cat. Cornell Vet 1976;66:14–26.
70. Caney SM, Holt PE, Day MJ, et al. Prostatic carcinoma in two cats. J Small Anim Pract 1998;39:140–3.
71. Tursi M, Costa T, Valenza F, et al. Adenocarcinoma of the disseminated prostate in a cat. J Feline Med Surg 2008;10:600–2.
72. Zambelli D, Cunto M, Raccagni R, et al. Successful surgical treatment of a prostatic biphasic tumour (sarcomatoid carcinoma) in a cat. J Feline Med Surg 2010; 12:161–5.
73. Hubbard BS, Vulgamott JC, Liska WD. Prostatic adenocarcinoma in a cat. J Am Vet Med Assoc 1990;197:1493–4.
74. LeRoy BE, Lech ME. Prostatic carcinoma causing urethral obstruction and obstipation in a cat. J Feline Med Surg 2004;6:397–400.
75. Patnaik AK, Schwarz PD, Greene RW. A histopathologic study of twenty urinary bladder neoplasms in the cat. J Small Anim Pract 1986;27:433–45.

76. Wilson HM, Chun R, Larson VS, et al. Clinical signs, treatments, and outcome in cats with transitional cell carcinoma of the urinary bladder: 20 cases (1990-2004). J Am Vet Med Assoc 2007;231:101–6.
77. Simpson CJ, Mansfield CS, Milne ME, et al. Central diabetes insipidus in a cat with central nervous system B cell lymphoma. J Feline Med Surg 2011;13:787–92.
78. Schwarz PD, Greene RW, Patnaik AK. Urinary-bladder tumors in the cat - a review of 27 cases. J Am Anim Hosp Assoc 1985;21:237–45.
79. Brearley MJ, Thatcher C, Cooper JE. Three cases of transitional cell carcinoma in the cat and a review of the literature. Vet Rec 1986;118:91–4.
80. Bommer NX, Hayes AM, Scase TJ, et al. Clinical features, survival times and COX-1 and COX-2 expression in cats with transitional cell carcinoma of the urinary bladder treated with meloxicam. J Feline Med Surg 2012;14:527–33.
81. Burk RL, Meierhenry EF, Schaubhut CW Jr. Leiomyosarcoma of the urinary bladder in a cat. J Am Vet Med Assoc 1975;167:749–51.
82. Pavia PR, Havig ME, Donovan TA, et al. Malignant peripheral nerve sheath tumour of the urinary bladder in a cat. J Small Anim Pract 2012;53:245–8.
83. Patnaik AK, Greene RW. Intravenous leiomyoma of the bladder in a cat. J Am Vet Med Assoc 1979;175:381–3.
84. Khodakaram-Tafti A, Shirian S, Vesal N, et al. Lipoma of the urinary bladder in a cat. J Comp Pathol 2011;144:212–3.
85. Benigni L, Lamb CR, Corzo-Menendez N, et al. Lymphoma affecting the urinary bladder in three dogs and a cat. Vet Radiol Ultrasound 2006;47:592–6.
86. Geigy CA, Dandrieux J, Miclard J, et al. Extranodal B-cell lymphoma in the urinary bladder with cytological evidence of concurrent involvement of the gall bladder in a cat. J Small Anim Pract 2010;51:280–7.
87. Sutherland-Smith M, Harvey C, Campbell M, et al. Transitional cell carcinomas in four fishing cats (*Prionailurus viverrinus*). J Zoo Wildl Med 2004;35:370–80.
88. Landolfi JA, Terio KA. Transitional cell carcinoma in fishing cats (*Prionailurus viverrinus*): pathology and expression of cyclooxygenase-1, -2, and p53. Vet Pathol 2006;43:674–81.
89. Buffington CA, Chew DJ, Kendall MS, et al. Clinical evaluation of cats with non-obstructive urinary tract diseases. J Am Vet Med Assoc 1997;210:46–50.
90. Sellon RK, Rottman JB, Jordan HL, et al. Hypereosinophilia associated with transitional cell carcinoma in a cat. J Am Vet Med Assoc 1992;201:591–3.
91. Walker DB, Cowell RL, Clinkenbeard KD, et al. Carcinoma in the urinary bladder of a cat: cytologic findings and a review of the literature. Vet Clin Pathol 1993;22:103–8.
92. Brace MA, Weisse C, Berent A. Preliminary experience with stenting for management of non-urolith urethral obstruction in eight cats. Vet Surg 2014;43:199–208.
93. Newman RG, Mehler SJ, Kitchell BE, et al. Use of a balloon-expandable metallic stent to relieve malignant urethral obstruction in a cat. J Am Vet Med Assoc 2009;234:236–9.
94. Lucroy MD, Bowles MH, Higbee RG, et al. Photodynamic therapy for prostatic carcinoma in a dog. J Vet Intern Med 2003;17:235–7.
95. L'Eplattenier HF, Klem B, Teske E, et al. Preliminary results of intraoperative photodynamic therapy with 5-aminolevulinic acid in dogs with prostate carcinoma. Vet J 2008;178:202–7.
96. Goldsmid SE, Bellenger CR. Urinary incontinence after prostatectomy in dogs. Vet Surg 1991;20:253–6.

97. L'Eplattenier HF, van Nimwegen SA, van Sluijs FJ, et al. Partial prostatectomy using Nd:YAG laser for management of canine prostate carcinoma. Vet Surg 2006;35:406–11.

98. Vlasin M, Rauser P, Fichtel T, et al. Subtotal intracapsular prostatectomy as a useful treatment for advanced-stage prostatic malignancies. J Small Anim Pract 2006;47:512–6.

99. Sorenmo KU, Goldschmidt M, Shofer F, et al. Immunohistochemical character-ization of canine prostatic carcinoma and correlation with castration status and castration time. Vet Comp Oncol 2003;1:48–56.

100. Teske E, Naan EC, van Dijk EM, et al. Canine prostate carcinoma: epidemiolog-ical evidence of an increased risk in castrated dogs. Mol Cell Endocrinol 2002; 197:251–5.

101. Obradovich J, Walshaw R, Goullaud E. The influence of castration on the devel-opment of prostatic carcinoma in the dog 43 cases (1978-1985). J Vet Intern Med 1987;1:183–7.

102. Lai CL, L'Eplattenier H, van den Ham R, et al. Androgen receptor CAG repeat polymorphisms in canine prostate cancer. J Vet Intern Med 2008;22:1380–4.

Interventional Urology

Endourology in Small Animal Veterinary Medicine

Allyson C. Berent, DVM

KEYWORDS

- Endourology • Ureteral obstruction • Ureteral stenting
- Subcutaneous ureteral bypass device (SUB) • Nephrolithiasis
- Endoscopic nephrolithotomy • Idiopathic renal hematuria
- Percutaneous cystolithotomy (PCCL)

KEY POINTS

- Minimally invasive treatment options for urologic disease are becoming more common in veterinary medicine.
- Ureteral obstructions should be considered an emergency, and decompression should be performed as quickly as possible using a procedure with the lowest morbidity and mortality.
- Azotemia in feline patients should be assessed for a ureteral obstruction as part of a minimum database workup, as it is being seen with far more frequency in the last decade, allowing for timely treatment to be considered.
- Current data suggest that some of the minimally invasive treatment options for feline and canine ureteral obstructions are met with lower morbidity and mortality rates than previously reported with traditional surgery, and this condition holds a better prognosis than previously reported.
- Proper training and expertise in these interventional techniques should be acquired before performing them on clinical patients for the best possible outcomes.

Endourology uses the combination of interventional radiology (IR) and interventional endoscopy (IE) techniques to provide image-guided interventions for the treatment of various urinary tract diseases. These techniques typically involve the use of fluoroscopy, endoscopy, and/or ultrasound to gain access to the kidney, ureter, bladder, and/or urethra. Over the past decade, these therapeutic and diagnostic modalities have become increasingly more accessible in veterinary medicine,[1] following the trend

Dr A.C. Berent is a consultant for Norfolk Vet Products and Infiniti Medical, LLC, both of which distribute various medical devices that are discussed in this article.
Department of Internal Medicine, Department of Surgery, The Animal Medical Center, 510 East 62nd Street, New York, NY 10065, USA
E-mail address: Allyson.Berent@amcny.org

Vet Clin Small Anim 45 (2015) 825–855
http://dx.doi.org/10.1016/j.cvsm.2015.02.003
vetsmall.theclinics.com

of what is considered standard of care in human medicine.[1-32] The traditional types of therapies using IR/IE techniques are associated with the relief of various urinary tract obstructions (ureteral stenting, subcutaneous ureteral bypass [SUB] device, urethral stenting), removal of urinary tract stones (lithotripsy, percutaneous nephrolithotomy [PCNL], percutaneous cystolithotomy [PCCL]), cessation of urinary tract bleeding (sclerotherapy, nephroscopy with electrocautery), and intra-arterial (IA) delivery of therapeutics to obtain higher local doses (stem cell therapy).

There are many advantages to IR/IE techniques when compared with traditional surgical alternatives. The reduced perioperative morbidity and mortality rates, shorter hospital stays, and availability of new therapeutic options when no treatments were traditionally safe or available are the main benefits of this technology. The main disadvantages are the requirement for proper technical training, the need for specialized equipment, and the steep learning curve.

With the high incidence of upper and lower urinary tract disease, combined with the invasiveness and morbidity associated with traditional techniques, the use of minimally invasive techniques is appealing. This article reviews some of the most common interventional procedures currently being performed in small animal veterinary patients. When possible, the reported outcomes, success rates, complications, and survival times are discussed using evidenced-based medicine.

KIDNEY
Interventional Approach to Nephrolithiasis

The need for nephrolith removal is rarely necessary in veterinary medicine. Nephroliths are considered problematic when they are (1) causing intractable pyelonephritis (despite appropriate medical management or stone dissolution diet when indicated), (2) causing a ureteral outflow tract obstruction associated with hydronephrosis, or (3) enlarging and overtaking the renal parenchyma resulting in progressive renal damage. It is important to note that it is suspected that most nephroliths do not cause pain or discomfort unless they are associated with pyelonephritis, pyonephrosis, or a ureteral outflow obstruction, so the need for removal is rare. There is some concern that dogs with progressive renal insufficiency may benefit from stone removal, but this is yet to be proven.

Traditional open surgical options to treat problematic nephroliths (nephrotomy or ureteronephrectomy) are associated with frequent complications and high long-term morbidity.[33,34] In a clinical study, approximately 43% of dogs had some stone fragments remaining after surgery with a 23% complication rate associated with the procedure.[33] In that same study, 67% of dogs developed renal azotemia following a nephrectomy. In a study of normal cats in which a nephrotomy was performed,[34] there was a 10% to 20% decrease in the glomerular filtration rate (GFR). In clinical patients, with prior renal injury associated with uroliths, compensatory mechanisms are often exhausted before diagnosis, so similar surgical interventions could have a more detrimental effect on renal function, emphasizing that one must be careful extrapolating these surgical results to clinical patients with upper tract uroliths, renal damage, and preexisting renal disease. In the author's opinion, open surgical nephrotomy is reserved for removal of large, obstructed nephroliths in dogs only when other options, such as extracorporeal shock-wave lithotripsy (ESWL) or PCNL, are not available. Open nephrotomy for removal of nonobstructive nephroliths in cats is not recommended particularly because the data confirming any benefit from nephrolith removal are lacking, and data confirming a negative effect on renal function exist.[34,35]

Extracorporeal shock-wave lithotripsy

ESWL refers to fragmentation of stones into small pieces using shocks generated outside of the body (**Fig. 1**). It is typically used for nephroliths and ureteroliths in dogs and not currently recommended in cats[3–5] because of their stone type, which is considered refractory to ESWL fragmentation,[36] and the small size of their ureteral lumen (0.3 mm), making stone fragments unlikely to pass. ESWL uses external shock waves that pass through a water medium, through the soft tissues of patients, and are directed onto the stone using fluoroscopic guidance. The stone is then shocked anywhere from 1000 to 3500 times at different energy levels to break up a stone into small fragments that are then allowed to pass down the ureter and into the urinary bladder passively. The debris is permitted to traverse the ureter over a 2- to 12-week period. ESWL is thought to be very safe for the kidney, though subclinical intrarenal hemorrhage does occur.[3–5] Studies have shown minimal effect on the GFR in both the short- and long-term after ESWL.[37,38] The availability of ESWL for veterinary patients in limited and currently only available at Purdue University (Dr Larry Adams) and The Animal Medical Center, New York City (Dr Allyson Berent).

In dogs, ESWL fragmentation is very successful, though up to 30% of dogs will require more than one treatment to achieve adequate fragmentation of nephroliths.[3–5] The mortality rate with ESWL is less than 1%, with the most common complication being the development of a transient ureteral obstruction in approximately 10% of cases.[3–5] The risk of ureteral obstruction may be minimized by placement of a ureteral stent before ESWL treatment to allow for passive ureteral dilation and prevent obstruction during fragment passage.[39] Pancreatitis is another possible complication with ESWL, which was documented in 2% to 3% of cases.[40]

For stones larger than 1.5 cm, endoscopic nephrolithotomy (ENL) is often recommended in both human and veterinary patients when possible (see later discussion).

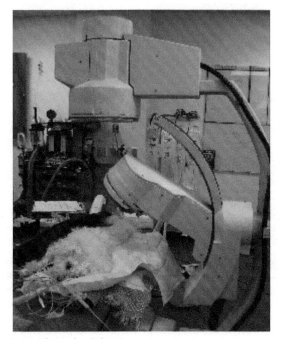

Fig. 1. ESWL in a dog with nephrolithiasis.

Endoscopic nephrolithotomy

ENL can either be performed percutaneously (PCNL) or surgically assisted (surgically assisted ENL [SENL]) and is available in veterinary medicine for problematic nephroliths larger than 1.5 cm or of cystine composition, which are ESWL resistant (**Fig. 2**).

This procedure has been shown to have minimal effect on renal function in both children and adults with large stone burdens, solitary kidneys, or renal insufficiency.[41] PCNL is reported to be the most renal sparing when compared with ESWL, laparoscopic-assisted nephrotomy, and traditional nephrotomy.[37,41,42] This finding is most likely because of the lack of nephron transection and the access point based on parenchymal dilation and spreading, sparing functional tissue.

PCNL/SENL was recently reported in an abstract of 9 dogs and 1 cat.[7] A combination of ultrasound, nephroscopy, fluoroscopy, and intracorporeal lithotripsy (electrohydraulic, ultrasonic, pneumatic and/or holmium:YAG [Hol:YAG] laser lithotripsy) is needed to remove the entire nephrolith. Patient size was not seen to be a factor in success, but proper training and appropriate equipment is needed for a successful outcome. The success rate of PCNL has been documented at 90% to 100% in both the adult and the pediatric human populations, and the author has experienced the same in veterinary patients.

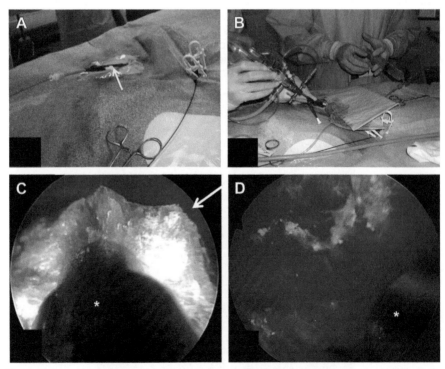

Fig. 2. ENL in a dog with large calcium oxalate nephroliths. (*A*) Percutaneous access into the renal pelvis with a sheath (*yellow arrow*). (*B*) Nephroscope through the sheath into the renal pelvis. (*C*) Lithotriptor (*white asterisk*), through the working channel of the nephroscope breaking the stone (*arrow*) inside the renal pelvis. (*D*) Renal pelvis after all stone fragments removed.

Idiopathic renal hematuria

Essential (idiopathic) renal hematuria (IRH) is a rare condition in which a focal area of bleeding in the upper urinary tract results in severe chronic hematuria and the potential for iron deficiency anemia and blood clot formation, which can ultimately result in a ureteral or urethral obstruction. In people, a hemangioma, angioma, or vascular malformation may be visualized ureteroscopically in the renal pelvis, and treatment via electrocautery can be accomplished.[43–47] IRH is diagnosed most commonly in very young large-breed dogs and occurs bilaterally in 25% to 33% of affected patients. For unilateral disease, usually confirmed by cystoscopy, ureteronephrectomy was previously recommended to minimize blood loss. Nephrectomy should be considered contraindicated because of the risk of progressive bilateral disease, the lack of disease of the functional renal tissue, and the availability and ease of kidney-sparing techniques.

Sclerotherapy can be performed with the use of silver nitrate and povidone-iodine as cauterizing agents that can be infused into the renal pelvis. This treatment can be done in any dog (male or female), regardless of size. Under cystoscopic and fluoroscopic guidance, the cauterizing agent is infused into the renal pelvis through a ureteral occlusion balloon catheter (**Fig. 3**). In a recent study[8] in which sclerotherapy was used for the treatment of IRH complete cessation of macroscopic hematuria occurred in 4 of 6 dogs within a median of 6 hours (range, postoperative to 7 days). Two additional dogs improved, one moderately and one substantially. None of the dogs required nephrectomy. To date the author has performed this procedure is more than 20 dogs with success rates at approximately 80%.

Ureteroscopy for electrocautery has only been performed in a small number of patients, and this is typically reserved for those that have failed sclerotherapy and have a large enough ureter to accept the 8-F ureteroscope (**Fig. 4**). There were no complications noted from the procedure when a stent was placed after infusion.

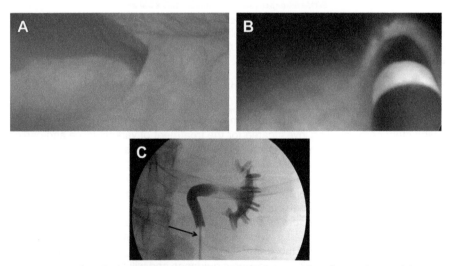

Fig. 3. IRH in a female dog during sclerotherapy. The dog is in dorsal recumbency. (*A*) Cystoscopic image of the left ureterovesicular junction with blood coming out of the ureter. (*B*) A ureteral catheter up the ureter visualized cystoscopically. (*C*) A ureteropyelogram through the UPJ balloon during sclerotherapy infusion. Not the balloon occluding the ureters (*black arrow*).

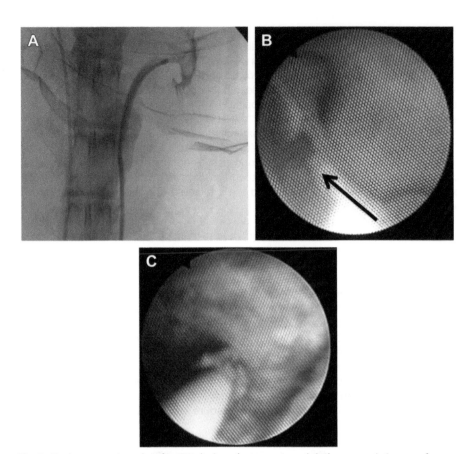

Fig. 4. Ureteroscopy in a dog for IRH during electrocautery. (*A*) Fluoroscopic image of a ureteroscope in the left ureter at the ureteropelvic junction. (*B*) Renal pelvis visualized during ureteroscopy visualizing the bleeding lesion (*black arrow*). (*C*) Electrocautery probe cauterizing the bleeding lesion in the renal pelvis.

Intra-arterial Stem Cell Delivery for Chronic Kidney Disease/Protein Losing Nephropathy

Infusion of autologous mesenchymal stem cells, an adipose stromal component containing stem cells, is being investigated for the treatment of various feline and canine renal diseases (**Fig. 5**). The goals of multipotent stem cell therapy are to decrease the inflammatory reaction and fibrosis associated with both glomerulonephritis and interstitial nephritis through paracrine mechanisms, with the aim to slow the progression of the disease.[48] Tissue regeneration has not yet been proven, but studies are showing very promising results in various animal models.

With intravenous infusion, the first-pass extraction of the cells occurs in the lungs, which are the first capillary bed to encounter the cells. Using interventional radiologic techniques directs delivery of the stem cells into the renal artery (via the femoral or carotid artery = IA delivery) using fluoroscopic guidance and will allow the glomeruli and vasa recta to be the first capillary bed to extract the cells, ultimately resulting in the highest engraftment rate. A phase I clinical trial evaluating the safety of IA delivery in both dogs and cats is completed, and the procedure was shown to be technically possible and safe. A randomized placebo-controlled study is currently under way

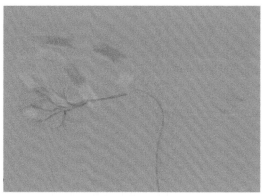

Fig. 5. Fluoroscopic image of a cat during digital subtraction angiography with a catheter in the renal artery infusing the kidney during stem cell delivery.

evaluating the efficacy of this approach in feline patients with International Renal Interest Society (IRIS) stage 3 chronic kidney disease (CKD). In the author's practice, more than 125 treatments have been performed in both dogs and cats. The efficacy to this point has been promising, though the studies are ongoing and the end points have not yet been met.[1]

URETERAL INTERVENTIONS

Ureteral diseases seem to be occurring in small animal veterinary patients with increased frequency over the past decade, with a ureteral obstruction being the most common disease in the upper urinary tract. The invasiveness and morbidity/mortality associated with traditional surgical techniques[49–51] makes the use of endourologic alternatives appealing (**Table 1**).

The physiologic response to a ureteral obstruction is very complex, with a rapid decrease in the GFR, resulting in progressive renal damage.[52,53] A ureteral obstruction necessitates timely and successful intervention for the best ultimate outcome. The composition of most ureteroliths in dogs (~50%) and cats (>95%) are calcium based, making dissolution completely contraindicated in cats, and should not be considered in dogs without concurrent decompression.[9,16,17,49,50] With medical management being effective in some feline cases (8%–13%)[49] and traditional surgical interventions being associated with a relatively high postoperative complication rate (31% in cats and ~7%–15% in dogs)[49–51] and perioperative mortality rate (18%–21% in cats and 6.25% in dogs),[49–51] short-term medical therapy should be considered before any intervention (24–48 hours). Interventional alternatives[2,9,10–18,54–60] are shown to result in immediate decompression, fewer perioperative complications, lower perioperative mortality rates, successful treatment of all causes of obstruction (stone, stricture, tumor), and a decreased recurrence rate of future obstructions, when compared with traditional options (see **Table 1**).[9–17]

Benign Ureteral Obstruction

Traditional ureteral surgery

Traditional ureteral surgery for obstructive ureterolithiasis is reported to include ureterotomy, neoureterocystostomy, ureteronephrectomy, or renal transplantation.[49–51] In a small study in dogs, results after a ureterotomy, pyelotomy, or ureteronephrectomy were associated with a surgical mortality rate of 6.25%, with 15% requiring an

Table 1
Potential outcomes of various ureteral interventions

Procedure	Operative	Postoperative (<1 wk)	Short-Term (1 wk to 1 mo)	Long-Term (>1 mo)	Follow-Up Time
Medical Management *Feline* Ureteral Obstructions[49] • Diuresis' • Mannitol therapy • Alpha-adrenergic blockade • Data on stones only • Will not help for the ~20% of strictures[9]	—	*Mortality:* 33% died or were euthanized before discharge[49]	Failure of renal function improvement (87%)[49]	If survived to discharge, 30% had an improvement in azotemia[49]	13% Had response to medical management with 7.7% documentation of stone passage[49]

Traditional Ureteral Surgery *Feline* (n = 153,[49] 47[50])
• Ureterotomy/reimplantation/ureteronephrectomy/renal transplantation[49]
• Ureterotomy/reimplantation[50]
• Data on ureteroliths only
	• Uroabdomen leakage (6%[50]–15%[49])
	• Presence of *abdominal effusion* postop (34%)[50]
		• Persistent ureteral obstruction (7%)[49] caused by stricture, edema, persistent stones
		• Failure of renal function improvement (17%)[49]
		• Require second surgery during hospitalization (13%)[49,50]
		• Other[49]: fluid overload (3%), septic peritonitis (2%), pancreatitis (1%)
		• *Mortality* (to discharge): 21%[49,50] (25% with ureterotomy/reimplant; 18% if include transplantation and ureteronephrectomy)[49]
			Failure to improve renal function: (17%)[49]
			Mortality (within 1 mo): 25%[49]
				• *Reobstruction* (40%)[49]
				  ○ ~ 1 y later
				  ○ 50% mortality
				  ○ In both medically and surgically managed cases[49]
					• Follow-up: 1–>2000 d
					• Major issue is postop complications: leakage, reobstruction, stricture formation, and long-term obstruction recurrence; few cases followed up long-term (~50%)[49]
					• 21% Perioperative mortality

Traditional Ureteral Surgery Canine (n = 16)[51]
• Ureterotomy/pyelotomy
• Ureteronephrectomy
• Data on ureteroliths only
	• Uroabdomen leakage
	• Stricture
		• Persistent ureteral obstruction
		• Failure of renal function improvement (21%)[51]
		• Worsening renal function (15%)[51]
		• *Mortality:* (to discharge) 6.25%
			• Reobstruction[51]
			  o Stone or surgical site stricture
			• Persistent renal dysfunction (43%)[51]
				• Recurrent or Persistent UTI (43%)[51]
				• Reobstruction (15%)[51]
				  o Stone or surgical site stricture
				  25% Died or euthanized because of renal-related diseases[51]
					Follow-up: 2–1876 d
					MST: 904 d (struvite MST 333 d; nonstruvite MST 1238 d)
					• Major issue is reobstruction and worsening of creatinine long-term; very few cases in this series

Feline Ureteral Stent[9,12] (n = 79,[9] 92[12])
• Data on 71%–79% ureteroliths, 21%–28% strictures, 1% obstructive pyelonephritis
	• Ureteral *penetration* with guidewire (17%) (little clinical consequence; no uroabdomen)
	• Leakage if concurrent ureterotomy needed (6.7%)
	• Eversion of ureteral mucosa during stent passage
	• Ureteral tear during stent passage (3.8%)
		• Fluid overload during postobstructive diuresis (17%)
		• Concurrent pancreatitis (6%)
		• Failure for creatinine to improve (5%)
		• *Mortality:* (to discharge) 7.5%[9]
		  o Caused by nonurinary causes (pancreatitis or CHF)
			• Inappetence (temporary) (25%)
			• Dysuria (self-limiting 7–14 d) <10%[9]
			• Stent migration[9,12] (3%)
				• Dysuria (38%)[9]
				  o Nearly all respond to prednisolone and/or prazosin (persistent 1.6% after steroid therapy)
				• UTI (13% postop vs 34% preop)[12]
				• Reobstruction (more than 3.5 y) (19%–26%)[9,12]
				  o Stricture (58% of strictures occluded the stent)
				  o Adhesions around ureter from ureterotomy
				  o Obstructive pyelonephritis
				  o Proliferative ureteritis
				  o Stent encrustation
				  o Chronic hematuria (18%)[9]
				• Stent migration[9] (6%)
				• Ureteral reflux[9] (<2%)
					Follow-up: 2–1278 d
					MST: 498 d
					MST for renal cause of death >1250 d
					21% of cats died of renal related causes
					Only predictor of long-term survival was the 3 mo postcreatinine[13]
					• Major issue is need for STENT EXCHANGE in 27% of cases because of migration or occlusion of ureter and DYSURIA caused by ureteral stent location in urinary bladder[9]
					• 7.5% Perioperative mortality (none related to surgical complications)

(continued on next page)

Table 1
(continued)

Procedure	Operative	Postoperative (<1 wk)	Short-Term (1 wk to 1 mo)	Long-Term (>1 mo)	Follow-Up Time
Canine Ureteral Stent (n = 13,[16] 57[17]) • Data on 55% ureteroliths, 40% tumors, and 5% strictures	• Endoscopic failure (~10% female; 30% male) • Ureteral perforation (<1%) • Leakage (<1%) • Ureteral tear (<1%)	• Hematuria (<5%) • Dysuria (<2%) • Migration (0%) • Occlusion with debris (0%) • *Mortality* (to discharge) <2%[17]	• Dysuria <2% • Persistent obstruction (<2%) • Hematuria (20%)	• Proliferative tissue at UVJ (5%–25%)[16,17] • Reobstruction (9%)[17] • UTIs (13%–59% after stent[16,17]; 59% before stent)[17] • Migration (6%)[17] • Encrustation (2%)[17] • Hematuria (7%)[17] • Stent fracture (<2%) • Dysuria (<2%)[16,17]	Follow-up: 30 d to 6 y (median 1158 d) • Major issue is reobstruction and RECURRENT UTIs, though rate is lower than before stent • <2% Perioperative mortality • All cases allowed for renal-sparing procedure
Feline SUB device[10,12,13] (n = 61,[10] 71[12]) • Data on 20% strictures (+/− ureteroliths), 76% ureteroliths, 4% obstructive ureteritis	• Kinking of catheters (3.5%) • Inability to place SUB (<1%)	• Leakage (5%)[10] resolved with new device • Fluid overload (<5%)[10,12] • Blockage of system (2%)[10,12] (blood clot, purulent material, device failure) • Failure for creatinine to improve (3%)[10,12] • *Mortality* (to discharge) 5.8%[12]	• Dysuria <2%[10,12] • Inappetence ~25% (temporary) • Seroma 1%[12]	• UTI[12] (15% postop; 35% preop) • Reobstruction[10] (18%) (0% strictures; 20% of stone cases) • Dysuria (<2%)[10,12]	Follow-up time: 2 d to 4.5 y Median: 762–923 d • Major issue is: (1) DEVICE OCCLUSION (10%), which requires serial flushing or exchange, usually caused by stone accumulation; (2) KINKING; and (3) LEAKAGE (is less of an issue with proper training) • 5.8% Perioperative mortality (none related to surgical complications)

Abbreviations: CHF, congestive heart failure; MST, median survival time; preop, preoperative; postop, postoperative; UTI, urinary tract infection; UVJ, ureterovesicular junction.

additional surgery for reobstruction within 30 days.[51] Additionally, 43% of dogs in this study had evidence of recurrent urinary tract infections after surgery, 21% remained azotemic, and 15% had worsening azotemia. In cats, the procedure-associated complication and mortality rates are reported to be 30% and 21%, respectively. Most complications associated with surgery are caused by ureterotomy site edema, nephroliths that pass from the renal pelvis to the surgery site, stricture formation, missed ureteroliths, and surgery-associated urine leakage.[49,50]

Subcutaneous ureteral bypass device in cats

The development of an indwelling *SUB* device[10] using a combination locking-loop nephrostomy catheter and cystostomy catheter connected to a subcutaneous shunting port has been used regularly in some practices for the last 5 to 6 years with high success (**Fig. 6**). In humans, a similar device has been shown to reduce complications associated with externalized nephrostomy tubes and improve quality of life as a long-term treatment modality.[55] The use of a SUB device has been described in abstract form in 25 cats and 2 dogs[10] and has been placed in more than 150 cats to date in the author's practice.

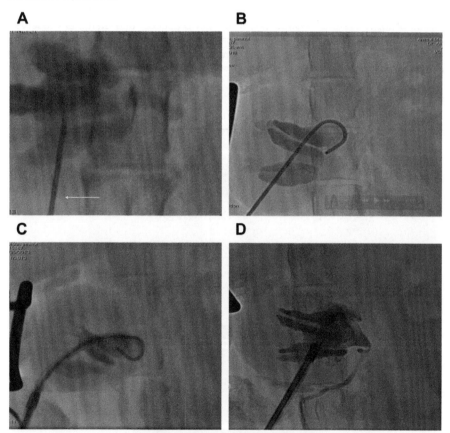

Fig. 6. Fluoroscopic images during placement of an SUB device in a cat with a right-sided ureteral obstruction. (*A*) An 18-gauge catheter (*white arrow*) in the renal pelvis during a pyelogram. (*B*) Guidewire in renal pelvis. (*C*) Nephrostomy catheter passed over the guide-wire into the renal pelvis. (*D*) Locking loop nephrostomy catheter coiled inside renal pelvis during pyelogram.

The SUB device (Norfolk Vet Products, Skokie, IL) is placed with surgical assistance using fluoroscopic guidance using the modified Seldinger technique (see **Fig. 6**). Then a multi-fenestrated catheter is placed into the urinary bladder at the apex. Each catheter is secured to the renal capsule and serosal surface of the bladder, respectively (**Fig. 7**). Once the catheters are in place, they are passed through the ventral body wall, just lateral to the abdominal incision, and connected to the shunting port securely (see **Fig. 7**). Contrast material is infused through the shunting port before closure to ensure patency and check for any leakage (**Fig. 8**).

With the commercially available device, 94% of patients survived to discharge[12]; no death was caused by a ureteral obstruction or procedure associated complications. The main short- and long-term complications were occlusion with stone material (~13%), occlusion with a blood clot (<3%), and kinking (<3%) of the tubing over a median follow-up period of 2.5 years (range, 1 month to >5 years).[12,13] Leakage of urine through the device is a rare complication with appropriate training and using the device properly. Because of the subcutaneous shunting port available for flushing and sampling of the device, management and maintenance has helped to maintain high patency rates. Initially the SUB device was reserved for feline patients with proximal ureteral strictures or ureteral stent failures; but more recently it has been used for all causes of feline ureteral obstructions in certain practices, and stents are reserved for canine ureteral obstructions. The outcome with the SUB device for feline patients has been shown to be superior to feline ureteral stents and traditional feline ureteral surgery (see **Table 1**).

Feline ureteral stenting

Ureteral stents are used in humans to divert urine from the renal pelvis into the urinary bladder for obstructions secondary to ureterolithiasis, ureteral stenosis/strictures,

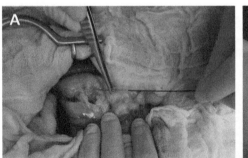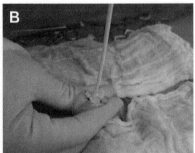
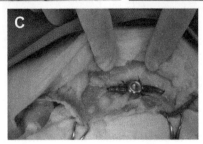

Fig. 7. Surgical images during placement of the SUB device. (*A*) Modified Seldinger technique during renal access. (*B*) Cystostomy tube placement. (*C*) Subcutaneous port connected to both catheters.

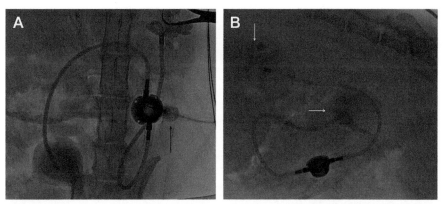

Fig. 8. Fluoroscopic images of a ventrodorsal view (*A*) and lateral (*B*) of the SUB device after placement. Notice the Huber needle (*black arrow*) during the SUB flush and the port (*red arrow*) and nephrostomy and cystostomy catheters (*white arrows*).

malignant neoplasia, or trauma.[54,56–59] The main type of ureteral stents used in both human and veterinary patients is an indwelling double-pigtail ureteral stent (**Fig. 9**). The double-pigtail stent is completely intracorporeal and is 2.5 F in diameter in feline patients and 3.7, 4.7, or 6.0 F in canine patients. In human medicine, it is recommended that the stents be removed or exchanged after 3 to 6 months[54,57,60]; but this does not seem to be necessary in feline or canine patients as they have remained patent and in place for more than 6 years in some patients. Stent placement may be considered a long-term treatment option for various causes of ureteral obstructions; however, potential side effects and long-term complications can exist (see **Table 1**).[2,9,11–14]

Feline ureteral stents are typically placed surgically assisted in an antegrade manner using the modified Seldinger technique under fluoroscopic guidance (**Fig. 10**). This technique is done over a guidewire using a ureteral dilation catheter.

In a recent study in 69 cats (79 ureters),[9] with both stone- and stricture-induced obstructions, stent placement was achieved in 95% of ureters. More than 60% of the cases in this study were considered poor ureterotomy candidates based on stone number, stone location, stricture location, and presence of concurrent nephroliths.

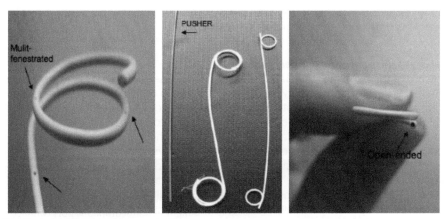

Fig. 9. A double-pigtail ureteral stent.

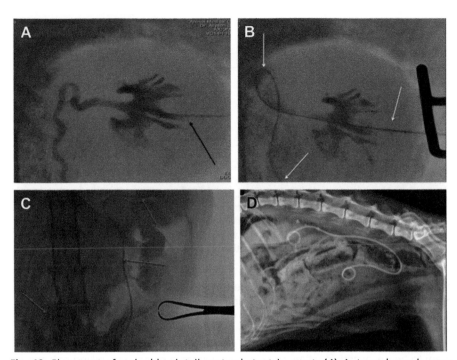

Fig. 10. Placement of a double-pigtail ureteral stent in a cat. (*A*) Antegrade pyelogram using a 22 Ga catheter (*black arrow*) under fluoroscopic guidance and surgical assistance. (*B*) Guidewire (*white arrows*) passing through the catheter and down the ureter. (*C*) Double-pigtail stent (*red arrows*) going from the renal pelvis, down the ureter, and into the urinary bladder. (*D*) Lateral radiograph of a cat with a double-pigtail ureteral stent.

There was a median of 4 stones per ureter, and 86% had concurrent nephroliths. About 25% of cats had a ureteral stricture (with or without a stone). After the stent was placed, 95% of cases had significant improvement in their azotemia; there was a perioperative mortality rate of 7.5%, none of which died of surgical complications or a persistent/recurrent ureteral obstruction.[9] The reported complications are outlined in **Table 1**. Because of these long-term complications, most commonly dysuria (up to 38%) and reocclusion (~25%), the SUB device is now recommended in cats, improving these long-term complication rates.[1,2,10–13]

Canine ureteral stenting for benign disease

The use of double-pigtail ureteral stents (**Fig. 11**) in dogs has been investigated as an alternative to traditional surgery, resulting in immediate ureteral decompression, stabilization of the associated azotemia, a decreased risk of ureteral stricture or ureteral leakage, and a decreased rate of ureteral obstruction recurrence.[15–17] Placement of a double-pigtail ureteral stent, via minimally invasive techniques (endoscopy and fluoroscopy or ultrasound and fluoroscopy) seems to have circumvented many of the complications of traditional surgery, avoiding the need for nephrotomy or ureteronephrectomy, and resulting in expedited stabilization and shorter hospital stays.[16,17,51] The main concerns with stents are typically seen months to years after placement. They are not usually life threatening and are relatively easy to address on an outpatient basis. These concerns include stent occlusion, migration,

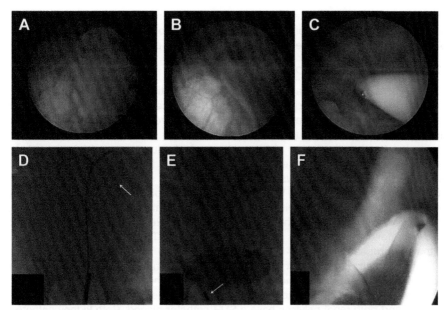

Fig. 11. Images during endoscopic placement of a double-pigtail ureteral stent in a female dog. (*A*) Cystoscopic image of the left ureterovesicular junction with the patient in dorsal recumbency. (*B*) Guidewire being advanced up the ureter. (*C*) Ureteral catheter advanced over the guidewire. (*D*) Guidewire (*white arrow*) and catheter (*black arrow*) coiling inside the renal pelvis using fluoroscopic guidance. (*E*) Stent (*blue arrow*) being pushed into the urinary bladder (*yellow arrow*). (*F*) Endoscopic image of the distal end of the stent in the urinary bladder.

encrustation, and proliferative tissue at the ureterovesicular junction. These problems are more common in cats than in dogs (see **Table 1**).

In dogs with ureterolithiasis, ureteral stenting is almost always performed noninvasively with endoscopic and fluoroscopic guidance (see **Fig. 11**) by gaining access to the ureter through the ureterovesicular junction cystoscopically. Once the renal pelvis is catheterized it is drained and lavaged, especially if this is associated with a pyonephrosis.[16] Then the ureteral length is measured using fluoroscopic guidance and an appropriately sized ureteral stent is placed over the guide wire through the working channel of the cystoscope. The patient is discharged the same day as the procedure.

This procedure has a reported mortality rate of less than 2%.[16,17] This procedure has been successful minimally invasively in more than 90% of dogs.[16,17] The stent-associated complications occur less in dogs compared with cats (see **Table 1**). The main issue in dogs long-term is the risk of recurrent urinary tract infections (15%–59% after stent vs ~60%–80% before stent),[16,17] which was also reported after traditional surgery. This issue is likely not associated with the presence of the stent but instead the concurrent stone disease, established pyelonephritis, decreased renal function, and concurrent immune dysfunction. In many cases when a ureteral stent is removed because of complete stone dissolution, in the case of struvite ureterolithiasis, chronic infections can still be seen months and years after stent removal. Careful monitoring of image findings, urinalysis, and cultures are required to avoid ascending pyelonephritis; owners should be aware of the potential for stent occlusion, migration, and the need for stent exchange. Cystoscopic-assisted ureteral stent placement is technically challenging and should not be attempted without endourology training.

For canine patients suspected of having struvite ureterolithiasis, successful dissolution after ureteral stent placement is documented; dissolution diet and long-term antibiotics should always be used in these cases (Berent, direct communication, 2015).

Canine Malignant Ureteral Obstruction

Ureteral stenting for the treatment of trigonal obstructive neoplasia is typically performed using both ultrasound and fluoroscopic guidance. Patients are placed in lateral recumbency, and an antegrade pyelogram is done percutaneously under ultrasound guidance (**Fig. 12**). Using fluoroscopic visualization, a guidewire is advanced down the ureter, through the tumor at the ureterovesicular junction, and into the urinary bladder. The wire is then passed down the urethra and through-and-through access is obtained. This access allows for retrograde ureteral stent placement. In a recent study[18] of 12 dogs (15 ureters) that had ureteral stents placed for ureteral obstructive neoplasia, 1 dog required surgical conversion. All patients survived to discharge, and the median survival time from the time of diagnosis was 285 days (range, 10–1571) and following stent placement was 57 days (range, 7–337). This procedure is typically an outpatient procedure.

A SUB can also be used for malignant ureteral obstructions but requires surgical placement. For cases when the tumor is localized to the urinary bladder and/or the proximal urethra, the entire bladder and urethra have been removed via a radical cystectomy and both renal pelvises have a SUB catheter placed. Both kidney catheters are then connected to a 3-way port (**Fig. 13**), and a third catheter is placed down the urethra or into the vagina. These dogs have been completely incontinent; but if done appropriately, only microscopic disease will remain.

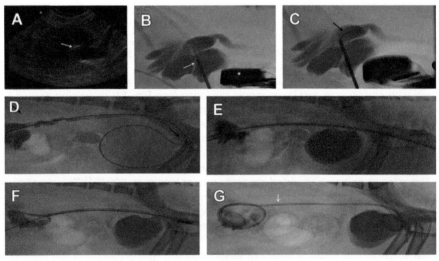

Fig. 12. Ureteral stenting in a dog with a malignant ureteral obstruction using antegrade access under ultrasound and fluoroscopic guidance. (*A*) Ultrasound image of a renal access needle inside the renal pelvis (*white arrow*). (*B*) Fluoroscopic image during antegrade pyelogram with needle (*white arrow*) seen in the renal pelvis and the ultrasound probe (*yellow asterisk*) guiding the renal puncture. (*C*) Guidewire (*black arrow*) being advanced down the ureter through the renal access needle. (*D*) Guidewire (*black arrows*) down the ureter, into the bladder, and out the urethra. (*E*) A ureteral dilation sheath being advanced over the guidewire into the renal pelvis in a retrograde fashion. (*F*) Stent being advanced up the ureter over the guidewire. (*G*) Stent (*white arrow*) coiled in the renal pelvis and urinary bladder.

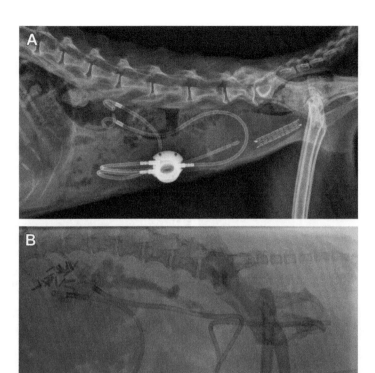

Fig. 13. SUB device used for malignant obstructions. (*A*) Feline patient with bilateral ureteral and a urethral obstruction. Notice the 3-way port connecting 2 nephrostomy catheters to a cystostomy catheter. Notice the urethral stent opening the urethra as well. (*B*) The patient also had a cystectomy done, so the cystostomy catheter is placed down the urethra.

Cystoscopic-guided laser ablation of ectopic ureters

Urinary incontinence caused by congenital ectopic ureters is a rare condition seen in various breeds of dogs and cats. Typically, with this condition the ureteral opening is found more caudal to the normal position in the trigone, most commonly within the urethra, prostate, or vestibule. This condition can be seen in both female and male patients (20:1 female to male).[61–63] More than 95% of ectopic ureters traverse intramurally and exit into the urethra making these patients candidates for a minimally invasive IE procedure involving Cystoscopic-guided laser ablation of ectopic ureters (CLA-EU).[62]

Endoscopic repair of ectopic ureters has been performed over the past 10 years in both male and female dogs and cats using a combination of fluoroscopy, cystoscopy, and a diode or Hol:YAG laser (**Figs. 14** and **15**).[20–22] The laser is applied to transect the medial side of the membrane of the ectopic ureter to separate the ureter from the normal trigone and urethra. The procedure can be performed on an outpatient basis at the same time as cystoscopic diagnosis of ectopic ureters is made, which avoids the need for more than one anesthetic procedure for fixation. During the CLA-EU

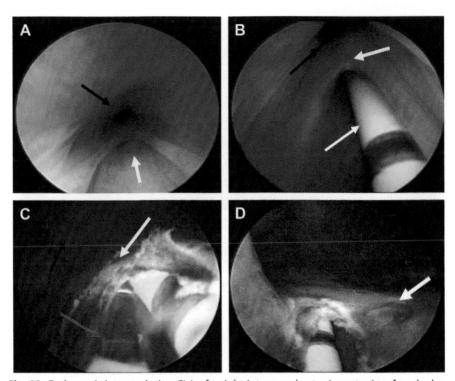

Fig. 14. Endoscopic images during CLA of a right intramural ectopic ureter in a female dog. The patient is in dorsal recumbency. (*A*) Urethral image showing the right ectopic ureteral opening (*yellow arrow*) and the urethral opening (*black arrow*). (*B*) Open-ended ureteral catheter (*white arrow*) inside the ureteral lumen. (*C*) Laser (*red arrow*) cutting the ureteral opening (*yellow arrow*) over the open-ended ureteral catheter. Cystoscopic image during laser ablation with the laser fiber (*red arrow*), ureteral opening (*yellow arrow*), and trigone of the bladder (*black arrow*) being shown. (*D*) Cystoscopic image after laser ablation. The normal left ureteral opening (*white arrow*) is visualized next to the neo-ureteral orifice on the right.

procedure various vaginal anomalies can be treated with laser therapy simultaneously (dual vagina, vaginal septum, persistent paramesonephric remnants), and this procedure is called endoscopic laser ablation of vaginal remnants (ELA-VR). A recent study showed that ELA-VR is a very effective procedure in maintaining a normal vaginal opening and may improve the risk of recurrent urinary tract infections, vaginitis, and vaginal pooling (**Fig. 16**).[23]

After CLA-EU the ureteral orifice has been shown to remain in a normal position at the trigone of the bladder, but many dogs have been shown[20] to have concurrent urethral incompetence and will require additional medication or procedures to maintain continence.[61] A prospective study of CLA-EU in 30 female dogs reported an overall urinary continence rate of 77% after CLA-EU with the addition of medical management, collagen injections, or placement of a urethral hydraulic occluder.[20,62] After laser ablation in male dogs the continence rate has been reported in a small group of dogs to be 100%[22]; in the author's experience, in a larger group of dogs, it remains approximately 85% (Berent, direct communication, 2015). The success rate of the CLA-EU procedure alone in female and male dogs is approximately

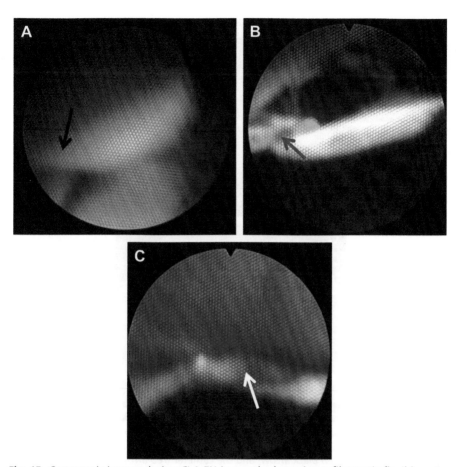

Fig. 15. Cystoscopic images during CLA-EU in a male dog using a fiberoptic flexible cysto-scope. (*A*) Guidewire (*black arrow*) in the ectopic ureteral orifice. (*B*) Laser fiber (*red arrow*) cutting the intramural ectopic ureteral wall. (*C*) New ureteral orifice after CLA-EU (*white arrow*). Notice the difficulty in visualization in male dogs when compared with female dogs.

56%. The addition of a hydraulic occluder has been reported to increase the conti-nence rate to 92%.[62]

URINARY BLADDER AND URETHRA
Bladder Stone Removal

Traditional surgical removal of stones via cystotomy or urethrotomy has been the traditional method of choice. Studies have shown that 10% to 20% of cases have incomplete surgical removal of stones, and this is likely caused by poor visualization, hemorrhage, and/or inappropriate technique (**Table 2**).[64] Recently, complications associated with traditional surgical cystotomy were reported in 37% to 50% of cases.[65] In addition, there is a suggestion of a 40% to 60% rate of stone recurrence, especially when dealing with calcium oxalate, urate, and cystine stones. Various mini-mally invasive stone-retrieval techniques are available in veterinary medicine; this has become more popular over the past few years, resulting in a high demand by the

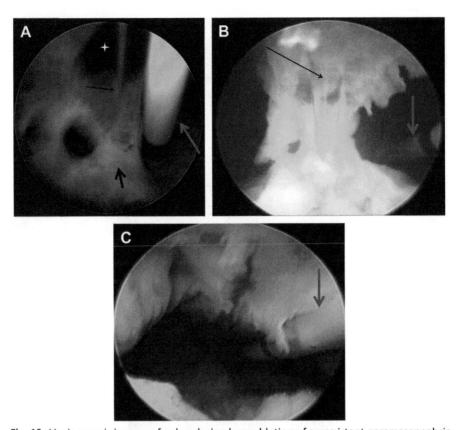

Fig. 16. Vaginoscopic images of a dog during laser ablation of a persistent paramesonephric remnant in dorsal recumbency. (*A*) Notice the vertical band (*thick black arrow*) of tissue being cut with the laser (*thin black arrow*) and the catheter (*red arrow*) in one of the vaginal compartments. The urethral opening is seen above (*yellow asterisk*) the vaginal opening. (*B*) Laser ablation of the band with the laser fiber cutting the tissue. The catheter (*red arrow*) and laser fiber (*black arrow*) are shown. (*C*) Vaginal opening after laser ablation showing the catheter (*red arrow*) is now in the vagina, and there is only one compartment.

veterinary clientele. These options include voiding urohydropropulsion (VUH), cystoscopic-guided stone basket retrieval, cystourethroscopy-guided laser lithotripsy, and PCCL.

Cystoscopic-Guided Stone Basket Retrieval

Cystoscopic-guided stone basket retrieval (**Fig. 17**) of bladder stones is performed routinely in both male and female dogs and female cats. This procedure is accomplished by transurethral cystourethroscopy and requires stringent size limitations of both the stone and the patients' urethra. Stones less than 4 mm in female dogs, 2 to 3 mm in most male dogs, and 2 mm in female cats can be routinely retrieved, in the author's experience. This procedure is typically done on an outpatient basis.

Laser Lithotripsy

Laser lithotripsy is a minimally invasive technique that fragments uroliths using intracorporeal cystoscopic guidance using a Hol:YAG laser until the stone fragments are

Table 2
Methods for bladder stone removal using IR/IE

Procedure	Stone Size Limit	Patient Size Limit	Equipment Required	Special Indications
VUH	Male dog: 2 mm Female dog: 3–4 mm Female cat: 2–3 mm Male cat: do not perform	Any size patient (not a male cat)	Urinary catheter for male dogs Rigid cystoscope or urinary catheter for female dogs and cats	The author finds it much easier to perform this procedure using a rigid cystoscope to fill the urinary bladder in female dogs and cats rather than repeat blind urethral catheterizations. If cystoscopy is not available, then urethral catheterization is used for bladder filling.
Basketing	Male dog: 2–3 mm Female dog: 4–5 mm Female cat: 2–3 mm Male cat: do not perform	Large enough to accept an appropriately sized cystoscope (not male cats)	Cystoscope and various sized stone baskets	The operator should be prepared for laser lithotripsy in the event the stone gets stuck in the urethra during removal. Do not apply excessive tension on the stone if it is not passively coming through the urethra with irrigation.
Laser Lithotripsy	Male dog: 5 mm Female dog: 10 mm Female cat: 5 mm Male cat: no not perform	Must be able to accept the cystoscope comfortably	Various cystoscopies Hol:YAG laser with appropriate fibers EHL	Operators have their own limits on which patients this is appropriate for. 1. Urethral stones 2. No more than 2–4 cystoliths that require fragmentation in female dogs 3. No more than 2 cystoliths that require fragmentation in female cats 4. No more than 2 cystoliths in a male dog
PCCL	All dogs and cats with any size or number of stones (male or female)	None	Screw trocar (6 mm +/− 10 mm for larger stones); 2.7-mm rigid cystoscope; 7.5- to 8.0-F flexible cystoscope	Cats are harder to distend and visualize, so the author recommends maintaining good apical traction to get the best visualization

Abbreviations: EHL, electrohydraulic lithotripsy; VUH, voiding urohydropropulsion.

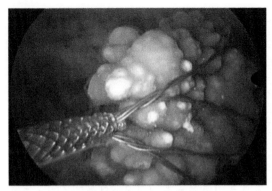

Fig. 17. A stone inside a stone retrieval basket during cystoscopy.

smaller than the urethra, in which case they can either be removed via VUH or stone basketing (**Fig. 18**). The Hol:YAG laser is a pulsed laser that emits light at an infrared wavelength of 2100 nm.[66] The energy is absorbed in less than 0.5 mm of fluid, making it safe to fragment uroliths in tight locations, as within the urethra or urinary bladder, with limited risk to the urothelial tissue. For stone fragmentation, laser energy is focused on the urolith surface, directed via cystoscopy. Pulsed laser energy is absorbed by water inside the urolith, resulting in a photothermal effect, which causes urolith fragmentation. The Hol:YAG laser effect on the calculus is by a vapor bubble created when the pulse of laser energy traveling through water from the tip of the fiber is trapped (Moses effect). With proper case selection, all uroliths can be fragmented by laser lithotripsy and removed in approximately 85% of male dogs and nearly all female dogs.[24–27]

In the author's experience this technique is best suited to female dogs with a small number of bladder or urethral uroliths and male dogs with ureteroliths. Animals with larger stone burdens are better suited for a PCCL procedure (see later discussion).

Percutaneous Cystolithotomy

PCCL is a new minimally invasive technique that combines cystic and urethral stone retrieval using cystoscopic and urethroscopic guidance in any size patient, sex, or species and is easy, fast, and highly effective (**Fig. 19**).[67] This technique is a

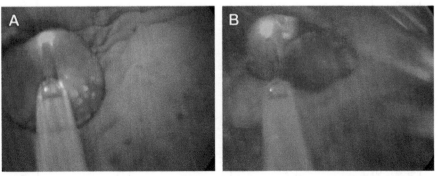

Fig. 18. Cystoscopic images of a calcium oxalate stone before (A) and after (B) laser lithotripsy.

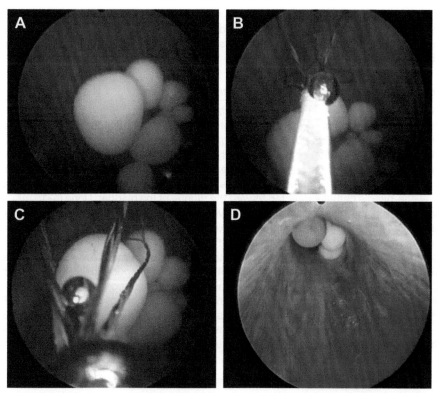

Fig. 19. Cystoscopic images during percutaneous cystolithotomy. (*A*) Antegrade cystoscopy visualizing bladder stones in the bladder. (*B*) Stone basket through the working channel of the endoscope before stone removal. (*C*) Stone retrieval. (*D*) Urethroscopic image during antegrade urethroscopy in a small male dog retrieving urethral stones, which are next to a red rubber catheter.

particularly useful endoscopic technique to assist in cystourethroscopy when retrograde access in not possible, as in small male dogs and male cats, for urethral stent placement in male cats, for evaluation of the ureterovesicular junction for upper tract hematuria/IRH, ureteral stenting in small male dogs, and to retrieve embedded urethral stones in the urethra of small male dogs and male or female cats.

This procedure is performed using a small 1- to 2-cm surgical incision to get access to the apex of the bladder. A 6-mm screw trocar is then used to cannulate the bladder apex, maintaining a seal to allow for both rigid and flexible antegrade cystoscopy. Slow saline irrigation is used to maintain bladder distension and visibility. A stone retrieval basket is advanced through the working channel of the cystoscope and guided to remove the uroliths. For any small remaining fragments that do not fit in the basket, suction is applied through the trocar as saline is irrigated through the urethral catheter. The proximal urethra is then visualized using the rigid, or semirigid, cystoscope in an antegrade manner. If more stones are identified they can be removed using a stone basket or flush until the entire urethra is deemed to be patent and catheter passage is smooth and easy. These patients are typically discharged the same day as their procedure, once adequate micturition is appreciated.

This is considered the most common minimally invasive bladder stone retrieval method in the author's practice to date and only 1 of 27 patients had a small fragment left behind on postoperative radiographs, showing improved surgical screening when compared with traditional cystotomy.[67]

Percutaneous Antegrade Urethral Catheterization

Percutaneous antegrade urethral catheterization (PAUC) may be needed for dogs or cats that are difficult or too small to catheterize, have a urethral tear, or have a distal urethral obstruction (**Fig. 20**). This technique can be performed under general anesthesia or heavy sedation and was recently reported in 9 cats.[28] For this procedure the abdomen and vulva/prepuce should be clipped and aseptically prepared. Patients are placed in lateral recumbency, and a cystocentesis is performed using an 18-gauge over-the-needle catheter directed toward the trigone of the bladder. Urine (5–15 mL) is drained from the bladder and replaced with an equal amount of contrast material diluted 50% with sterile saline until the proximal urethra is identified and visualized under fluoroscopic guidance. A hydrophilic guidewire (0.018 in for male cats and 0.035 in for dogs or female cats) is advanced into the bladder and aimed toward the bladder trigone, down the urethra, and passed out of the vulva/prepuce, using fluoroscopic guidance, which allows for through-and-through guidewire access. Once the guidewire is outside the urethra, a urinary catheter (open ended; red rubber [3.5–5.0 F male cats, 5.0–12 F dogs, and 5–8 F female cats], a locking-loop pigtail catheter [5 F male cats; 6–8 F female cats], or a nonlocking pigtail catheter) is advanced over the wire in a retrograde manner, within the urethral lumen and into the urinary bladder.

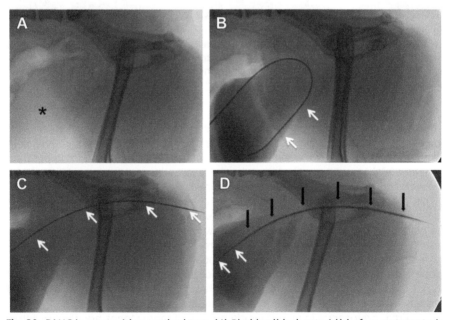

Fig. 20. PAUC in a cat with a urethral tear. (*A*) Bladder (*black asterisk*) before cystocentesis. (*B*) Guidewire coiled inside the bladder (*white arrows*). (*C*) Guidewire (*white arrows*) through-and-through from the bladder, down the urethra, and outside the prepuce. (*D*) Catheter (*black arrows*) advanced over the wire (*white arrows*) in a retrograde manner. (*Courtesy of* Dr Elaine Holmes.)

This procedure is highly effective for male cats with urethral tears, as the tears are typically made in a longitudinal retrograde direction, making antegrade passage easy. Longitudinal urethral tears will usually heal within 5 to 10 days without surgical intervention, and the catheter should be maintained for that length of time using clean/sterile technique.[68]

Percutaneous Cystostomy Tube Placement

Percutaneous cystostomy tube placement can be considered to bypass a urethral obstruction or as a bridge while a urethral, trigonal, or bladder lesion is healing or awaiting a more definitive treatment. A urethral obstruction can be secondary to obstructive urethral reflex dyssynergia, malignant neoplasia, aggressive bladder surgeries, severe urethritis, urethral strictures, urethral tears, or urethral stones that are difficult to remove surgically. With the advent of urethral stents (see later discussion), the use of cystostomy tubes has declined in the author's practice; but the ease and success of placement of these tubes make them a viable option when necessary. Cystostomy tubes can be placed percutaneously using fluoroscopic guidance. With the locking-loop pigtail catheter (**Fig. 21**), percutaneous cystostomy tube placement is a fast, safe, and highly effective technique.

Using the modified Seldinger technique, a stab incision is made through the skin and abdominal musculature over the area of puncture. Then, an 18-gauge over-the-needle catheter is advanced into the urinary bladder via cystocentesis (paramedian at the bladder body) until urine is draining. The stylet is removed, and a sterile urine sample is obtained for culture and analysis. Then a cystogram is performed using a 50% mixture of contrast and sterile saline to fill the bladder (approximately total volume bladder holds is 5–15 mL/kg). Next, through the catheter, a 0.035-in hydrophilic angle-tipped guidewire is advanced though the catheter and coiled within the urinary bladder. The guidewire can be advanced down the urethra using fluoroscopic guidance if antegrade catheterization is desired (see PAUC later), using this same technique.

For placement of the cystostomy tube, the locking-loop catheter is cannulated with the stiff hollow trocar and is advanced over the wire. This catheter is then punctured through the body and urinary bladder wall. Once it is well within the urinary bladder, the hollow trocar is withdrawn as the catheter is advanced over the guidewire to ensure the entire distal end of the catheter is within the bladder lumen. Then the locking string is engaged as the trocar and guidewire are removed creating a loop of the pigtail catheter. The bladder is then drained and filled to ensure the entire pigtail is

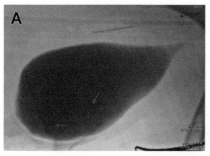
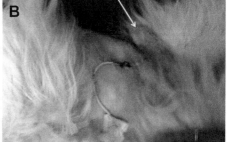

Fig. 21. Percutaneous cystostomy tube in a dog. (*A*) Lateral fluoroscopic image of the locking-loop pigtail tube (*red arrows*) within the urinary bladder. (*B*) Tube externalized in the dog (*red arrow*) in dorsal recumbency. Notice the location to the prepuce (*white arrow*).

appropriately positioned in the bladder lumen and is functioning well. The loop of the catheter should be within the lumen of the bladder, extending approximately 1 to 2 cm from the wall, so that it is not too snug against the bladder wall, allowing movement when the bladder is full or empty. The catheter is carefully secured to the body wall using a purse-string suture and Chinese-finger trap suture pattern. This tube should remain in place or at least 2 to 4 weeks before removal. Catheter care and cleanliness should be emphasized, as cystostomy tubes are commonly associated with secondary infections (86% in one study) because of the external nature of the tube.[69] Additional complications with cystostomy tubes have been reported in as high as 49% of patients, involving inadvertent tube removal, eating of the tube by the patients, fistulous tract formation, and mushroom tip breakage during removal.[69]

Urethral Stenting for Urethral Obstructions

Urethral stenting for urethral obstructions are most commonly used for the relief of benign or malignant obstructions in the trigone or urethra of dogs and cats.[29–32] The most common cause of malignant obstructions in dogs and cats is transitional cell carcinoma.[29,30] Benign obstructions are less common and are most typically associated with urethral strictures from either urethral tears, vehicular trauma, or chronic obstructive stone disease.[31,32]

When signs of obstruction occur, more aggressive therapy is indicated, with euthanasia commonly ensuing because of a lack of good alternative options. Placement of surgical cystostomy tubes, debulking surgery, and surgical diversionary procedures are invasive and often associated with undesirable outcomes.[70–74] Placement of self-expanding metallic stents under fluoroscopic guidance via a transurethral approach can be a fast, reliable, and safe alternative to establish urethral patency regardless of the benign or malignant nature and is an outpatient procedure.[29–32] This technique has been performed in more than 100 canine and 15 feline patients in the author's practice (**Fig. 22**). Benign urethral strictures may resolve with balloon dilation alone and have also been successful in a small number of patients.

To place a urethral stent, patients are placed in lateral recumbency and a marker catheter is placed inside the colon to allow for urethral measurement and determination of stent size. The bladder is maximally distended with contrast, and a pullout urethrogram is performed to allow for maximal distension of the urethra. Measurements of the normal urethral diameter and the length of the associated obstruction are obtained, and an appropriately sized self-expanding metallic urethral stent is chosen (approximately 10%–15% greater than the normal urethral diameter and 3–5 mm longer than the obstruction on both the cranial and caudal ends). The stent is deployed under fluoroscopic guidance, and a repeat contrast cystourethrogram is performed to document restored urethral patency. The procedure is considered an outpatient procedure, and the animals are typically discharged the same day. In some cases with trigonal transitional cell carcinoma, bilateral concurrent ureteral obstructions may be present, so an ultrasound should be evaluated and followed regularly. When this is encountered, it is typically recommended to have bilateral SUBs placed or percutaneous antegrade ureteral stents (see earlier discussion). These procedures can be highly successful when necessary.

For urethral strictures, balloon dilation alone can be performed using fluoroscopic guidance. After balloon dilation is complete (using a balloon size similar to that measured for stent placement), topical mitomycin C (MMC) can be applied to decrease the risk of stricture reformation. MMC is an antibiotic that is produced by *Streptomyces caespitosus*. Aside from being an antibiotic, it is an antineoplasticlike alkylating agent, causing single-band breakage and cross-linking of DNA at the

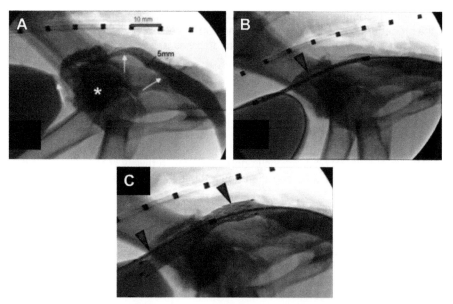

Fig. 22. Fluoroscopic images in lateral recumbency during urethral stent placement in a male dog with prostatic transitional cell carcinoma. (*A*) Cystourethrogram. Notice extravasation of contrast into the prostate (*white asterisk*) and the obstructive lesions in the urethra (*yellow arrows*). (*B*) Urethral stent (*blue arrowhead*) compressed on delivery system over a guidewire, across the obstruction. (*C*) Stent (*blue arrowhead*) after it is deployed. Notice the small amount of tumor behind the stent (*red asterisk*).

adenosine and guanine molecules. It inhibits RNA and protein synthesis and inhibits fibroblast proliferation, hence, decreasing scar tissue formation.[75,76]

In a recent study evaluating the use of urethral stents for malignant obstructions in dogs, the median survival time after stent placement was 78 days; but for those patients treated with chemotherapy, it was 251 days.[29] Resolution of urinary tract obstruction was achieved in 97.6% of dogs, and 26% were severely incontinent.[29] Another study evaluating urethral stents in 11 dogs for benign urethral obstructions found 100% of dogs had clinical relief of their urethral obstruction with a stent with only 12.5% of dogs being severely incontinent after stent placement, when not incontinent before stent placement.[31] Another study[32] evaluating 9 cats after urethral stent placement for benign and malignant obstruction also had a 100% success in obstruction relief, with a 25% severe incontinence rate following stenting. Palliative stenting for urethral obstructions in dogs and cats can provide a rapid, effective, and safe alternative to more traditional and invasive options; long-term survival times can be achieved.

SUMMARY/DISCUSSION

Interventional options for the treatment of urinary tract disease in veterinary medicine have dramatically expanded over the past decade and are continuing to do so. The aforementioned procedures are only a small handful of the most common procedures performed in veterinary medicine to date, and these have become more popular in both academic and private practice settings in the last few years. This popularity is following the trend that has been occurring in human medicine over the past 25 years and will likely continue to grow as such.

It is highly recommended that operators get proper training before considering most of the procedures described as the learning curve is steep, and complications should be avoided whenever possible. Training laboratories are available to further develop interventional skills if desired.

REFERENCES

1. Berent A. New techniques on the horizon: interventional radiology and interventional endoscopy of the urinary tract ('endourology'). J Feline Med Surg 2014; 16(1):51–65.
2. Berent A. Ureteral obstructions in dogs and cats: a review of traditional and new interventional diagnostic and therapeutic options. J Vet Emerg Crit Care 2011; 21(2):86–103.
3. Adams LG, Goldman CK. Extracorporeal shock wave lithotripsy. In: Polzin DJ, Bartges JB, editors. Nephrology and urology of small animals. Ames (IA): Blackwell Publishing; 2011. p. 340–8.
4. Adams LG. Nephroliths and ureteroliths: a new stone age. N Z Vet J 2013;61:1–5.
5. Block G, Adams LG, Widmer WR, et al. Use of extracorporeal shock wave lithotripsy for treatment of nephrolithiasis and ureterolithiasis in five dogs. J Am Vet Med Assoc 1996;208:531–6.
6. Donner GS, Ellison GW, Ackerman N, et al. Percutaneous nephrolithotomy in the dog: an experimental study. Vet Surg 1987;16:411–7.
7. Berent A, Weisse C, Bagley D, et al. Endoscopic nephrolithotomy for the treatment of complicated nephrolithiasis in dogs and cats [abstract]. San Antonio (TX): ACVS; 2013.
8. Berent A, Weisse C, Bagley D, et al. Renal sparing treatment for idiopathic renal hematuria (IRH): endoscopic-guided sclerotherapy. J Am Vet Med Assoc 2013; 242(11):1556–63.
9. Berent A, Weisse C, Bagley D. Ureteral stenting for benign feline ureteral obstructions: technical and clinical outcomes in 79 ureters (2006–2010). J Am Vet Med Assoc 2014;244:559–76.
10. Berent A, Weisse C, Bagley D, et al. The use of a subcutaneous ureteral bypass device for the treatment of feline ureteral obstructions. Seville (Spain): ECVIM; 2011.
11. Zaid M, Berent A, Weisse C, et al. Feline ureteral strictures: 10 cases (2007–2009). J Vet Intern Med 2011;25(2):222–9.
12. Steinhaus J, Berent A, Weisse C, et al. Presence of circumcaval ureters and ureteral obstructions in cats. J Vet Intern Med 2015;29(1):63–70.
13. Horowitz C, Berent A, Weisse C, et al. Predictors of outcome for cats with ureteral obstructions after interventional management using ureteral stents or a subcutaneous ureteral bypass device. J Feline Med Surg 2013;15(12): 1052–62.
14. Nicoli S, Morello E, Martano M, et al. Double-J ureteral stenting in nine cats with ureteral obstruction. Vet J 2012;194(1):60–5.
15. Lam N, Berent A, Weisse C, et al. Ureteral stenting for congenital ureteral strictures in a dog. J Am Vet Med Assoc 2012;240(8):983–90.
16. Kuntz J, Berent A, Weisse C, et al. Double pigtail ureteral stenting and renal pelvic lavage for renal-sparing treatment of pyonephrosis in dogs: 13 cases (2008–2012). J Am Vet Med Assoc 2015;246(2):216–25.
17. Pavia P, Berent A, Weisse C, et al. Canine ureteral stenting for benign ureteral obstruction in dogs [abstract]. San Diego (CA): ACVS; 2014.

18. Berent A, Weisse C, Beal M, et al. Use of indwelling, double-pigtail stents for treatment of malignant ureteral obstruction in dogs: 12 cases (2006–2009). J Am Vet Med Assoc 2011;238(8):1017–25.
19. Weisse C, Berent A. Percutaneous fluoroscopically-assisted perineal approach for rigid cystoscopy in 9 male dogs. Barcelona (Spain): ECVS; 2012.
20. Berent A, Weisse C, Mayhew P, et al. Evaluation of cystoscopic-guided laser ablation of intramural ectopic ureters in 30 female dogs. J Am Vet Med Assoc 2012;240:716–25.
21. Smith AL, Radlinsky MG, Rawlings CA. Cystoscopic diagnosis and treatment of ectopic ureters in female dogs: 16 cases (2005–2008). J Vet Med Assoc 2010; 237(2):191–5.
22. Berent AC, Mayhew PD, Porat-Mosenco Y. Use of cystoscopic-guided laser ablation for treatment of intramural ureteral ectopia in male dogs: four cases (2006–2007). J Am Vet Med Assoc 2008;232(7):1026–34.
23. Burdick S, Berent A, Weisse C, et al. Endoscopic-guided laser ablation of vestibulovaginal defects in 36 dogs. J Am Vet Med Assoc 2014;244(8):944–9.
24. Defarges A, Dunn M. Use of electrohydraulic lithotripsy to treat bladder and urethral calculi in 28 dogs. J Vet Intern Med 2008;22:1267–73.
25. Adams LG, Berent AC, Moore GE, et al. Use of laser lithotripsy for fragmentation of uroliths in dogs: 73 cases (2005–2006). J Am Vet Med Assoc 2008;232:1680–7.
26. Grant DC, Werre SR, Gevedon ML. Holmium:YAG laser lithotripsy for urolithiasis in dogs. J Vet Intern Med 2008;22:534–9.
27. Lulich JP, Osborne CA, Albasan H, et al. Efficacy and safety of laser lithotripsy in fragmentation of urocystoliths and urethroliths for removal in dogs. J Am Vet Med Assoc 2009;234(10):1279–85.
28. Holmes ES, Weisse C, Berent AC. Use of fluoroscopically guided percutaneous antegrade urethral catheterization for the treatment of urethral obstruction in male cats: 9 cases (2000–2009). J Am Vet Med Assoc 2012;241(5):603–7.
29. Blackburn AL, Berent AC, Weisse CW, et al. Evaluation of outcome following urethral stent placement for the treatment of obstructive carcinoma of the urethra in dogs: 42 cases (2004–2008). J Am Vet Med Assoc 2013;242(1):59–68.
30. McMillan SK, Knapp DW, Ramos-Vara JA, et al. Outcome of urethral stent placement for management of urethral obstruction secondary to transitional cell carcinoma in dogs: 19 cases (2007–2010). J Am Vet Med Assoc 2012;241(12): 1627–32.
31. Hill TL, Berent AC, Weisse CW. Evaluation of urethral stent placement for benign urethral obstructions in dogs. J Vet Intern Med 2014;28:1384–90.
32. Brace MA, Weisse C, Berent A. Preliminary experience with stenting for management of non-urolith urethral obstruction in eight cats. Vet Surg 2014;43:199–208.
33. Gookin JL, Stone EA, Spaulding KA, et al. Unilateral nephrectomy in dogs with renal disease: 30 cases (1985–1994). J Am Vet Med Assoc 1996;208:2020–6.
34. King M, Waldron D, Barber D, et al. Effect of nephrotomy on renal function and morphology in normal cats. Vet Surg 2006;35(8):749–58.
35. Ross SJ, Osborne CA, Lekcharoensuk C, et al. A case-control study of the effects of nephrolithiasis in cats with chronic kidney disease. J Am Vet Med Assoc 2007; 230:1854–9.
36. Adams LG, Williams JC Jr, McAteer JA, et al. In vitro evaluation of canine and feline urolith fragility by shock wave lithotripsy. Am J Vet Res 2005;66:1651–4.
37. Chen KK, Chen MT, Yeh SH, et al. Radionuclide renal function study in various surgical treatments of upper urinary stones. Zhonghua Yi Xue Za Zhi (Taipei) 1992;49(5):319–27.

38. Reis LO, Zani EL, Ikari O, et al. Extracorporeal lithotripsy in children - the efficacy and long-term evaluation of renal parenchyma damage by DMSA-99mTc scintigraphy. Actas Urol Esp 2010;34(1):78–81 [in Spanish].

39. Hubert KC, Palmar JS. Passive dilation by ureteral stenting before ureteroscopy: eliminating the need for active dilation. J Urol 2005;174(3):1079–80.

40. Daugherty MA, Adams LG, Baird DK, et al. Acute pancreatitis in two dogs associated with shock wave lithotripsy [abstract]. J Vet Intern Med 2004;18:441.

41. Meretyk S, Gofrit ON, Gafni O, et al. Complete staghorn calculi: random prospective comparison between extracorporeal shock wave lithotripsy monotherapy and combined with percutaneous nephrostolithotomy. J Urol 1997;157:780–6.

42. Al-Hunayan A, Khalil M, Hassabo M, et al. Management of solitary renal pelvic stone: laparoscopic retroperitoneal pyelolithotomy versus percutaneous nephrolithotomy. J Endourol 2011;25(6):975–8.

43. Tawfiek ER, Bagley DH. Ureteroscopic evaluation and treatment of chronic unilateral hematuria. J Urol 1998;160:700–2.

44. Bagley DH, Allen J. Flexible ureteropyeloscopy in the diagnosis of benign essential hematuria. J Urol 1990;143:549–53.

45. Nandy P, Dwivedi US, Vyas N, et al. Povidone iodine and dextrose solution combination sclerotherapy in chyluria. Urology 2004;64(6):1107–9.

46. Bahnson RR. Silver nitrate irrigation for hematuria from sickle cell hemoglobinopathy. J Urol 1987;137:1194–5.

47. Diamond DA, Jeffs RD, Marshall FF. Control of prolonged, benign, renal hematuria by silver nitrate instillation. Urology 1981;18(4):337–41.

48. Villanueva S, Carreño JE, Salazar L. Human mesenchymal stem cells derived from adipose tissue reduce functional and tissue damage in a rat model of chronic renal failure. Clin Sci (Lond) 2013;125(4):199–210.

49. Kyles A, Hardie E, Wooden E, et al. Management and outcome of cats with ureteral calculi: 153 cases (1984–2002). J Am Vet Med Assoc 2005;226(6):937–44.

50. Roberts S, Aronson L, Brown D. Postoperative mortality in cats after ureterolithotomy. Vet Surg 2011;40:438–43.

51. Snyder DM, Steffey MA, Mehler SJ, et al. Diagnosis and surgical management of ureteral calculi in dogs: 16 cases (1990–2003). N Z Vet J 2004;53(1):19–25.

52. Kerr WS. Effect of complete ureteral obstruction for one week on kidney function. J Appl Physiol 1954;6:762.

53. Vaughan DE, Sweet RE, Gillenwater JY. Unilateral ureteral occlusion: pattern of nephron repair and compensatory response. J Urol 1973;109:979.

54. Mustafa M. The role of stenting in relieving loin pain following ureteroscopic stone therapy for persisting renal colic with hydronephrosis. Int Urol Nephrol 2007;39(1):91.

55. Berent A, Weisse C, Todd K, et al. The use of locking-loop nephrostomy tubes in dogs and cats: 20 cases (2004–2009). J Am Vet Med Assoc 2012;241(3):348–57.

56. Zimskind PD. Clinical use of long-term indwelling silicone rubber ureteral splints inserted cystoscopically. J Urol 1967;97:840.

57. Uthappa MC. Retrograde or antegrade double-pigtail stent placement for malignant ureteric obstruction? Clin Radiol 2005;60:608.

58. Goldin AR. Percutaneous ureteral splinting. Urology 1977;10(2):165.

59. Lennon GM. Double pigtail ureteric stent versus percutaneous nephrostomy: effects on stone transit and ureteric motility. Eur Urol 1997;31(1):24.

60. Yossepowitch O. Predicting the success of retrograde stenting for managing ureteral obstruction. J Urol 2001;166:1746.

61. Lane IF, Lappin MR, Seim HB III. Evaluation of results of preoperative urodynamic measurements in nine dogs with ectopic ureters. J Am Vet Med Assoc 1995;206: 1348–57.
62. Holt PE, Moore AH. Canine ureteral ectopia: an analysis of 175 cases and comparison of surgical treatments. Vet Rec 1995;136:345–9.
63. Currao RL, Berent A, Weisse C, et al. Use of a percutaneously controlled urethral hydraulic occluder for treatment of refractory urinary incontinence in 18 female dogs. Vet Surg 2013;42(4):440–7.
64. Grant DC, Harper TA, Werre SR. Frequency of incomplete urolith removal, complications, and diagnostic imaging following cystotomy for removal of uroliths from the lower urinary tract in dogs: 128 cases (1994–2006). J Am Vet Med Assoc 2010;236(7):763–6.
65. Thieman-Mankin KM, Ellison GW, Jeyapaul CJ, et al. Comparison of short-term complication rates between dogs and cats undergoing appositional single-layer or inverting double-layer cystotomy closure: 144 cases (1993–2010). J Am Vet Med Assoc 2012;240(1):65–8.
66. Wollin TA, Denstedt JD. The holmium laser in urology. J Clin Laser Med Surg 1998;16(1):13.
67. Runge JJ, Berent AC, Mayhew PD. Transvesicular percutaneous cystolithotomy for the retrieval of cystic and urethral calculi in dogs and cats: 27 cases (2006–2008). J Am Vet Med Assoc 2011;239:344–9.
68. Meige F, Sarrau S, Autefage A. Management of traumatic urethral rupture in 11 cats using primary alignment with a urethral catheter. Vet Comp Orthop Traumatol 2008;21:76–84.
69. Beck AL, Grierson JM, Ogden DM, et al. Outcome of and complications associated with tube cystostomy in dogs and cats: 76 cases (1995–2006). J Am Vet Med Assoc 2007;230:1184.
70. Knapp DW, Glickman NW, Widmer WR, et al. Cisplatin versus cisplatin with piroxicam in a canine model of human invasive urinary bladder cancer. Cancer Chemother Pharmacol 2000;46(3):221.
71. Norris AM, Laing EJ, Valli VE, et al. Canine bladder and urethral tumors: a retrospective study of 115 cases (1980–1985). J Vet Intern Med 1992;16:145.
72. Liptak JM, Brutscher SP, Monnet E, et al. Transurethral resection in the management of urethral and prostatic neoplasia in 6 dogs. Vet Surg 2004;33:505.
73. Fries CL, Binnington AG, Valli VE, et al. Enterocystoplasty with cystectomy and subtotal intracapsular prostatectomy in the male dogs. Vet Surg 1991;20(2):104.
74. Stone EA, Withrow SJ, Page RL, et al. Ureterocolonic anastomosis in ten dogs with transitional cell carcinoma. Vet Surg 1998;17:147.
75. Ayyildiz A, Nuhoglu B, Gulerkaya B, et al. Effect of intraurethral mitomycin-C on healing and fibrosis in rats with experimentally induced urethral stricture. J Urol 2004;11(12):1122.
76. Mazdak H, Meshki I, Ghassami F. Effect of mitomycin C on anterior urethral stricture recurrence after internal urethrotomy. Eur Urol 2006;51(4):1089.

Complementary and Integrative Therapies for Lower Urinary Tract Diseases

Donna M. Raditic, DVM, CVA

KEYWORDS

- Complementary and alternative medicine • Integrative medicine
- Lower urinary tract disease (LUTD) • Urinary tract infection • Urolithiasis
- Urinary tract tumor • Supplement • Herbs

KEY POINTS

- There is a growing demand for the use of integrative medicine in veterinary medicine.
- Evidence-based research using integrative medicine in veterinary patients with lower urinary tract diseases is scarce.
- Translational research with animal models of human lower urinary tract disease (LUTD) is an opportunity to expand our knowledge of etiopathogenesis and identifying complementary treatments.
- Translational evidence-based research is needed to accelerate the use of integrative health care in both human and veterinary medicine where there is a concern for antimicrobial resistance.

In 2014, the National Center for Complementary and Alternative Medicine changed its name to the National Center for Complementary and Integrative Health (NCCIH). Complementary approaches have grown in use to where they are no longer considered an alternative to medical care. For example, more than half of Americans report using a dietary supplement and spend nearly $4 billion annually on spinal manipulation therapy. Large population-based surveys have been done and found that the use of alternative medicine, which has been defined as unproven practices used in place of conventional medicine, is actually rare. The NCCIH defines integrative health care as the combination of complementary approaches into conventional treatment plans and has widespread use in human medicine. The goal of an integrative approach is to enhance overall health, prevent disease, and to alleviate debilitating symptoms, which often affect patients with chronic diseases and affect outcomes. The NCCIH states that despite the widespread use of integrative health care, the scientific evidence for many complementary approaches is still needed.[1]

The author has no financial disclosures to acknowledge.
Integrative Medicine, Nutrition Service, Department of Small Animal Clinical Sciences, College of Veterinary Medicine, University of Tennessee, 2407 River Drive, Knoxville, TN 37996, USA
E-mail address: draditic@utk.edu

Complementary approaches can include herbs, supplements, acupuncture, and other modalities that are rational and supported by evidence to alleviate physical symptoms, improve quality of life, and also prevent diseases in veterinary patients. There is a growing consumer demand for an integrative health care approach, and veterinarians are being challenged to know more about these nontraditional therapies.[2,3] In recognition and response to these demands, the American Veterinary Medicine Association admitted the American Veterinary Holistic Medical Association and the American Academy of Veterinary Acupuncture into the House of Delegates as constituent allied veterinary organizations.[4,5]

URINARY TRACT INFECTIONS

Veterinarians frequently manage patients with simple lower urinary tract diseases (LUTD), such as bacterial urinary tract infections (UTIs), with conventional therapies with good outcomes. Most simple infections resolve with an approximate 2-week course of oral antimicrobials, but persistent or recurrent UTIs (RUTIs) that involve refractory bacterial isolates can be difficult to treat using conventional antimicrobial therapy alone.[6] UTIs develop when there is a breach in host defense mechanisms, which allows virulent microbes to adhere, multiply, and persist within the urinary tract. Bacterial UTIs may affect 14% of all dogs during their lifetimes, and they are more common in females. Although less common in cats, bacterial UTIs usually occur in those older than 10 years, with incidence increasing with age. In these patients, repeated courses of antimicrobials are typically ineffective at achieving long-term bladder sterility and a nonantimicrobial preventative strategy is needed.[7] The bacteria that most commonly cause UTIs are similar in dogs and cats; *Escherichia coli* infections account for more than one-half of all positive urine cultures.[6,7]

In the human literature, the efficacy of different forms of nonantimicrobial prophylaxis are being assessed for effectiveness and tolerability in adults with recurrent UTIs. UTIs are more common in women, accounting for nearly 25% of all infections, with around 50% to 60% developing UTIs in their lifetimes. Similar to veterinary patients it has been shown that *E coli* is the organism that causes UTIs in most human patients, and RUTIs are reinfection by the same pathogen.[8] In human medicine managing, RUTI is primarily done with repeated or continuous antimicrobial therapy, and resistance in common urinary pathogens is increasing because of the overuse and misuse of antimicrobials. It has been shown that resistance patterns vary by geographic location but are rising nationwide and globally.[9]

Because of the growing concern for antimicrobial resistance, nonantimicrobial, unconventional treatments evaluated in the human literature include vaginal vaccines, behavioral modifications, vaginal and oral estrogens, oral immunostimulant *E coli* fractions OM-39 (Uro-Vaxom), cranberry supplements, oral and vaginal probiotics, herbs or herbal preparations, mannose, and acupuncture.[8–13]

A systematic review and meta-analysis of randomized controlled trials (RCTs) in human research included 17 studies with data for 2165 patients, and the Jadad score was used to assess the risk of bias (0–2, high risks and 3–5, low risks). The Jadad scale assigns scores for the best-quality trial from 0 to 5 based on the following: (1) the study is randomized; (2) the intervention is double blind; (3) study withdrawals are accounted for and described; (4) the randomization procedure is adequately performed using an appropriate method; and (5) the blinding is adequately performed using placebo. An assessment of effectiveness, tolerability, and safety of nonantibiotic prophylaxis in adults with recurrent UTIs was reported. The oral immunostimulant OM-89 (Uro-Vaxom), an extract of 18 different serotypes of heat-killed uropathogenic *E coli*, decreased the rate of UTI recurrence (Jadad score 3, relative risk [RR] 0.61, 95% confidence interval [CI] 0.48–0.78). A vaginal vaccine Urovac was shown to reduce UTI recurrence (Jadad score 3, RR 0.81, 95% CI 0.68–0.96), whereas vaginal estrogens demonstrated a trend toward preventing UTI recurrence (Jadad score 2.5, RR 0.42, 95% CI 0.16–1.10). Cranberries and acupuncture were reported to decrease recurrent UTIs (Jadad score 4, RR 0.53, 95% CI 0.33–0.83) and (Jadad score 2, RR 0.48, 95% CI 0.29–0.79) respectively, whereas oral estrogens and lactobacilli prophylaxis did not decrease the rate of UTI recurrence.[12]

The evidence base for the use of relevant and practical nonantimicrobial treatments of UTIs in veterinary medicine was assessed via a literature search in dog/cat, in vitro using dog/cat cells, in vivo other species especially humans, and in vitro cell lines. From this review of the current literature, consideration of common nonantimicrobial treatments that could be relevant, safe, and practical for UTI in dogs and cats included cranberry supplements, mannose, oral probiotics, acupuncture, herbs, or herbal preparations.

Cranberry (Vaccinium Macrocarpon)

Cranberries have been used in the prevention of UTIs for many years. The mechanism of action has not been elucidated completely, but cranberries contain an A type proanthocyanidins (PAC), which may inhibit the adherence of P fimbriae of *E coli* to uroepithelial cells. There is no meta-analysis or RCTs evaluating the use of cranberry (*Vaccinium* species) juice or extracts and UTIs in dogs or cats. A small study using the mannose-resistant hemagglutination urine assay was used for detecting antiadhesion activity both in vitro and ex vivo following ingestion of a cranberry product in 6 beagle dogs. After one Crananidin (Nutramax Laboratories, Inc, Lancaster, SC) tablet containing 16 mg of bioactive PACs (mean dose 1.14 mg/kg body weight) was administered daily for 3 weeks, collected urine samples were tested in an in vitro assay for the ability of P-fimbriated *E coli* to agglutinate human red blood cells. Control urine demonstrated hemagglutination activity. Antiadhesive activity appeared within 3 hours of Crananidin administration, peaked on day 7 at 80 ± 26.5% and remained elevated on day 21 at 73 ± 28.5% over the 24-hour period. The investigators suggested that this study demonstrates metabolites of the extract in the urine of 6 healthy dogs is sufficient to reduce adhesion of Pf *E coli* and may be beneficial in preventing *E coli*–associated UTIs in dogs. Reported is the need for further studies of this extract in a clinical trial of affected dogs.[14]

Numerous studies in humans report that UTIs are one of the most commonly treated outpatient diseases, and complications from persistent or repeated infections result in more than a million hospital admissions annually in the United States. A 2012 updated review of 24 RCTs with 4473 participants (using cranberry juice, concentrate, tablets, or capsules to treat or prevent UTIs compared with placebo, no treatment, water, methenamine hippurate, antibiotics, or lactobacillus) was published. Compared with placebo, water, or no treatment, cranberry products did not significantly reduce the occurrence of symptomatic UTIs overall (RR 0.86, 95% CI 0.71–1.04). No significant difference in adverse effects from cranberry products compared with those of placebo/no treatment (RR 0.83, 95% CI 0.31–2.27) was noted. It was noted that the cranberry products may not have had enough potency to be effective, and the concentration of the active ingredient or type A PAC was often unknown in these studies.[15]

In a double-blind, double-dummy noninferiority trial, 221 premenopausal women with RUTIs were randomized to 12-month prophylaxis use of trimethoprim-sulfamethoxazole (TMP-SMX) 480 mg once daily or cranberry capsules 500 mg twice daily. Unlike most studies, 1 capsule with 500 mg cranberry extract (Cran-Max) was used; the amount of type A PACs in the cranberry extract was 9.1 mg/g, quantified using a high-performance liquid chromatography (HPLC) method coupled with fluorescence and mass detection. The proportion of patients with at least 1 symptomatic UTI was higher in the cranberry group than in the TMP-SMX group (78.2% vs 71.1%), and median time to first recurrence was 8 months for the TMP-SMX and 4 months for the cranberry group ($P = .03$, log-rank test). The study also compared the effects of 2 different forms of prophylaxis, TMP-SMX and cranberry prophylaxis, on antimicrobial resistance among indigenous and uropathogenic E coli (UPEC) isolates; high resistance rates occurred after 1 month of TMP-SMX prophylaxis use. An increase in resistance to amoxicillin and the quinolones was demonstrated during use of TMP-SMX prophylaxis. A high percentage (95%) of TMP-SMX–resistant microorganisms in the feces and urine of TMP or TMP-SMX recipients was reported after only 2 weeks. In summary, in premenopausal women with RUTIs, TMP-SMX, 480 mg once daily, is more effective than cranberry capsules, 500 mg twice daily, for the prevention of RUTIs; but it should be weighed against the greater development of antimicrobial resistance.[16]

In vitro studies have identified the role of PAC with A-type linkages in cranberries. These studies show specific PAC inhibits P-fimbriae synthesis and induces a bacterial deformation, on both antimicrobial-susceptible and antibiotic-resistant UPEC. It has been suggested that cranberry PAC prevent bacteria from adhering to the uroepithelium of the bladder, therefore, blocking the ability of E coli to infect the urinary mucosa.[17–19]

An in vitro study of antiadhesion activity of A2-linked proanthocyanidins from cranberry on UPEC and Proteus mirabilis strains and their possible influence on urease activity of the latter reported a significant reduction of UPEC adhesion (up to 75%) on the HT1376 cell line versus control. A reduction of adhesion (up to 75%) compared with controls as well as a reduction in motility and urease activity in the strains of Proteus was demonstrated. These results suggest that A2-type cranberry proanthocyanidins could aid in maintaining urinary tract health.[20]

In summary, studies evaluating cranberry juice, capsules, and extract suggest a role in the prevention of UTIs in susceptible populations but may not be as effective in RUTIs. Standardization of A2-type proanthocyanidins is needed to perform double-blind, placebo-controlled clinical trials that can determine the role of this nonantibiotic therapy for UTIs and RUTIs as well as appropriate dosing.[13,21,22]

Mannose

E coli is the major causative agent of UTIs and the most nonepidemic bacterial infection in humans and domestic animals. UTIs are primarily caused by UPEC (70%–95% of cases) expressing type 1 pili. At the tip of these pili, the lectin fimbriae H (FimH) is located; it enables the bacteria to adhere to oligomannosides of the glycoprotein uroplakin Ia, which is located on the uroepithelium. This initial adhesion is required for infection because it prevents the rapid clearance from the urinary tract by the bulk flow of urine enabling the invasion of the host cells.[23,24]

The interaction of the lectin FimH, at the tip of bacterial pili, with mannose structures is critical for the ability of UPEC to colonize and invade the bladder. Synthesis and in vitro/in vivo evaluation of R-D-mannosides with the ability to block this bacteria/host cell interaction, described as FimH antagonists, have been reported. Initially, FimH antagonists were directly instilled into the bladder concomitantly with uropathogenic; but more recent studies in mice have evaluated nanomolar FimH antagonists as α-D-mannosides exhibiting appropriate pharmacokinetic properties for intravenous and oral treatment of UTIs.[25]

More recent in vivo mice studies indicate the potential of orally available FimH antagonists for the prevention and treatment of UTIs, with a higher therapeutic effect compared with antimicrobials. Furthermore, antagonists applied together with antimicrobials were reported to have a synergistic effect on treatment outcomes. In the UTI mouse model, treatment with FimH antagonists prevented invasion of UPECs into bladder cells leading to a reduction of biofilm formation. The oral α-D-mannopyranosides tested in the UTI mouse model, including biphenyl α-D-mannopyranoside, diamidobiphenyl α-D-mannopyranoside, and monoamidobiphenyl α-D-mannopyranoside, are promising; but they still present challenging pharmacokinetics, such as low solubility and short exposure in plasma and urine, and require further study.[26]

The reported FimH antagonists are α-D-mannosides and act as potential ligands of mannose receptors of the human host system; therefore, target selectivity of these FimH antagonists is a safety concern. Mammalian mannose receptors are present on many tissues throughout the whole body and are involved in cell-cell adhesion and serum glycoprotein homeostasis, and they intervene in the innate and the adaptive immune response by recognizing molecular patterns on pathogens. A study investigated the selectivity range of 5 FimH antagonists belonging to different compound families by comparing their affinities for FimH and 8 human mannose receptors. From this study using cell-free competitive binding assay, no adverse side effects from nonselective binding to human receptors were reported. It was concluded that FimH antagonists should be further considered as a nonantimicrobial therapy for the treatment of UTIs.[24]

D-mannose powder is available and has been used to treat UTIs in horses, cats, and dogs, although there are no RCTs or case studies published or validated. It has been shown that in vitro D-mannose applied locally reduces the adherence of *E coli*, *Pseudomonas aeruginosa*, and *Streptococcus zooepidemicus* to endometrial epithelial cells in mares. It is marketed for UTI prevention in human beings as a food supplement. In 2012, a clinical trial that included 308 women greater than 18 years of age with acute UTI and a history of recurrent UTIs was reported. Patients were initially treated with ciprofloxacin 500 mg twice daily for 1 week for their UTI and then randomly allocated to one of 3 equal groups: prophylaxis with 2 g of D-mannose powder daily, 50 mg of nitrofurantoin once a day, or no prophylaxis. During the 6-month study period, there was 32% RUTIs, with the rate of RUTI significantly higher in the no-prophylaxis group (60%) compared with the groups receiving D-mannose (15%) and nitrofurantoin (20%). The risk of recurrent UTI episodes was significantly higher in the no-prophylaxis group compared with the groups that received active prophylaxis (RR 0.24 and 0.34). Diarrhea (8%) was the only adverse effect noted with the D-mannose, but it did not require discontinuation of the supplement. This study reported no difference between patients taking nitrofurantoin or D-mannose. Another study in humans with a history of uroliths and UTI evaluated a D-mannose–containing supplement and determined the supplement was well tolerated, but more RCTs and pharmacokinetics are needed to ensure efficacy and safety.[27,28]

Studies of proximal tubular reabsorption in dogs demonstrated a separate binding site for D-mannose from D-glucose, D-deoxyglucose, and D-galactose.[29] Studies of mannose metabolism have been evaluated in other mammals as well as tissue distribution in rats demonstrating rapid uptake with oral administration, incorporation into plasma glycoproteins and organ glycoprotein, and are referenced in FimH antagonist research.[30]

The author has used D-mannose in select cases of RUTIs in dogs and cats with no adverse effects and positive outcomes. Using the same laboratory for all sampling, pathogens were cultured and found resistant to an antimicrobial panel; a specific D-mannose supplement was given orally; and follow-up culture and sensitivity of urine was performed. It was noted that the same bacterium was present but with different antimicrobial sensitivity pattern. Appropriate antimicrobial therapy was initiated with continuation of the D-mannose supplement, and the infection was eliminated as demonstrated by follow-up negative urine cultures.

Probiotics

The use of probiotics for disease treatment and prevention is growing rapidly as research explores the role of normal microbial flora and the gastrointestinal tract's role in host immune function. Data regarding probiotic use for the prevention or treatment of lower urinary tract diseases in cats and dogs is lacking. Research has primarily examined the role of probiotics in gastrointestinal diseases, with a recent small study comparing probiotic with traditional therapy for inflammatory bowel disease in dogs.[31,32]

Proposed mechanisms in the human literature for prevention of urogenital infection by probiotics include modulating host immunity, preventing adherence of pathogenic organisms to the urogenital epithelium, and modulating growth and/or the colonization of pathogens.[9] In woman, vaginal colonization with lactic acid–producing bacteria (LAB) is associated with a reduction in RUTIs. The role of LAB vaginal colonization was evaluated in 35 healthy spayed female dogs with no history of UTI. In this study dogs, were given an oral probiotic containing Lactobacillus, Bifidobacterium, and Bacillus species once daily for either 14 days or 28 days in a prospective, controlled study. A vaginal tract culture was obtained from each dog before and after oral probiotic administration. Twenty-three dogs received oral probiotic supplement for a period of 14 days, and 12 dogs received the oral probiotic for 28 days. LAB were isolated from 7 of the 35 dogs before probiotic administration, and only 6 of 35 dogs had LAB isolated after the treatment course. Administration of this oral probiotic for a 2- or 4-week period did not increase the prevalence of vaginal LAB in healthy dogs, and it was concluded that LAB are not common isolates from the vaginal vault of dogs.[33] A more recent study by the same investigator compared the vaginal microbiota of dogs with historical RUTIs to dogs with no history of UTIs. The vaginal microbial population was reported to be the similar in the two groups.[34]

A systematic review of the human research included data from 5 different studies (294 patients) and reported no statistically significant difference in the risk for recurrent UTIs in patients receiving lactobacillus versus controls. In the 2013 review, when studies using ineffective strains and studies testing for safety were excluded, a marginally statistically significant decrease in recurrent UTI was found in patients on lactobacillus (RR 0.51, 95% CI 0.26 to 0.99, $P = .05$).[35] In a randomized trial comparing Lactobacillus and TMP-SMX in 252 postmenopausal women with recurrent UTIs, the 12 months' prophylaxis using probiotic did not meet the noninferiority criteria in the prevention of UTIs when compared with TMP-SMX. It was noted that unlike TMP-SMX, lactobacilli probiotic do not increase antimicrobial resistance, which is problematic in RUTIs. The investigators agreed that more research is needed to explore the role of probiotics in UTIs especially with growing pathogen resistance to antibiotic therapies.[36,37]

Acupuncture

Human studies indicate that the UTIs in susceptible women treated with acupuncture were reduced by one-third compared with untreated woman and half the rate among woman treated by sham acupuncture.[8,38] Human studies have looked at interstitial cystitis in woman with inconclusive results.[39–41] Sacral acupuncture in an acetic acid bladder irritation rat model suggested a positive effect perhaps through inhibition of capsaicin-sensitive C-fiber activation.[42]

UROLITHIASIS

Urolithiasis is a common and often challenging disorder in dogs and cats. Many factors contribute to saturation of urine with solutes that contribute to the formation of crystal formation, aggregation, and growth into uroliths. Urinary factors include concentration of solutes, urine volume, pH, concentration of solutes, and uroliths promoters and inhibitors.[31] It has been reported in human studies that urolithiasis is the third most common urinary problem with an estimated risk factor of 8% to 15% in America and Europe and a reoccurrence rate of 10% to 23% per year, 50% in 5 to 10 years, and 75% in 20 years.[43] Because of the multifactorial contributors, variable response, and high rate of reoccurrence in both veterinary and human urolithiasis, complementary therapies and prevention are being investigated.

D,L-*Methionine*

A study evaluated use of the urinary acidifier (D,L-methionine) and an appropriate antimicrobial agent to dissolve spontaneously occurring, infection-induced struvite urocystoliths in dogs within 8 to 12 weeks. Conventional treatment of canine struvite uroliths involves appropriate antimicrobial therapy with a concurrent therapeutic diet formulated for struvite dissolution. Fourteen client-owned dogs with presumed infection-induced struvite urocystoliths were administered antimicrobials based on the culture and sensitivity results; antimicrobial therapy was continued during medical dissolution and for 2 weeks beyond radiographic evidence of urocystolith dissolution. The urinary acidifier D,L-methionine was administered during medical dissolution and for 2 weeks beyond radiographic evidence of urocystolith dissolution at an initial dosage of 100 mg/kg by mouth every 12 hours. Plasma biochemical analysis, urinalysis, urine culture, venous blood gas analysis, and abdominal radiography were performed every 4 weeks until radiographic evidence of dissolution or until uroliths did not change over 2 successive reevaluations at which time they were removed surgically. Three dogs dropped out of the study as the owners could not administer the acidifier. Urocystoliths dissolution occurred in 8 of 11 dogs with a median time of 2 months and range of 1 to 4 months. The average final dose of the D,L-methionine in which urocystoliths dissolution occurred (n = 8) was 97.3 ± 25.6 with a median of 104.2 and range of 56.8 to 125.0 mg/kg by mouth every 12 hours. In 3 dogs, urolith dissolution failed; surgery was performed; and analysis of the urocystoliths revealed calcium oxalate (CaOx) urocystoliths.[44]

Probiotics

Cats and dogs are prone to oxalate uroliths similar to humans. In the human literature, hyperoxaluria complicated by urinary tract uroliths are an important clinical problem; the lifetime reoccurrence rate can be 50%. Mammals do not have the enzyme required to metabolize oxalate and depend on oxalate-degrading bacteria in the gut for this function.[45] Currently, there is no successful medical dissolution protocol published in either the human or veterinary literature; similarly uroliths are removed by physical methods, and dietary management for prevention is not always successful.[31,46]

The interest in probiotics to reduce the CaOx urolithiasis risk is based on the link between the reduced prevalence of *Oxalobacter formigenes*, an oxalate-degrading bacterium in stone-forming populations. This oxalate-degrading bacterium has been detected by quantitative polymerase chain reaction in 25% of dogs with CaOx uroliths compared with 50% of clinically healthy, age-, breed-, and sex-matched dogs and 75% in non–stone-forming breeds.[31,45]

The use of oxalate-degrading bacteria as probiotics have demonstrated the potential for microbial metabolic interactions that may support oxalate degradation.[45] A study evaluating oxalate degradation in dogs and cats reported intestinal microflora play an important role in the regulation of intestinal oxalate, oxalate absorption, urinary excretion, and in possible oxalate urolith formation. The study evaluated the ability of the lactic acid bacteria (LAB) component of canine and feline feces to degrade oxalate in vitro. Oxalate degradation by individual canine-origin LAB was also evaluated, and the effects of various prebiotics on in vitro oxalate degradation by selected oxalate-degrading canine LAB were also evaluated.[47]

A study evaluated oxalate degradation by *Bifidobacteria* species and *Lactobacillus* species isolated from the canine and feline gastrointestinal tract in vitro and selected strains in vivo in rats. *Bifidobacteria* species and *Lactobacillus* species that degraded oxalate in vitro were shown to survive gastric transit and were selected for further examination. In vitro degradation was detected for 11 of 18 of the *Lactobacillus* species, whereas oxalate degradation was not detected for any of the 13 *Bifidobacterium* species tested. A 4-week in vivo rat study demonstrated urinary oxalate levels were significantly reduced ($P<.05$) in rats fed *L animalis* 5323 and *L animalis* 223C but were unaltered when fed *L murinus* 1222, *L murinus* 3133, or placebo. It was reported that probiotic organisms vary widely in their capacity to degrade oxalate, and in vitro degradation does not uniformly translate to in vivo effect. The results have therapeutic implications and may influence the research of probiotics and oxalate metabolism.[48]

Several human studies have assessed the role of probiotics with oxalate-degrading potential and reducing the risk of developing CaOx uroliths. Studies have mixed results and suggest that the ability of chronic probiotic ingestion to reduce urinary oxalate excretion may be primarily confined to individuals with absorptive (enteric) hyperoxaluria.[49]

A recent study, using an oxalate-rich diet, induced in 20 healthy human subjects persistent dietary hyperoxaluria and increased plasma oxalate concentration. After 2 weeks of the oxalate-rich diet, the subjects were administered a LAB preparation (Oxadrop, VSL Pharmaceuticals, Rome, Italy) containing 3.6×10^{11} colony-forming unit (*Lactobacillus acidophilus*, *Bifidobacterium infantis*, *Streptococcus thermophiles*, and *Lactobacillus brevis*). There was no change in urinary oxalate excretion; therefore, it was concluded that it is unlikely that the LAB preparation decreased the intestinal oxalate concentration and/or absorption. The study reported the preparation may be altered in the future to select for LAB strains with the highest oxalate-degrading activity.[50]

Another study assessed the oxalate-degrading ability of bacterium from human feces and fermented food to isolated 3 strains: *L fermentum* AB1, *L fermentum* TY5, and *L salivarius* AB11 with efficient oxalate degradation. These strains were evaluated and demonstrated desirable properties for probiotic applications, such as good adherence to human colonic cell line HT-29 cells, tolerance to acid and bile, strong inhibition against pathogens, and absence of transferable antibiotic resistance. The reported strains survived well during gastrointestinal transit and reduced the coliform counts in feces with good a fecal recovery rate in the rat model; the study concluded that these isolates should be considered for prophylaxis of CaOx uroliths.[51] It is evident because of the prevalence, incidence, and similar mammalian oxalate metabolism that a need for translational research in the use of probiotics and CaOx uroliths in human and veterinary medicine is needed.[45]

N-3 Fatty Acids in Urolithiasis and Urinary Tract Tumors

Inflammation is characteristic of urolithiasis, interstitial cystitis, and urinary tract tumors (UTT). It has been noted that in cultures eating cold-water fish, urolithiasis is rare and has been attributed to the dietary intake of eicosapentaenoic acid (EPA) content in the diet. The N-6 fatty acid, arachidonic acid (AA), is a precursor for proinflammatory and pro-aggregatory prostaglandin E_2 (PGE_2), which influences renal calcium excretion and hypercalciuria. Both EPA and docosahexaenoic acid (DHA) are known to be precursors of less inflammatory precursors, such as PGE_3. High EPA intake competitively inhibits conversion of AA to PGE_2 and other proinflammatory cytokines.[46,52]

A study of 10 cats with a history of urolithiasis or with current urolithiasis were fed a dry food with 0.65% total omega 3 fatty acids on a dry matter basis (DMB) and an N-6 to N-3 ratio or a top-selling over-the-counter diet for 4 weeks. Blood samples were analyzed using HPLC demonstrating that EPA and DHA from the fish oil sources were readily absorbed by the cats and appear in the serum at a ratio similar to the diet fed; therefore, there is therapeutic potential of dietary EPA and DHA in cats as well as dogs.[46,53]

A human study investigated the effects of an N-6 fatty acid, γ-linolenic acid (γ-LA), in the form of evening primrose oil (EPO) in 2 ethnic groups. Eight healthy white and 8 healthy black men were given a single 1000-mg capsule of EPO for 20 days. During the study baseline, day 10, day 20, and day 24 (4 days after cessation of EPO), 24-hour urine collections were obtained and analyzed. Calcium excretion decreased significantly in both groups by day 20, and citrate excretion increased and was statistically significant at day 20 for the black men and day 10 in white men. A statically significant decrease in the CaOx stone formation Tiselius risk index occurred in both groups. AA is released by the key enzyme phospholipase A2, which increases anion-carried phosphorylation and potentially calcium excretion. It was speculated in this study that EPO may modulate the action of fatty acid desaturases, inhibit production of AA and PGE_2, thereby decreasing calcium excretion.[52] In a more recent study of N-3 polyunsaturated fatty acid (PUFA), 15 health human subjects were given 30 days of a 900-mg EPA and 600-mg DHA capsule once a day. Relative supersaturation of CaOx decreased 23% from a mean $\pm$ SD of 2.01 $\pm$ 1.26 to 1.55 $\pm$ 0.83 because of a significant decrease in oxalate excretion ($P = .023$). It was concluded that CaOx formers may benefit from N-3 fatty acid supplementation, although more studies are needed.[54]

Abnormal PUFA metabolism may occur in humans, which is not only related to the complex metabolic syndrome, such as diabetes and obesity, but also to urolithiasis and UTIs. In human patients with urolithiasis, an anomalous phospholipid metabolism of N-6 PUFA was recorded; in plasma and the erythrocyte phospholipid membrane of stone subjects, the observed AA/LA (N-6 to N-3) acid ratio was increased. Phospholipase A2 increases the erythrocyte anion-carrier protein phosphorylation and the oxalate exchange, revealing that idiopathic nephrolithiasis is related to abnormal phospholipid-AA metabolism. Fish oil supplementation was shown to lower calcium and oxalate urinary excretion and normalize the erythrocyte oxalate exchange.[55]

There is cumulative evidence in the literature linking the low-grade chronic inflammatory state of the urinary tract mucosa, calculi, and UTTs. UTTs are the 10th cause of human cancer worldwide; similar to veterinary medicine, direct mortality is not high, but morbidity and recurrence of these tumors is challenging. In human UTTs, the death rate caused by bladder neoplasia has not diminished over decades; we have also not seen significant advancement in veterinary medicine with bladder neoplasia. Evidence strongly suggests that moderate, long-standing consumption of dietary supplementation of N-3 PUFAs may improve the chances of avoiding recurrent CaOx uroliths as well as the development of UTT.[55]

Acrylamide (ACR) is a vinyl monomer that improves the aqueous solubility, adhesion, and cross-linking of polymers. The International Agency for Research on Cancer classified ACR in 1994 as probably carcinogenic to humans (group 2A) from sufficient evidence for carcinogenicity in experimental animals and concluded that current ACR levels in food items may indicate a human health concern. A study investigated whether various dietary fats affected preneoplastic lesions of the urinary tract in ACR-treated mice.

Eighty Kunming mice were initiated with ACR at dose 10 mg/kg and fed with 6% or 10% of the following PUFA: fish oil (enriched N-3), corn oil (enriched N-6), olein (enriched N-9 or essential fatty acids [EFA] deficiency inducer), and a commercial chow. After 22 weeks the mice were euthanized and macroscopic and biochemical evaluation of liver shoed fatty acid tissue profiles correlated closely with dietary source. In the ACR mice with olein, both macroscopic and biochemical evaluations demonstrated EFA-deficient (EFAD) characteristics. The corn oil (N-6) and olein (EFAD) diet had a significant promoting effect on urothelial lesions induced by ACR, with a greater number of mice developing simple hyperplasia without atypia or dysplasia/carcinoma in situ lesions, in comparison with fish oil and commercial dietary groups. It was concluded longer investigations are necessary to induce full-blown invasive carcinomas in the ACR mice model as well as to study the role of different dietary PUFA.[56]

As naturally occurring canine transitional cell carcinoma (TCC) of the urinary bladder is very similar to human invasive bladder cancer, spontaneous canine TCC has been applied as a relevant animal model of humans in a translational study using metabolomics to identify early makers for screening and monitoring treatments. Metabolomics is an emerging research used to analyze a large number of small molecules in a single step and promises immense potential for discovering metabolite markers for disease detection, monitoring, and evaluating treatments. In this study, nuclear magnetic resonance (NMR) combined with statistical analysis was used to profile and compare the urine metabolites from dogs with TCC and healthy control dogs with no bladder disease; the approach was proven to be a powerful method for TCC biomarker discovery. Six individual metabolites (urea, choline, methylguanidine, citrate, acetone, and β-hydroxybutyrate) between samples from dogs with TCC and the control group based on the Student t-test were selected to build a separate partial least square-discriminant analysis model. The results showed good classification between TCC and control groups; the sensitivity and specificity of the model were 86% and 78%, respectively. In the translational model, it was concluded that urine metabolic profiling may have potential for early detection of bladder cancer and of bladder cancer recurrence following treatment and may enhance our understanding of the mechanisms involved.[57]

HERBS AND LOWER URINARY TRACT DISEASES

Herbal medicines are in great demand in both developed and developing countries because of their wide biological activities and lesser costs. With Internet and increased emphasis on a global economy, consumers have a greater access to herbal products from anywhere in the world. There is much research evaluating the use of herbs and to develop new conventional drugs by isolating bioactive compounds in herbs. Although benefits can be derived from herbs alone, the areas of concern include product contamination and/or adulteration, potential toxicity, and herb/drug interactions. In many countries, including the United States, herbal medicines are not regulated as extensively; the 1994 Dietary Supplement Act classifies herbal products as dietary supplements. Other countries attempt to prove efficacy and safety of herbal medicines are superior to the United States. The Commission E monographs in Germany are an example combining the scientific, health care, and industry leaders producing guidelines grounded in evidence-based knowledge. Prescribing of herbal medicines among health care providers in Germany is common. With the cost implications of a worldwide herbal medicine market estimated at $83 billion, implementation of standards for growing, selecting, manufacturing, conducting appropriate clinical trials and treating patients with herbal medicines is necessary. The World Health Organization (WHO) has provided technical guidelines to standardize herbal medicines.[58]

With an increasing popularity of herbal remedies by consumers, research has advanced to develop analytical techniques, as there is a need to identify and maintain uniform quality, quantification, and standardize these products. Advanced analysis techniques to characterize chemical structure, bioactivity, quality control, safety, and efficacy are available and include mass spectrometry (MS), NMR, HPLC, gas chromatography-MS, capillary electrophoresis, liquid chromatography beam MS, fluorescence detector, and flame ionization detector. These analytical techniques, although not recognized by pertinent authorities (the Food and Drug Administration), have identified many potential bioactive substances, including glycosides, saponins, phenolic compounds, flavones, quinones, xanthones, alkaloids, benzopyrone derivatives, and terpenes in foods, plants, and herbal preparations.[59–62]

It is known that more than 80% of drug substances are either directly derived from natural products or developed from natural compounds, such as antimicrobial, cardiovascular, immunosuppressive, and anticancer drugs. Active ingredients in herbal extracts for potential drug targets are identified by using comparative gene profiling studies. Metabolomics studies can also be used to screen herbs and identify mechanisms of action. Bioactive compound from transgenic plants or microbes for therapeutic application reduces the cost of drug development by applying genetic engineering.[63–66]

It should be noted, despite advanced techniques for drug discovery, understanding plant/herbs has formed the basis of traditional medicine systems, which have existed and been used for thousands of years. For example, the first drug-screening experiments of the antimalarial activity of *Artemisia annua* extracts were poor, and scientists ignored the results. Later cold-water extracts demonstrated complete inhibition of mouse malaria as Artemisinin, a novel antimalarial drug that is heat labile, was finally discovered in China. Knowledge accumulated in traditional medicine plays an important role in increasing the success rate of drug discovery. It has been estimated that the success rate of a synthetic route for developing new drugs may be 1 per 10,000, whereas the success rate based on medicinal plants used in traditional medicinal systems can be as high as one-quarter or more.[63]

Plants can have antimicrobial, antiinflammatory, and diuretic properties, which may be beneficial in lower urinary tract diseases. These important properties of plants provide a role in the treatment and/or prevention of lower urinary diseases, such as UTIs, RUTIs, and urolithiasis. Currently the WHO reports about 80% of the world population relies on plant-based medicine; there is a move toward the use of natural products for the prevention and treatment of diseases in humans and animals in developed countries.[59,67]

Herbs and Urinary Tract Infections

Herbs and herbal formulas have been used in traditional medicine for the treatment of lower urinary tract diseases in many cultures, but there is little research in dog or cat lower urinary diseases. Studies of the Japanese formula, choreito was evaluated in vitro and in vivo in cat and cat urine. An in vivo study reported improvement of struvite-related lower urinary tract signs in 12 cats fed the herbal formula.[68–70] Another study evaluated 3 commonly used herbal treatments recommended for use in cats with lower urinary tract disease (LUTD) including 2 formulas (1) San Ren Tang (SRT) and (2) Wei Ling Tang (WLT) and the single herb (3) Alisma (A). It was hypothesized that these 3 herbal preparations would induce increased urine volume and decreased urine saturation for CaOx and struvite. In this study, 6 healthy, spayed female, adult cats were evaluated in a placebo-controlled, randomized, crossover design study randomized to 1 of 4 treatments, including placebo, SRT, WLT, or A. Treatment was for 2 weeks each with a 1-week washout period between treatments. At the end of each treatment period, a 24-hour urine sample was collected with urine volume and urine biochemistries measured. Urine saturation for struvite and CaOx was estimated using EQUIL 1.5b (College of Medicine, The University of Florida, Gainesville, FL). Analysis of variance was used to analyze data statistically if distributed normally, and Kruskal-Wallis was used to analyze data statistically if data were not distributed normally. No differences were found in 24-hour urinary analyte excretions, 24-hour urine volume, urine pH, or 24-hour urinary saturation for CaOx or struvite between treatments. Results did not support the use of SRT, WLT, or A for increasing urine volume or for decreasing urine saturation for CaOx or struvite in cats; but no adverse events occurred during the study; therefore, these herbal compounds seem safe in cats.[71]

There are published studies in vivo in humans and rats and in vitro evaluating the antibacterial activity of selective plants and herbal formulas. Mechanisms of action include bioactive compounds in these plants having antiadhesive properties or direct cytotoxic activity. An in vitro study of 20 herb extracts against UPEC and T24 human bladder carcinoma cells reported that none of the herbs demonstrated direct cytotoxic effects. Two extracts prepared from Agropyron repens L and Zea mays decreased bacterial adhesion by interacting with bacterial outer membrane proteins. Three herb extracts, Betula spp, Orthosiphon stamineus, and Urtica spp, showed antiadhesive effects by interacting with T24 cell surface.[72]

Arctostaphylos uva ursi folium (bearberry leaf) has traditionally been used for medicinal purposes in Europe and America for the treatment of UTIs and may have direct antibacterial effects. The bioactive substance arbutin is rapidly absorbed and undergoes hepatic conjugation to hydroquinone (HQ) conjugates. The proposed mechanism of action is via HQ conjugates carried to the kidneys for excretion followed by decomposition, releasing the HQ to act as a direct antimicrobial agent.[73,74] Women (n = 57) with recurrent cystitis volunteered for a double-blind trial and were randomized to take placebo or an uva ursi extract for 1 month. Women in the uva ursi group had no episodes of cystitis in the following year compared with 23% of women who took placebo. No adverse effects were reported in this study; but there have been concerns as free HQ used in cosmetic products has nephrotoxic, hepatotoxic, or carcinogenic potential.[73]

A recent review of HQ toxicity noted arbutin metabolism forms primarily HQ conjugates, HQ glucuronide and sulfate, which are nontoxic and have rapid excretion via the urine. It is concluded that extracts of uva ursi folium are a safe therapeutic option for the treatment of lower UTIs, and no human case reports have been published regarding toxicity of this herb. Herbal medicinal preparations of bearberry leaves have been standardized or quantified to the content of arbutin and is one of the herbs monographed in Germany's Commission E.[75,76]

In a current study of Aframomum melegueta, bacteriocidal activity was evaluated against E coli, L monocytogenes, methicillin-resistant Staphylococcus aureus, and S aureus. Using NMR and MS, diterpenes were isolated and tested for their antibacterial effects. Two of the diterpenes exhibited more potent antibacterial activity compared with current clinically used antibiotics.[77] Other plant extracts have been evaluated for use in UTIs with the bioactive compound berberines, including *Mahonia aquifolium* (Oregon grape), *Hydrastis canadensis* (goldenseal), and *Coptis chinensis* (goldthread).[73]

Other plant extracts have been evaluated for their activity against uropathogens with elucidation of the bioactive compound and/or mechanism of action. P and type 1 fimbriae play a particular role in the adhesiveness of UPECs and bacterial binding is also mediated by the hydrophobic interactions between uropathogenic rods and uroepithelial cell surfaces. Correlation of bacterial adherence and increasing cell surface hydrophobicity of the microorganism has been demonstrated as another mechanism for infection. Studies of herbs and their metabolites interfering with UPECs by preventing bacterial adherence, increasing hydrophobicity, and development of biofilm rather than direct cytotoxic mechanisms are considered in vitro studies.[78–83]

Mechanisms of resistance is important in the development of integrative strategies for resolving RUTIs. Active efflux of antibiotics is one of the major mechanisms of drug resistance in bacteria. Multidrug-resistant (MDR) pathogens express and overproduce efflux pumps that expel and extrude of the antibiotics from inside the cell. Combining efflux-pump inhibitors (EPIs) together with antibiotics can reduce the invasiveness of these drug-resistant pathogens. In vitro studies have demonstrated herbs and/or metabolites that may be effective contain EPI properties such as seen with hydroalcoholic extract of *Terminalia chebula* fruits, which exhibited strong antibacterial activity against MDR uropathogens.[79,80]

Herbs and Urolithiasis

Diet manipulation to influence the volume, pH, and solute concentration has been the conventional treatment of urolithiasis in veterinary medicine. Besides the in vivo and in vitro studies discussed previously, herbal medicine has not been evaluated by RCTs in veterinary urolithiasis. A published case series between 2001 and 2009 identified 33 dogs and 13 cats with radiographic or ultrasonographic evidence of urolithiasis that were treated with Chinese herbal supplement, CrystaClair, a proprietary blend[84] developed by the investigators. Patients were administered CrystaClair at a dosage 0.5 g per 15 lb body weight twice a day and were monitored with abdominal radiographs to assess uroliths number and size on presentation and periodically during herbal treatment until uroliths dissolution or treatment was discontinued. No adverse effects were reported, and the overall duration of treatment and end point was defined as uroliths resolution or herbal medicine discontinued. Dissolution was reported in 56.5% of patients (58% of dogs and 54% of cats) over 4 to 60 weeks with CrystaClair. The investigators stated this case series was not ideal with unknown uroliths but that this was similar to clinical practice whereby uroliths composition is often unknown. Problems with study design, definition of known prior (surgery and crystalluria), and the use of diet therapy make it difficult to interpret this study.[85]

Fourteen Kampo extracts (10 mg/mL) were examined in vitro by assessing whether they could inhibit 2 critical steps in the early process of CaOx stone formation, namely, crystal aggregation and adhesion to the renal tubular epithelium of Madin-Darby canine kidney cells. The inhibitory effect of the extracts on stone formation was examined by using an ethylene glycol (EG) rat model. Sanshishi (Gardeniae Fructus) and Takusha (Alismatis Rhizoma) inhibited CaOx monohydrate crystal aggregation (84.5% and 64.2%, respectively) and crystal adhesion to Madin-Darby canine kidney cells (88.2% and 54.6%, respectively). The combination of these two herbs in a Kampo formula, known as Gorin-san, showed significantly stronger inhibitory activities; the study concluded Gorin-san may be a prophylaxis for CaOx urolithiasis.[86]

It is estimated that 12% of the world population experiences renal stone disease with a recurrence rate of 70% to 80% in men and 47% to 60% in women. The pathophysiological mechanisms of urolithiasis are still not well understood, and it is currently the third most common urologic disease after UTIs and prostatic disease in human medicine.[87] In traditional human medicine systems, herbs have been used for thousands of years to manage urolithiasis especially CaOx. Herbs and herbal preparations have been evaluated for their antiurolithic properties in vivo in humans and in the EG-induced nephrocalcinosis rat model. A traditional Chinese formula, Wu ling san (WLS), using the EG-induced nephrocalcinosis rat model used 41 male Sprague-Dawley (SD) rats divided into 4 groups: normal, placebo (EG and starch), low-dose 375 mg/kg of WLS and EG, and high-dose WLS 1.125 mg/kg and EG. Biochemical data of urine and serum were collected; at the end of 4 weeks, the rats were euthanized and renal tissues examined by polarized light microscopy and the crystal deposits evaluated by a semiquantitative scoring method using computer software (*ImageScoring*). In summary, WLS inhibited the deposition of CaOx crystal and lowered the incidence of stones in rats ($P = .035$) as well as reduced the severity of CaOx crystal deposits in rat kidneys demonstrating antiurolithic properties.[88]

A prospective RCT to investigate the effect of WLS in recurrent CaOx nephrolithiasis human patients reported urine output increased after treatment with WLS group, and this increase was significant when compared with the change in urine output in patients treated with placebo without causing electrolyte imbalance. The study limitations of this study are the small number of subjects (28) and that urine oxalate and citrate levels were not measured. Another limitation was using the daily amount of urine output as a marker of drug efficacy, as the environment temperature, the water content of meal, and the amount of insensible water losses will affect urine output.[89] A study evaluated WSL and doxorubicin hydrochloride (Adriamycin [ADR]) nephrotoxicity in rats demonstrating that WSL ameliorates ADR-induced nephrotic syndrome in rats. The results suggested that WLS ameliorates ADR-induced proteinuria and podocyte injury, whereas gene analysis demonstrated a suppression of renal overexpression of nephrin mRNA and protein by WLS. Radioimmunoassay showed that WLS suppressed ADR-induced increased renal angiotensin II content in rats. Some of these nephron-protective mechanisms of WSL may be involved in its antiurolithic mechanisms.[90]

There are other proprietary herbal formulas for the treatment and prevention of urolithiasis, including Cystone.[91] Recurrent kidney stone formers with documented CaOx stones were recruited into a 2-phased study to assess safety and effectiveness of Cystone, an herbal treatment used for the prevention of kidney stones. In the first phase, a randomized double-blinded 12-week crossover study assessed the effect of Cystone versus placebo on urinary supersaturation, whereas the second phase was an open-label 1-year study of Cystone to determine if renal stone burden decreased, as assessed by quantitative and subjective assessment of computed tomography. The results revealed no statistically significant effect of Cystone on short (6 weeks) or long (52 weeks) urinary composition, and average renal stone burden increased rather than decreased. This study did not support the efficacy of the herbal formula Cystone to treat human CaOx stone formers.[92] An in vitro crystallization study of 5 herbs (*Folium pyrrosiae*, *Desmodium styracifolium*, *Phyllanthus niruri*, *Orthosiphon stamineus*, and Cystone) in synthetic urine concluded all extracts decreased the rate of crystal growth, but Cystone had the greatest impact on all risk factors measured.[93]

The single herbs *Poria cocos* and *Alisma orientalis* found in many traditional herbal formulas have been evaluated with numerous rat in vivo studies to determine the bioactive compounds and mechanism of action as diuretic, antiurolithic, and renal protective. These herbs contain tetracyclic triterpenes and steroids, which have a similar structure to aldosterone nucleus structure and may exert diuretic effect through competitive inhibition of aldosterone receptors in different parts of tubular reabsorption to increase urine output.[94] Studies of different fractions of *Poria cocos* administered to rats all demonstrate its diuretic effects while trying to elucidate its mechanism of action. One study suggested at least 2 mechanisms for its observed diuretic activity with the potassium ion–saving diuretic effect related to the triterpenoid components. A metabonomic study of *Poria* reported by partial least squares-discriminate analysis 15 biomarkers in rat urine were identified and 11 of them were related to the pathway of adenine metabolism and amino acid metabolism.[95]

Extracts of *Alismatis rhizoma* (AR) or *Alisma orientale* ("Zexie" in Chinese) are well-known traditional Chinese medicines and are used as agents for diuresis. It has been reported using the EG rat model for urolithiasis that similar to *Poria cocos*, total triterpenoids are the antiurolithiatic active constituents of AR.[96] An in vivo study evaluated different fractions orally administered to rats measuring urinary excretion rate, pH and electrolyte excretion were measured in the urine. AR fractions demonstrated diuretic activity and inhibiting diuretic activity. The components with strong polarities in AR may have antidiuretic activities, which might be an effect of promoting the sodium-chloride cotransporter in the distal tubule.[97] In another in vivo study, the ethanol extract (EE) and the aqueous extract of AR were orally administered to rats to further elucidate the diuretic mechanisms of this herb. This study identified that EE but not AE presents a notable diuretic effect, and EE had diuretic and antidiuretic effects, which seems to be related to the sodium-chloride cotransporter in the renal distal convoluting tubule.[97] A study to investigate the subchronic toxicity of triterpene-enriched extract from AR (TEAR), as a 90-day oral toxicity study, was conducted in rats. No mortality or obvious treatment-related clinical signs, hematology, urinalysis parameters, and macroscopic or microscopic examinations were observed; it was concluded that the no-observed-adverse-effect level for TEAR was 1440 mg/kg/d in both sexes.[98]

Another herbal preparation that has been evaluated is Canephron N (CAN) the main ingredients of which are centaury (*Centaurium erythraea*), lovage (*Levisticum officinale*), and rosemary (*Rosmarinus officinalis*). The active ingredients are phenolic glycosides, phenolcarboxylic acids, phthalides, secoiridoids, essential oils, and flavonoids. In the Community of Independent States, CAN is registered for prophylaxis against and after removal of uroliths as well as RUTIs, pyelonephritis, glomerulonephritis, and interstitial nephritis. Because of its diuretic, spasmolytic, antiinflammatory, antioxidative, antibacterial, and nephroprotective properties, CAN seems to have a positive clinical impact on infectious and inflammatory processes within the urinary tract. Studies indicate this herbal remedy may have a positive effect in patients with urolithiasis and after stone removal and on spontaneous elimination of small CaOx stones. It may also reduce the risk of uroliths. Adult and children dosing is reported, and no adverse events were reported in the 1762 pregnant women treated with the compound demonstrating the safety of this herbal preparation.[99,100]

Urolithiasis is the third most common urinary problem sparing no geographic, racial, or cultural boundaries; reoccurrence is common. As herbs and herbal formulas have been used by many cultures, numerous studies using the in vivo EG antiurolithiatic rat model of CaOx have been published.[101–118] These studies suggest that herbs could provide integrative therapy for urolithiasis treatment and prevention. Attention to the knowledge accumulated through traditional herbal medicine will improve the development of effective therapies. Ecological ethics should be upheld to preserve biodiversity while we explore and use natural therapies and drug discovery.[63]

REFERENCES

1. https://nccih.nih.gov/news/press/12172014. Accessed January 20, 2015.
2. Budgin JB, Flaherty MJ. Alternative therapies in veterinary dermatology. Vet Clin North Am Small Anim Pract 2013;43:189–204.
3. Memon MA, Sprunger LK. Survey of colleges and schools of veterinary medicine regarding education in complementary and alternative veterinary medicine. J Am Vet Med Assoc 2011;239:619–23.
4. https://www.avma.org/news/pressroom/pages/acupuncture-group-HOD-release.aspx. Accessed January 20, 2015.
5. https://www.avma.org/About/Governance/Documents/2013S_Resolution12_AHVMA.pdf. Accessed January 20, 2015.
6. Thompson MF, Litster AL, Platell JL, et al. Canine bacterial urinary tract infections: new developments in old pathogens. Vet J 2011;190:22–7.
7. Litster A, Thompson M, Moss S, et al. Feline bacterial urinary tract infections: an update on an evolving clinical problem. Vet J 2011;187:18–22.
8. Al-Badr A, Al-Shaikh G. Recurrent urinary tract infections management in women: a review. Sultan Qaboos Univ Med J 2013;13:359–67.
9. Shepherd AK, Pottinger PS. Management of urinary tract infections in the era of increasing antimicrobial resistance. Med Clin North Am 2013;97:737–57.
10. Dineshkumar B, Krishnakumar K, Menon JS, et al. Natural approaches for treatment of urinary tract infections: a review. Scholars Academic J Pharmacy 2013; 2:442–4.
11. Head KA. Natural approaches to prevention and treatment of infections of the lower urinary tract. Altern Med Rev 2008;13:227–44.
12. Beerepoot MA, Geerlings SE, van Haarst EP, et al. Nonantibiotic prophylaxis for recurrent urinary tract infections: a systematic review and meta-analysis of randomized controlled trials. J Urol 2013;190:1981–9.
13. Geerlings SE, Beerepoot MA, Prins JM. Prevention of recurrent urinary tract infections in women: antimicrobial and nonantimicrobial strategies. Infect Dis Clin North Am 2014;28:135–47.
14. Howell AB, Griffin D, Whalen MO. Inhibition of P-fimbriated Eschericia coli adhesion in an innovational e-vivo model in dogs receiving a bioactive cranberry tablet (Crananidin). Anaheim, CA: ACVIM 2010; 2010.
15. Jepson RG, Williams G, Craig JC. Cranberries for preventing urinary tract infections. Cochrane Database Syst Rev 2012;(10):CD001321.
16. Beerepoot MA, ter Riet G, Nys S, et al. Cranberries vs antibiotics to prevent urinary tract infections: a randomized double-blind noninferiority trial in premenopausal women. Arch Intern Med 2011;171:1270–8.
17. Howell AB. Bioactive compounds in cranberries and their role in prevention of urinary tract infections. Mol Nutr Food Res 2007;51:732–7.
18. Lavigne JP, Bourg G, Botto H, et al. Cranberry (Vaccinium macrocarpon) and urinary tract infections: study model and review of literature. Pathol Biol (Paris) 2007;55:460–4.
19. Perez-Lopez FR, Haya J, Chedraui P. Vaccinium macrocarpon: an interesting option for women with recurrent urinary tract infections and other health benefits. J Obstet Gynaecol Res 2009;35:630–9.

20. Nicolosi D, Tempera G, Genovese C, et al. Anti-adhesion activity of A2-type proanthocyanidins (a cranberry major component) on uropathogenic E. coli and P. mirabilis strains. Antibiotics 2014;3:143–54.
21. Vasileiou I, Katsargyris A, Theocharis S, et al. Current clinical status on the preventive effects of cranberry consumption against urinary tract infections. Nutr Res 2013;33:595–607.
22. Davidson E, Zimmermann BF, Jungfer E, et al. Prevention of urinary tract infections with vaccinium products. Phytother Res 2014;28:465–70.
23. Cavallone D, Malagolini N, Monti A, et al. Variation of high mannose chains of Tamm-Horsfall glycoprotein confers differential binding to type 1-fimbriated Escherichia coli. J Biol Chem 2004;279:216–22.
24. Scharenberg M, Schwardt O, Rabbani S, et al. Target selectivity of FimH antagonists. J Med Chem 2012;55:9810–6.
25. Klein T, Abgottspon D, Wittwer M, et al. FimH antagonists for the oral treatment of urinary tract infections: from design and synthesis to in vitro and in vivo evaluation. J Med Chem 2010;53:8627–41.
26. Abgottspon D, Ernst B. In vivo evaluation of FimH antagonists - a novel class of antimicrobials for the treatment of urinary tract infection. Chimia (Aarau) 2012; 66:166–9.
27. Papeš D, Altarac S. Use of d-mannose in prophylaxis of recurrent urinary tract infections (UTIs) in women. BJU Int 2013;113:9–10.
28. Proietti S, Giannantoni A, Luciani LG, et al. Cystoman (R) and calculi: a good alternative to standard therapies in preventing stone recurrence. Urolithiasis 2014;42:285–90.
29. Silverman M, Aganon MA, Chinard FP. Specificity of monosaccharide transport in dog kidney. Am J Physiol 1970;218:743–50.
30. Alton G, Hasalik M, Niehues R, et al. Direct utilization of mannose for mammalian glycoprotein biosynthesis. Glycobiology 1998;8:285–95.
31. Kerr KR. Companion animals symposium: dietary management of feline lower urinary tract symptoms. J Anim Sci 2013;91:2965–75.
32. Rossi G, Pengo G, Caldin M, et al. Comparison of microbiological, histological, and immunomodulatory parameters in response to treatment with either combination therapy with prednisone and metronidazole or probiotic VSL#3 strains in dogs with idiopathic inflammatory bowel disease. PLoS One 2014;9:e94699.
33. Hutchins RG, Bailey CS, Jacob ME, et al. The effect of an oral probiotic containing lactobacillus, bifidobacterium, and bacillus species on the vaginal microbiota of spayed female dogs. J Vet Intern Med 2013;27:1368–71.
34. Hutchins RG, Vaden SL, Jacob ME, et al. Vaginal microbiota of spayed dogs with or without recurrent urinary tract infections. J Vet Intern Med 2014;28:300–4.
35. Grin PM, Kowalewska PM, Alhazzan W, et al. Lactobacillus for preventing recurrent urinary tract infections in women: meta-analysis. Can J Urol 2013;20: 6607–14.
36. Beerepoot MA, ter Riet G, Nys S, et al. Lactobacilli vs antibiotics to prevent urinary tract infections: a randomized, double-blind, noninferiority trial in postmenopausal women. Arch Intern Med 2012;172:704–12.
37. Beerepoot M, Ter Riet G, Geerlings SE. Lactobacilli vs Antibiotics to prevent recurrent urinary tract infections: an inconclusive, not inferior, outcome-reply. Arch Intern Med 2012;172:1690–4.
38. Alraek T, Soedal LI, Fagerheim SU, et al. Acupuncture treatment in the prevention of uncomplicated recurrent lower urinary tract infections in adult women. Am J Public Health 2002;92:1609–11.

39. Katayama Y, Nakahara K, Shitamura T, et al. Effectiveness of acupuncture and moxibustion therapy for the treatment of refractory interstitial cystitis. Hinyokika Kiyo 2013;59:265–9.

40. O'Hare PG 3rd, Hoffmann AR, Allen P, et al. Interstitial cystitis patients' use and rating of complementary and alternative medicine therapies. Int Urogynecol J 2013;24:977–82.

41. Leong FC. Complementary and alternative medications for chronic pelvic pain. Obstet Gynecol Clin North Am 2014;41:503–10.

42. Hino K, Honjo H, Nakao M, et al. The effects of sacral acupuncture on acetic acid-induced bladder irritation in conscious rats. Urology 2010;75:730–4.

43. Kahn A, Bashir S, Khan S, et al. Antiurolithic activity of Origanum vulgare is mediated through multiple pathways. BMC Complement Altern Med 2011;11:96.

44. Bartges JW, Moyers TM. Evaluation of d,l-methionine and antimicrobial agents for medical dissolution of spontaneously occurring infection-induced struvite urocystoliths in dogs. Anaheim, CA: ACVIM 2010; 2010.

45. Aaron Miller DD. The metabolic and ecological interactions of oxalate-degrading bacteria in the mammalian gut. Pathogens 2013;2:636–52.

46. Yu SG, Gross KL. Dietary management of the three most common lower urinary tract diseases in cats. Topeka (KS): Hill's Pet Nutrition Inc; 2007.

47. Weese JS, Weese HE, Yuricek L, et al. Oxalate degradation by intestinal lactic acid bacteria in dogs and cats. Vet Microbiol 2004;101:161–6.

48. Murphy C, Murphy S, O'Brien F, et al. Metabolic activity of probiotics-oxalate degradation. Vet Microbiol 2009;136:100–7.

49. Liebman M, Al-Wahsh IA. Probiotics and other key determinants of dietary oxalate absorption. Adv Nutr 2011;2:254–60.

50. Siener R, Bade DJ, Hesse A, et al. Dietary hyperoxaluria is not reduced by treatment with lactic acid bacteria. J Transl Med 2013;11:306.

51. Gomathi S, Sasikumar P. Screening of indigenous oxalate degrading lactic acid bacteria from human faeces and South Indian fermented foods: assessment of probiotic potential. ScientificWorldJournal 2014;2014:648059.

52. Rodgers A, Lewandowski S, Allie-Hamdulay S, et al. Evening primrose oil supplementation increases citraturia and decreases other urinary risk factors for calcium oxalate urolithiasis. J Urol 2009;182:2957–63.

53. Bauer JE. Therapeutic use of fish oils in companion animals. J Am Vet Med Assoc 2011;239:1441–51.

54. Siener R, Jansen B, Watzer B, et al. Effect of n-3 fatty acid supplementation on urinary risk factors for calcium oxalate stone formation. J Urol 2011;185:719–24.

55. Eynard AR, Navarro A. Crosstalk among dietary polyunsaturated fatty acids, urolithiasis, chronic inflammation, and urinary tract tumor risk. Nutrition 2013;29:930–8.

56. Zhang X, Zhao C, Jie B. Various dietary polyunsaturated fatty acids modulate acrylamide-induced preneoplastic urothelial proliferation and apoptosis in mice. Exp Toxicol Pathol 2010;62:9–16.

57. Zhang J, Wei S, Liu L, et al. NMR-based metabolomics study of canine bladder cancer. Biochim Biophys Acta 2012;1822:1807–14.

58. Ceballos R, Loya AM. Use of herbal medicines and implications for conventional drug therapy medical sciences. Altern Integr Med 2013;02.

59. Bernal J, Mendiola JA, Ibanez E, et al. Advanced analysis of nutraceuticals. J Pharm Biomed Anal 2011;55:758–74.

60. Steinmann D, Ganzera M. Recent advances on HPLC/MS in medicinal plant analysis. J Pharm Biomed Anal 2011;55:744–57.

61. Li SP, Zhao J, Yang B. Strategies for quality control of Chinese medicines. J Pharm Biomed Anal 2011;55:802–9.
62. Wu H, Guo J, Chen S, et al. Recent developments in qualitative and quantitative analysis of phytochemical constituents and their metabolites using liquid chromatography-mass spectrometry. J Pharm Biomed Anal 2013;72:267–91.
63. Pan S, Zhou S, Gao S, et al. New perspectives on how to discover drugs from herbal medicines: CAM's outstanding contribution to modern therapeutics. Evid Based Complement Alternat Med 2013;2013:627375.
64. Wang X, Sun H, Zhang A, et al. Potential role of metabolomics approaches in the area of traditional Chinese medicine: as pillars of the bridge between Chinese and Western medicine. J Pharm Biomed Anal 2011;55:859–68.
65. Sun H, Zhang A, Wang X. Potential role of metabolomic approaches for Chinese medicine syndromes and herbal medicine. Phytother Res 2012;26:1466–71.
66. Xie G, Zhang S, Zheng X, et al. Metabolomics approaches for characterizing metabolic interactions between host and its commensal microbes. Electrophoresis 2013;34:2787–98.
67. Bag A, Bhattacharyya SK, Chattopadhyay RR. Medicinal plants and urinary tract infections: an update. Pharmacogn Rev 2008;2:277–84.
68. Buffington CA, Blaisdell JL, Komatsu Y, et al. Effects of choreito consumption on struvite crystal growth in urine of cats. Am J Vet Res 1994;55:972–5.
69. Buffington CA, Blaisdell JL, Kawase K, et al. Effects of choreito consumption on urine variables of healthy cats fed a magnesium-supplemented commercial diet. Am J Vet Res 1997;58:146–9.
70. Buffington CA, Blaisdell JL, Komatsu Y, et al. Effects of choreito and takushya consumption on in vitro and in vivo struvite solubility in cat urine. Am J Vet Res 1997;58:150–2.
71. Daniels M, Bartges JW, Raditic DM, et al. Evaluation of 3 herbal compounds used for management of lower urinary tract disease in cats. J Vet Intern Med 2011;25:721–2.
72. Rafsanjany N, Lechtenberg M, Petereit F, et al. Antiadhesion as a functional concept for protection against uropathogenic Escherichia coli: in vitro studies with traditionally used plants with antiadhesive activity against uropathogenic Escherichia coli. J Ethnopharmacol 2013;145:591–7.
73. Yarnell E. Botanical medicines for the urinary tract. World J Urol 2002;20: 285–93.
74. de Arriba SG, Stammwitz U, Pickartz S, et al. Changes in the urine pH-value have no effect on the efficacy of 'Uvae ursi folium' Änderungen des Urin-pH-Werts haben keinen Einfluss auf die Wirksamkeit von Uvae ursi folium. Z Phytother 2010;31:95–7.
75. de Arriba SG, Naser B, Nolte KU. Risk assessment of free hydroquinone derived from Arctostaphylos Uva-ursi folium herbal preparations. Int J Toxicol 2013;32:442–53.
76. DiPasquale R. Effective use of herbal medicine in urinary tract infections. J Diet Suppl 2008;5:219–28.
77. Ngwoke KG, Chevallier O, Wirkom VK, et al. In vitro bactericidal activity of diterpenoids isolated from Aframomum melegueta K. Schum against strains of Escherichia coli, Listeria monocytogenes and Staphylococcus aureus. J Ethnopharmacol 2014;151:1147–54.
78. Shukla N, Panda CS, Satapathy KB, et al. Evaluation of antibacterial efficacy of Clerodendrum serratum Linn. and Clerodendrum viscosum Vent. Leaves against some human pathogens causing UT and GIT infection. Res J Pharm Biol Chem Sci 2014;5:621–6.

79. Bag A, Bhattacharyya SK, Chattopadhyay RR. Isolation and identification of a gallotannin 1,2,6-tri-O-galloyl-beta-D-glucopyranose from hydroalcoholic extract of Terminalia chebula fruits effective against multidrug-resistant uropathogens. J Appl Microbiol 2013;115:390–7.
80. Bag A, Chattopadhyay RR. Efflux-pump inhibitory activity of a gallotannin from Terminalia chebula fruit against multidrug-resistant uropathogenic Escherichia coli. Nat Prod Res 2014;28:1280–3.
81. Issam A, Alharbi AE. Antimicrobial activity of Hibiscus sabdariffa extract against uropathogenic strains isolated from recurrent urinary tract infections. Asian Pac J Trop Dis 2014;4:317–22.
82. Wojnicz D, Kucharska AZ, Sokol-Letowska A, et al. Medicinal plants extracts affect virulence factors expression and biofilm formation by the uropathogenic Escherichia coli. Urol Res 2012;40:683–97.
83. Devi AS, Rajkumar J, Beenish TK. Detection of antibacterial compound of Avicennia marina against pathogens isolated from urinary tract infected patients. Asian J Chem 2014;26:458–60.
84. http://www.naturalsolutionsvet.com. Accessed January 20, 2015.
85. Wen JJ, Johnston K. Treatment of urolithiasis in 33 dogs and 13 cats with a novel Chinese herbal medicine. Am J Traditional Chinese Veterinary Medicine 2012;7: 39–45.
86. Nishihata M, Kohjimoto Y, Hara I. Effect of Kampo extracts on urinary stone formation: an experimental investigation. Int J Urol 2013;20:1032–6.
87. Sumalatha G, Tanuja M, Chandu BR, et al. Antiurolithiatic and in vitro antioxidant activity of leaves of Ageratum conyzoides in rat. World J Pharmacy Pharmaceutical Sciences (WJPPS) 2013;2:636–49.
88. Tsai C, Chen Y, Chen L, et al. A traditional Chinese herbal antilithic formula, Wulingsan, effectively prevents the renal deposition of calcium oxalate crystal in ethylene glycol-fed rats. Urol Res 2008;36:17–24.
89. Lin E, Ho L, Lin M, et al. Wu-Ling-San formula prophylaxis against recurrent calcium oxalate nephrolithiasis - a prospective randomized controlled trial. Afr J Tradit Complement Altern Med 2013;10:199–209.
90. He L, Rong X, Jiang J, et al. Amelioration of anti-cancer agent Adriamycin-induced nephrotic syndrome in rats by Wulingsan (Gorei-San), a blended traditional Chinese herbal medicine. Food Chem Toxicol 2008;46:1452–60.
91. Anubhav N, Singla RK. Herbal resources with antiurolithiatic effects: a review. Indo Global J Pharmaceutical Sciences 2013;3:6–14.
92. Erickson SB, Vrtiska TJ, Lieske JC. Effect of Cystone on urinary composition and stone formation over a one year period. Phytomedicine 2011;18:863–7.
93. Rodgers AL, Webber D, Ramsout R, et al. Herbal preparations affect the kinetic factors of calcium oxalate crystallization in synthetic urine: implications for kidney stone therapy. Urolithiasis 2014;42:221–5.
94. Zhao Y, Tang D, Chen D, et al. Progress on chemical components and diuretic mechanisms of traditional Chinese diuretic medicines Porta cocos, Cortex Poriae, Polyporus umbellatus and Alisma orientalis. Chinese J Pharmacology Toxicology 2014;28:594–9.
95. Zhao Y, Li H, Feng Y, et al. Urinary metabonomic study of the surface layer of Poria cocos as an effective treatment for chronic renal injury in rats. J Ethnopharmacol 2013;148:403–10.
96. Ou S, Su Q, Peng K. Effects of the total triterpenoids extract of Alismatis rhizoma on calcium oxalate urinary stone formation in rats. Acta Medicinae Universitatis Scientiae et Technologiae Huazhong 2011;40:634–9.

97. Chen D, Feng Y, Tian T, et al. Diuretic and anti-diuretic activities of fractions of Alismatis rhizoma. J Ethnopharmacol 2014;157:114–8.
98. Huang M, Xu W, Wu S, et al. A 90-day subchronic oral toxicity study of triterpene-enriched extract from Alismatis rhizoma in rats. Food Chem Toxicol 2013;58:318–23.
99. Gaybullaev AA, Kariev SS. Effects of the herbal combination Canephron N on urinary risk factors of idiopathic calcium urolithiasis in an open study. Z Phytother 2013;34:16–20.
100. Naber KG. Efficacy and safety of the phytotherapeutic drug Canephron (R) N in prevention and treatment of urogenital and gestational disease: review of clinical experience in Eastern Europe and Central Asia. Res Rep Urol 2013;5:39–46.
101. Argal A, Saxena N. Ameliorative antiurolithiatic effect of a polyherbal suspension. J Drug Delivery Therapeutics 2014;4:83–7.
102. Ghaeni FA, Amin B, Hariri AT, et al. Antilithiatic effects of crocin on ethylene glycol-induced lithiasis in rats. Urolithiasis 2014;42:549–58.
103. Cho H, Bae W, Kim S, et al. The inhibitory effect of an ethanol extract of the spores of Lygodium japonicum on ethylene glycol-induced kidney calculi in rats. Urolithiasis 2014;42:309–15.
104. Soundararajan M. Antiurolithiatic effect of various whole plant extract of Ageratum conzoides Linn. on ethylene glycol induced urolithiasis in male wistar albino rats. Int J Pharm Sci Res 2014;5:4499–505.
105. Hardik KS, Vrushali VP, Jitendra DV, et al. Pharmacological evaluation of antiurolithiatic activity of UCEX01-a herbo-mineral Ayurvedic formulation. J Pharm Biomed Sci 2013;1834–9.
106. Kameshwaran S, Thenmozhi S, Vasuki K, et al. Antiurolithiatic activity of aqueous and methanolic extracts of Tecoma stans flowers in rats. Int J Pharmaceutical Biological Archives 2013;4:446–50.
107. Prathibhakumari PV, Prasad G. Efficacy of Andrographis paniculata on ethylene glycol induced nephrolithiasis in Albino rats. J Pharmaceutical Scientific Innovation (JPSI) 2013;2:50.
108. Vijayakumar S, Velmurugan C, Kumar PR, et al. Anti-urolithiatic activity of methanolic extract of roots of "Carica papaya" Linn in ethylene glycol induced urolithiatic rats. World J Pharm Res 2013;2:2816–26.
109. Sailaja B, Bharathi K, Prasad KV. Role of Tridax procumbens Linn. in the management of experimentally induced urinary calculi and oxidative stress in rats. Indian J Nat Prod Resour 2012;3:535–40.
110. Lin W, Lai M, Chen H, et al. Protective effect of Flos carthami extract against ethylene glycol-induced urolithiasis in rats. Urol Res 2012;40:655–61.
111. Sathya M, Kokilavani R. Antilithiatic activity of Saccharum spontaneum Linn. on ethylene glycol-induced lithiasis in rats. Int J Pharmaceutical Research Bio-Science 2012;1:338–50.
112. Manjula K, Rajendran K, Eevera T, et al. Effect of Costus igneus stem extract on calcium oxalate urolithiasis in albino rats. Urol Res 2012;40:499–510.
113. Patel PK, Patel MA, Vyas BA, et al. Antiurolithiatic activity of saponin rich fraction from the fruits of Solanum xanthocarpum Schrad. & Wendl. (Solanaceae) against ethylene glycol induced urolithiasis in rats. J Ethnopharmacol 2012;144:160–70.
114. Gadge NB, Jalalpure SS. Curative treatment with extracts of Bombax ceiba fruit reduces risk of calcium oxalate urolithiasis in rats. Pharm Biol 2012;50:310–7.
115. Samra B, Gilani AH. Antiurolithic effect of berberine is mediated through multiple pathways. Eur J Pharmacol 2011;651:168–75.

116. Hosseinzadeh H, Khooei AR, Khashayarmanesh Z, et al. Antiurolithiatic activity of Pinus eldarica Medw. Fruits aqueous extract in rats. Urol J 2010;7:232–7.
117. Samra B, Gilani AH. Antiurolithic effect of Bergenia ligulata rhizome: an explanation of the underlying mechanisms. J Ethnopharmacol 2009;122:106–16.
118. Mi J, Duan J, Zhang J, et al. Evaluation of antiurolithic effect and the possible mechanisms of Desmodium styracifolium and Pyrrosiae petiolosa in rats. Urol Res 2012;40:151–61.

Index

Note: Page numbers of article titles are in **boldface** type.

Vet Clin Small Anim 45 (2015) 879–894
http://dx.doi.org/10.1016/S0195-5616(15)00055-8
0195-5616/15/$ – see front matter © 2015 Elsevier Inc. All rights reserved.

vetsmall.theclinics.com

Moving?

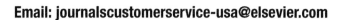

Make sure your subscription moves with you!

To notify us of your new address, find your **Clinics Account Number** (located on your mailing label above your name), and contact customer service at:

Email: journalscustomerservice-usa@elsevier.com

800-654-2452 (subscribers in the U.S. & Canada)
314-447-8871 (subscribers outside of the U.S. & Canada)

Fax number: 314-447-8029

Elsevier Health Sciences Division
Subscription Customer Service
3251 Riverport Lane
Maryland Heights, MO 63043

*To ensure uninterrupted delivery of your subscription, please notify us at least 4 weeks in advance of move.

Printed and bound by CPI Group (UK) Ltd, Croydon, CR0 4YY

14/10/2024

01773722-0002